O9-ABF-200

AIDS/HIV

DATE DUE

DEMCO, INC. 38-2931

ISSN 1532-2718

RA
643.75
.A37
2012

AIDS/HIV

Barbara Wexler

INFORMATION PLUS® REFERENCE SERIES
Formerly Published by Information Plus, Wylie, Texas

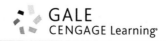

GALE
CENGAGE Learning·

Detroit • New York • San Francisco • New Haven, Conn • Waterville, Maine • London

KVCC
KALAMAZOO VALLEY
COMMUNITY COLLEGE
LIBRARY
WITHDRAWN

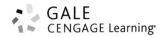
GALE
CENGAGE Learning®

AIDS/HIV

Barbara Wexler

Kepos Media, Inc.: Paula Kepos and Janice Jorgensen, Series Editors

Project Editors: Elizabeth Manar, Kathleen J. Edgar, Kimberley McGrath

Rights Acquisition and Management: Jacqueline Flowers, Kimberly Potvin, Christine Myaskovsky

Composition: Evi Abou-El-Seoud, Mary Beth Trimper

Manufacturing: Cynde Lentz

© 2012 Gale, Cengage Learning

ALL RIGHTS RESERVED. No part of this work covered by the copyright herein may be reproduced, transmitted, stored, or used in any form or by any means graphic, electronic, or mechanical, including but not limited to photocopying, recording, scanning, digitizing, taping, Web distribution, information networks, or information storage and retrieval systems, except as permitted under Section 107 or 108 of the 1976 United States Copyright Act, without the prior written permission of the publisher.

This publication is a creative work fully protected by all applicable copyright laws, as well as by misappropriation, trade secret, unfair competition, and other applicable laws. The authors and editors of this work have added value to the underlying factual material herein through one or more of the following: unique and original selection, coordination, expression, arrangement, and classification of the information.

For product information and technology assistance, contact us at
Gale Customer Support, 1-800-877-4253.
For permission to use material from this text or product,
submit all requests online at **www.cengage.com/permissions.**
Further permissions questions can be e-mailed to
permissionrequest@cengage.com

Cover photograph: Image copyright Sebastian Kaulitzki, 2011. Used under license from Shutterstock.com.

While every effort has been made to ensure the reliability of the information presented in this publication, Gale, a part of Cengage Learning, does not guarantee the accuracy of the data contained herein. Gale accepts no payment for listing; and inclusion in the publication of any organization, agency, institution, publication, service, or individual does not imply endorsement of the editors or publisher. Errors brought to the attention of the publisher and verified to the satisfaction of the publisher will be corrected in future editions.

Gale
27500 Drake Rd.
Farmington Hills, MI 48331-3535

ISBN-13: 978-0-7876-5103-9 (set)   ISBN-10: 0-7876-5103-6 (set)
ISBN-13: 978-1-4144-8130-2   ISBN-10: 1-4144-8130-6

ISSN 1532-2718

This title is also available as an e-book.
ISBN-13: 978-1-4144-9632-0 (set)
ISBN-10: 1-4144-9632-X (set)
Contact your Gale sales representative for ordering information.

Printed in the United States of America
1 2 3 4 5 6 7 16 15 14 13 12

WITHDRAWN

TABLE OF CONTENTS

PREFACE

AIDS/HIV is part of the *Information Plus Reference Series*. The purpose of each volume of the series is to present the latest facts on a topic of pressing concern in modern American life. These topics include the most controversial and studied social issues of the 21st century: abortion, capital punishment, care for senior citizens, crime, the environment, health care, immigration, minorities, national security, social welfare, sports, women, youth, and many more. Even though this series is written especially for high school and under-graduate students, it is an excellent resource for anyone in need of factual information on current affairs.

By presenting the facts, it is the intention of Gale, Cengage Learning to provide its readers with everything they need to reach an informed opinion on current issues. To that end, there is a particular emphasis in this series on the presentation of scientific studies, surveys, and statistics. These data are generally presented in the form of tables, charts, and other graphics placed within the text of each book. Every graphic is directly referred to and carefully explained in the text. The source of each graphic is pre-sented within the graphic itself. The data used in these graphics are drawn from the most reputable and reliable sources, such as from the various branches of the U.S. government and from private organizations and associa-tions. Every effort has been made to secure the most recent information available. Readers should bear in mind that many major studies take years to conduct and that addi-tional years often pass before the data from these studies are made available to the public. Therefore, in many cases the most recent information available in 2012 is dated from 2008 to 2011. Older statistics are sometimes presented as well if they are landmark studies or of particular interest and no more-recent information exists.

Even though statistics are a major focus of the *Informa-tion Plus Reference Series*, they are by no means its only content. Each book also presents the widely held positions and important ideas that shape how the book's subject is discussed in the United States. These positions are explained in detail and, where possible, in the words of their propo-nents. Some of the other material to be found in these books includes historical background, descriptions of major events related to the subject, relevant laws and court cases, and examples of how these issues play out in American life. Some books also feature primary documents or have pro and con debate sections that provide the words and opinions of prominent Americans on both sides of a controversial topic. All material is presented in an even-handed and unbiased manner; readers will never be encouraged to accept one view of an issue over another.

HOW TO USE THIS BOOK

The spread of acquired immunodeficiency syndrome (AIDS) has become a global epidemic. As of 2009, an estimated 33.3 million people worldwide were living with human immunodeficiency virus (HIV), according to the Joint United Nations Program on HIV/AIDS. That same year there were 2.6 million new HIV cases diagnosed and 1.8 million HIV-related deaths. This book includes information on the nature of HIV/AIDS and the HIV/AIDS epidemic; symptoms and transmittal; patterns and trends in surveillance; popula-tions at risk; children, adolescents, costs, and treatment; peo-ple living with HIV/AIDS; testing, prevention, and education; HIV/AIDS worldwide; and knowledge, awareness, behavior, and opinion of those affected by HIV/AIDS.

AIDS/HIV consists of 10 chapters and three appen-dixes. Each chapter is devoted to a particular aspect of HIV/AIDS. For a summary of the information that is covered in each chapter, please see the synopses provided in the Table of Contents. Chapters generally begin with an overview of the basic facts and background informa-tion on the chapter's topic, then proceed to examine subtopics of particular interest. For example, Chapter 4: Populations at Risk, begins with a description of how prevalence rates are estimated and how they reveal trends such as the geographic distribution of the disease or changes in how the disease is transmitted. The chapter then goes on to provide information regarding the increase in the number and proportion of HIV/AIDS cases among heterosexuals, which signals a major shift in the pattern of the epidemic. The chapter also describes HIV/AIDS in injection drug users and explains how HIV is transmitted through injection drug use. It provides the epidemiology of HIV in terms of specific populations by examining differences based on age, race, geography, and sex and addresses the epidemic among prison inmates. Readers can find their way through a chapter by looking for the section and subsection headings, which are clearly set off from the text. They can also refer to the book's extensive Index if they already know what they are looking for.

Statistical Information

The tables and figures featured throughout *AIDS/HIV* will be of particular use to readers in learning about this issue. These tables and figures represent an extensive collection of the most recent and important statistics on HIV/AIDS and related issues—for example, graphics cover clinical categories of AIDS infection; adult and adolescent HIV infection and AIDS cases; pediatric AIDS cases; AIDS-defining conditions; syringe exchange statistics; states with confidential HIV reporting; and the percentage of high school students tested for HIV. Gale, Cengage Learning believes that making this information available to readers is the most important way to fulfill the goal of this book: to help readers understand the issues and controversies surrounding HIV/AIDS in the United States and to reach their own conclusions.

Each table or figure has a unique identifier appearing above it, for ease of identification and reference. Titles for the tables and figures explain their purpose. At the end of each table or figure, the original source of the data is provided.

To help readers understand these often complicated statistics, all tables and figures are explained in the text. References in the text direct readers to the relevant statistics. Furthermore, the contents of all tables and figures are fully indexed. Please see the opening section of the Index at the back of this volume for a description of how to find tables and figures within it.

Appendixes

Besides the main body text and images, *AIDS/HIV* has three appendixes. The first is the Important Names and Addresses directory. Here, readers will find contact information for a number of government and private organizations that can provide further information on HIV/AIDS. The second appendix is the Resources section, which can also assist readers in conducting their own research. In this section, the author and editors of *AIDS/HIV* describe some of the sources that were most useful during the compilation of this book. The final appendix is the detailed Index. It has been greatly expanded from previous editions and should make it even easier to find specific topics in this book.

ADVISORY BOARD CONTRIBUTIONS

The staff of Information Plus would like to extend its heartfelt appreciation to the Information Plus Advisory Board. This dedicated group of media professionals provides feedback on the series on an ongoing basis. Their comments allow the editorial staff who work on the project to make the series better and more user-friendly. The staff's top priority is to produce the highest-quality and most useful books possible, and the Information Plus Advisory Board's contributions to this process are invaluable.

The members of the Information Plus Advisory Board are:

- Kathleen R. Bonn, Librarian, Newbury Park High School, Newbury Park, California

- Madelyn Garner, Librarian, San Jacinto College, North Campus, Houston, Texas

- Anne Oxenrider, Media Specialist, Dundee High School, Dundee, Michigan

- Charles R. Rodgers, Director of Libraries, Pasco-Hernando Community College, Dade City, Florida

- James N. Zitzelsberger, Library Media Department Chairman, Oshkosh West High School, Oshkosh, Wisconsin

COMMENTS AND SUGGESTIONS

The editors of the *Information Plus Reference Series* welcome your feedback on *AIDS/HIV*. Please direct all correspondence to:

Editors
Information Plus Reference Series
27500 Drake Rd.
Farmington Hills, MI 48331-3535

CHAPTER 1
THE NATURE OF HIV/AIDS

The acquired immunodeficiency syndrome (AIDS) is the late stage of an infection that is caused by the human immunodeficiency virus (HIV). HIV is a retrovirus that attacks and destroys certain white blood cells. The targeted destruction weakens the body's immune system and makes the infected person susceptible to infections and diseases that ordinarily would not be life threatening. AIDS is considered a bloodborne, sexually transmitted disease because HIV is spread through contact with blood, semen, or vaginal fluids from an infected person.

Before 1981 AIDS was virtually unknown in the United States. In that year, testing of blood and other samples for HIV began, and reporting of the disease became mandatory. In 1983 a research team at the Pasteur Institute in Paris, France, that was led by Luc Montagnier (1932–), Françoise Barré-Sinoussi (1947–), and Harald zur Hausen (1936–) first isolated HIV. Montagnier, Barré-Sinoussi, and zur Hausen were awarded the Nobel Prize in physiology or medicine for this discovery in 2008.

Over time, awareness grew as the annual number of diagnosed cases and deaths steadily increased. In "First 500,000 AIDS Cases—United States, 1995" (*Morbidity and Mortality Weekly Report*, vol. 44, no. 46, November 24, 1995), the Centers for Disease Control and Prevention (CDC) stated that the number of U.S. AIDS cases reported since 1981 reached the half-million mark in 1995. Indeed, in 1995 HIV infection was the leading cause of death among Americans aged 25 to 44 years.

By 1998, however, HIV/AIDS deaths among this age group had fallen dramatically, and HIV infection was the fifth most common cause of death among people in the United States between 25 and 44 years old. HIV/AIDS deaths fell to sixth place in 2001. This rank was the same in 2009, the most recent year for which data were available as of August 2011, with the disease claiming 3,326 people aged 25 to 44 years. (See Table 1.1.)

By 2009 HIV disease was no longer among the 15 leading causes of death among people of all ages in the United States. In "Deaths: Preliminary Data for 2009" (*National Vital Statistics Reports*, vol. 59, no. 4, March 16, 2011), Kenneth D. Kochanek et al. of the CDC observe that the age-adjusted death rate for HIV disease decreased by 9.1% from 2008 to 2009. Among people aged 15 to 24 years, HIV disease was the 12th leading cause of death in 2009, and among those aged 45 to 64 years, HIV disease dropped from the 12th leading cause in 2008 to the 13th leading cause of death in 2009.

Overall, HIV mortality (death) rates plateaued in 1995 and began to decline in 1996, even before the widespread use of new and effective drug treatments such as protease inhibitors. In 1997 HIV infection was the 14th leading cause of death overall in the United States. By 1999 HIV infection no longer ranked among the 15 leading causes of death in the United States. Figure 1.1 shows the sharp decline in deaths from HIV disease since the mid-1990s and the subsequent stabilization in the number of deaths attributable to HIV/AIDS between 1985 and 2008.

When examined at a general level, the overall decline in HIV/AIDS deaths between 1995 and 2000 was a positive trend for people infected with HIV and those suffering from AIDS. Nonetheless, the reality is that the actual number of people living with HIV/AIDS increased during this period. In other words, even though not as many people were dying from HIV/AIDS, more people were living with the disease due to the success of new therapies. These people require ongoing treatment and care.

The observed decline in HIV/AIDS deaths is no reassurance to the estimated 40,000 people who are diagnosed with an HIV infection each year in the United States. The CDC indicates in *HIV Surveillance Report: Diagnoses of HIV Infection and AIDS in the United States and Dependent*

TABLE 1.1

Deaths and death rates for the 10 leading causes of death by age groups, preliminary 2009

Rank[a]	Cause of death and age	Number	Rate
All ages[b]			
...	All causes	2,436,652	793.7
1	Diseases of heart	598,607	195.0
2	Malignant neoplasms	568,668	185.2
3	Chronic lower respiratory diseases	137,082	44.7
4	Cerebrovascular diseases	128,603	41.9
5	Accidents (unintentional injuries)	117,176	38.2
...	Motor vehicle accidents	36,284	11.8
...	All other accidents	80,892	26.3
6	Alzheimer's disease	78,889	25.7
7	Diabetes mellitus	68,504	22.3
8	Influenza and pneumonia	53,582	17.5
9	Nephritis, nephrotic syndrome and nephrosis	48,714	15.9
10	Intentional self-harm (suicide)	36,547	11.9
...	All other causes	600,280	195.5
1–4 years			
...	All causes	4,448	26.1
1	Accidents (unintentional injuries)	1,446	8.5
...	Motor vehicle accidents	462	2.7
...	All other accidents	984	5.8
2	Congenital malformations, deformations and chromosomal abnormalities	485	2.8
3	Assault (homicide)	385	2.3
4	Malignant neoplasms	349	2.0
5	Diseases of heart	154	0.9
6	Influenza and pneumonia	132	0.8
7	Septicemia	70	0.4
8	Chronic lower respiratory diseases	60	0.4
9	Certain conditions originating in the perinatal period	58	0.3
10	In situ neoplasms, benign neoplasms and neoplasms of uncertain or unknown behavior	51	0.3
...	All other causes	1,258	7.4
5–14 years			
...	All causes	5,628	13.9
1	Accidents (unintentional injuries)	1,667	4.1
...	Motor vehicle accidents	950	2.3
...	All other accidents	717	1.8
2	Malignant neoplasms	893	2.2
3	Congenital malformations, deformations and chromosomal abnormalities	350	0.9
4	Assault (homicide)	319	0.8
5	Intentional self harm (suicide)	266	0.7
6	Influenza and pneumonia	230	0.6
7	Diseases of heart	200	0.5
8	Chronic lower respiratory diseases	116	0.3
9	In situ neoplasms, benign neoplasms and neoplasms of uncertain or unknown behavior	84	0.2
10	Cerebrovascular diseases	69	0.2
...	All other causes	1,434	3.5
15–24 years			
...	All causes	30,252	70.2
1	Accidents (unintentional injuries)	12,351	28.7
...	Motor vehicle accidents	7,648	17.8
...	All other accidents	4,703	10.9
2	Assault (homicide)	4,820	11.2
3	Intentional self harm (suicide)	4,341	10.1
4	Malignant neoplasms	1,659	3.9
5	Diseases of heart	1,010	2.3
6	Congenital malformations, deformations and chromosomal abnormalities	451	1.0
7	Influenza and pneumonia	410	1.0
8	Pregnancy, childbirth and the puerperium	202	0.5
9	Cerebrovascular diseases	198	0.5
10	Chronic lower respiratory diseases	182	0.4
...	All other causes	4,628	10.7

TABLE 1.1

Deaths and death rates for the 10 leading causes of death by age groups, preliminary 2009 [CONTINUED]

Rank[a]	Cause of death and age	Number	Rate
25–44 years			
...	All causes	116,830	140.6
1	Accidents (unintentional injuries)	28,844	34.7
...	Motor vehicle accidents	11,033	13.3
...	All other accidents	17,811	21.4
2	Malignant neoplasms	16,236	19.5
3	Diseases of heart	14,053	16.9
4	Intentional self harm (suicide)	11,871	14.3
5	Assault (homicide)	6,883	8.3
6	Human immunodeficiency virus (HIV) disease	3,326	4.0
7	Chronic liver disease and cirrhosis	2,931	3.5
8	Cerebrovascular diseases	2.432	2.9
9	Diabetes mellitus	2,429	2.9
10	Influenza and pneumonia	2,052	2.5
...	All other causes	25,773	31.0
45–64 years			
...	All causes	490,145	617.5
1	Malignant neoplasms	157,544	198.5
2	Diseases of heart	103,704	130.6
3	Accidents (unintentional injuries)	32,357	40.8
...	Motor vehicle accidents	9,818	12.4
...	All other accidents	22,539	28.4
4	Chronic lower respiratory diseases	18,651	23.5
5	Chronic liver disease and cirrhosis	17,499	22.0
6	Diabetes mellitus	17,052	21.5
7	Cerebrovascular diseases	16,663	21.0
8	Intentional self harm (suicide)	14,192	17.9
9	Influenza and pneumonia	7,069	8.9
10	Nephritis, nephrotic syndrome and nephrosis	7,047	8.9
...	All other causes	98,367	123.9
65 years and over			
...	All causes	1,762,494	4,454.1
1	Diseases of heart	479,046	1,210.6
2	Malignant neoplasms	391,855	990.3
3	Chronic lower respiratory diseases	117,048	295.8
4	Cerebrovascular diseases	109,055	275.6
5	Alzheimer's disease	78,058	197.3
6	Diabetes mellitus	48,811	123.4
7	Influenza and pneumonia	43,433	109.8
8	Nephritis, nephrotic syndrome and nephrosis	40,341	101.9
9	Accidents (unintentional injuries)	39,316	99.4
...	Motor vehicle accidents	6,259	15.8
...	All other accidents	33,057	83.5
10	Septicemia	26,810	67.8
...	All other causes	388,721	982.3

...Category not applicable.
[a]Rank based on number of deaths.
[b]Includes deaths under 1 year of age.
Notes: For certain causes of death such as unintentional injuries, homicides, suicides, and respiratory diseases, preliminary and final data differ because of the truncated nature of the preliminary file. Data are subject to sampling or random variation.

SOURCE: Adapted from Kenneth D. Kochanek et al., "Table 7. Deaths and Death Rates for the 10 Leading Causes of Death in Specified Age Groups: United States, Preliminary 2009," in "Deaths: Preliminary Data for 2009," *National Vital Statistics Reports*, vol. 59, no. 4, March 16, 2011, http://www.cdc.gov/nchs/data/nvsr59/nvsr59_04.pdf (accessed June 1, 2011)

Areas, 2009 (February 2011, http://www.cdc.gov/hiv/surveillance/resources/reports/2009report/pdf/2009SurveillanceReport.pdf) that in 2009 there were 42,959 new cases of HIV infection in adults, adolescents, and children in the 40 states and five dependent areas with long-term, confidential name-based HIV reporting. Because not all states report HIV/AIDS cases, the CDC developed a method for estimating the incidence (the number of newly diagnosed cases during a specific time period) of HIV infection in the United States each year. Using this method, H. Irene Hall et al. note in "Estimation of HIV Incidence in the United

FIGURE 1.1

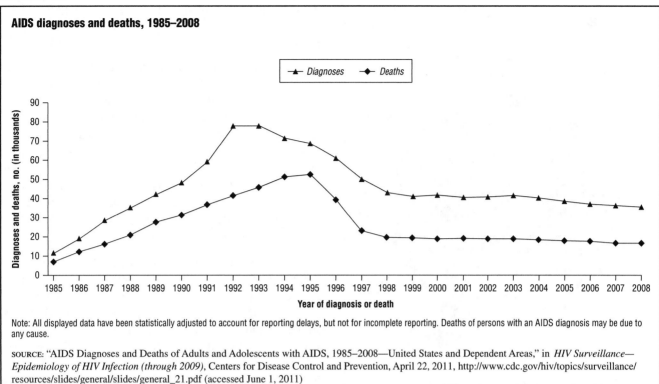

AIDS diagnoses and deaths, 1985–2008

Note: All displayed data have been statistically adjusted to account for reporting delays, but not for incomplete reporting. Deaths of persons with an AIDS diagnosis may be due to any cause.

SOURCE: "AIDS Diagnoses and Deaths of Adults and Adolescents with AIDS, 1985–2008—United States and Dependent Areas," in *HIV Surveillance—Epidemiology of HIV Infection (through 2009)*, Centers for Disease Control and Prevention, April 22, 2011, http://www.cdc.gov/hiv/topics/surveillance/resources/slides/general/slides/general_21.pdf (accessed June 1, 2011)

States" (*Journal of the American Medical Association*, vol. 300, no. 5, August 6, 2008) that there were 55,400 new infections each year between 2003 and 2006. The researchers estimate that approximately 56,300 people were newly infected with HIV in 2006.

In *Changing Patterns of HIV Epidemiology United States—2011* (2011, http://www.acthiv.org/2011_presentations/opening_plenary_040711/John%20T.%20Brooks.pdf), John T. Brooks of the CDC indicates that in 2011 HIV incidence was stable at an estimated 50,000 to 60,000 new infections per year and the prevalence of HIV infection (an estimate of the number of people living with an HIV infection) was 1.1 million people.

Between 1996 and 1997 the number of AIDS deaths declined by 42%. This dramatic decrease was the result of the introduction and use of effective antiretroviral drugs that slow the progression of an HIV infection. This decline continued but slowed to 20% between 1997 and 1998, and to 8% between 1998 and 1999. This may be due to a combination of several factors: resistance to the drug treatments developed in some patients, complicated drug treatment regimens that are difficult for patients to maintain, and a possible lack of access to prompt testing or treatment. The CDC reports in "HIV Surveillance—United States, 1981–2008" (*Morbidity and Mortality Weekly Report*, vol. 60, no. 21, June 3, 2011) that a cumulative estimate of 1,178,350 people in the United States were living with HIV infection at the end of 2008, including 236,400 people

with undiagnosed HIV infection. Through the end of 2008, 594,496 people had died from AIDS.

The AIDS epidemic is by no means strictly a U.S. phenomenon. According to the Joint United Nations Program on HIV/AIDS, in *Global Report: UNAIDS Report on the Global AIDS Epidemic, 2010* (2010, http://www.unaids.org/globalreport/documents/20101123_GlobalReport_full_en.pdf), an estimated 33.3 million people worldwide were living with HIV/AIDS in 2009. In that year alone, an estimated 2.6 million people became infected and 1.8 million people worldwide died of AIDS. In 2009 the countries of sub-Saharan Africa continued to have the world's highest annual rates of HIV infection and deaths.

THE HUMAN IMMUNODEFICIENCY VIRUS

A virus is a tiny infectious agent composed of genes that are surrounded by a protective coating. Until a virus contacts a host cell, it is essentially an inert bag of genetic material. Viruses are parasites. They must invade other cells and commandeer the host cell's replication machinery to reproduce. A frequent outcome of viral infection is the destruction of the host cell, as the newly made virus particles burst out of the cell. The host cell destruction can harm the host (in the case of HIV, a human). The common cold, influenza (flu), and some forms of pneumonia are also caused by specific, non-HIV viruses.

HIV belongs to a group of viruses known as retroviruses. The name arises from the presence of a special enzyme—

FIGURE 1.2

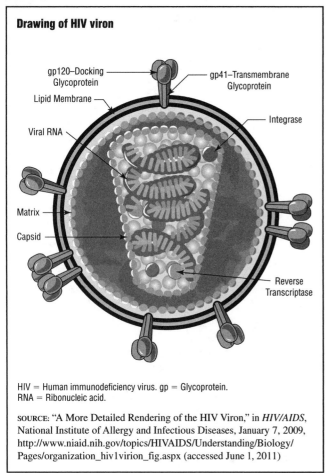

Drawing of HIV viron

gp120–Docking Glycoprotein
gp41–Transmembrane Glycoprotein
Lipid Membrane
Viral RNA
Integrase
Matrix
Capsid
Reverse Transcriptase

HIV = Human immunodeficiency virus. gp = Glycoprotein.
RNA = Ribonucleic acid.

SOURCE: "A More Detailed Rendering of the HIV Viron," in *HIV/AIDS*, National Institute of Allergy and Infectious Diseases, January 7, 2009, http://www.niaid.nih.gov/topics/HIVAIDS/Understanding/Biology/Pages/organization_hiv1virion_fig.aspx (accessed June 1, 2011)

reverse transcriptase—that reverses the usual pattern of translating the genetic message. (See Figure 1.2.) In animals the genetic units of information that are called genes consist of deoxyribonucleic acid (DNA). DNA is the blueprint from which another type of genetic material called ribonucleic acid (RNA) is made, in a process called transcription. In turn, the RNA serves as the blueprint for the various proteins that are the structural building blocks of the virus. In contrast to animals, retroviruses have their genes stored in RNA. After HIV infects a human cell, the viral reverse transcriptase works to transcribe HIV RNA into DNA. The viral DNA then becomes part of the host DNA—a process called integration—and is replicated along with the host DNA to produce new HIV particles.

Before 1980 retroviruses had been found in some animals. Indeed, as far back as 1911 Francis Peyton Rous (1879–1970) isolated an infectious and debilitating virus from a chicken. The Rous sarcoma virus was later shown to be both an oncogenic (cancer-causing) virus and the first known retrovirus. The first known human retroviruses, human T cell leukemia virus (HTLV-I) and the closely related human T cell lymphotropic virus (HTLV-II), were discovered in 1980 by Robert C. Gallo (1937–) and his colleagues at the U.S. National Cancer Institute (NCI). This

breakthrough provided the groundwork for the discovery of the virus that would eventually be known as HIV.

Identifying the Virus

In September 1983 Montagnier and his colleagues at the Pasteur Institute took a sample from a lymph node biopsy of a hospitalized patient in Paris and identified a retrovirus they named lymphadenopathy-associated virus (LAV). Eight months later Gallo's group at the NCI isolated the same virus in AIDS patients, which they called HTLV-III. LAV and HTLV-III were found to be identical and are now referred to as HIV. A conflict arose about which researcher should be credited with the discovery. In 1991, in an intense, politically charged atmosphere, Gallo dropped his claim to the discovery of HIV.

The original HIV is now known as HIV-1. This is due to the 1986 discovery by scientists at the Pasteur Institute of a new AIDS-causing virus in West Africans, which was labeled as HIV-2. Even though the two forms of HIV have similar modes of transmission, the symptoms of HIV-2 were found to be milder than those of HIV-1. Furthermore, HIV-2 was shown to differ in molecular structure from HIV-1 in a way that ties it more closely to a virus that causes AIDS in macaque monkeys. Antoine Benard et al. indicate in "Immunovirological Response to Triple Nucleotide Reverse-Transcriptase Inhibitors and Ritonavir-Boosted Protease Inhibitors in Treatment-Naive HIV-2–Infected Patients: The ACHIEV2E Collaboration Study Group" (*Clinical Infectious Diseases*, vol. 52, no. 10, May 2011) that HIV-2 is generally diagnosed in western Africa, and only small numbers of cases are diagnosed in Europe and North America each year. (Unless otherwise specified, the term *HIV* in the remainder of this edition refers to HIV-1.)

The Origins of the Virus

Montagnier and Gallo, along with other investigators, believed that HIV had been present in Central Africa and other regions for some time, and at some point the virus crossed the species barrier from primates to humans. The rural nature of these societies and the limited access to the outside world by those infected with the virus may have confined the spread of HIV for many decades. However, once the migration of tribal Central Africans to urban areas began, the more liberated sexual practices there promoted the spread of HIV. Within a comparatively short time, the once rare and remote disease was spread by globe-trotting HIV-infected people.

It was long speculated that HIV evolved from simian immunodeficiency virus (SIV), a retrovirus that infects monkeys. The theory was that HIV evolved from a human infection with a mutated form of SIV that was infectious to humans. Consistent with this theory was the finding that HIV is a part of the lentivirus family, which includes SIV.

In 1982 Isao Miyoshi (1932–) of Kochi University identified an HTLV-related virus in Japanese macaque monkeys. Genetically similar to HTLV, it was designated as the simian T-lymphotropic virus (STLV). Further studies identified STLV in both Asian and African monkeys and apes, with an infection rate ranging from 1% to 40%.

In 1988 Myron Essex (1939–) and Phyllis Jean Kanki (1956–) of the Harvard School of Public Health discovered that the simian virus found in African chimpanzees and African green monkeys was more homologous (related in primitive origin) to the human virus than to the simian virus in Asian macaques. This discovery provided strong support for an evolved version of African STLV as being the origin of human HTLV.

In 1999 an international team of researchers working at the University of Alabama announced its determination that the genetic sequence of a simian virus isolated from a tissue sample obtained from a chimpanzee was virtually identical to the HIV discovered by Montagnier. Interestingly, chimpanzees are only rarely infected with SIV. This implies that the chimpanzee may be a temporary carrier of the virus, which normally resides in some other, as yet unidentified, primate species. A common chimpanzee subspecies, *Pan troglodytes troglodytes*, which along with the bonobo is the closest living species to humans, naturally harbors HIV-1, and there have been documented occurrences of cross-species transmission from them to humans. Because these chimpanzees are still poached for bushmeat, humans may be at risk for continued exposure. A complete understanding of the mechanisms of cross-species transmission and the ability of these chimpanzees to resist infection may help researchers develop strategies to protect humans from HIV as well as from other viruses such as H1N1, SARS coronavirus, hantaviruses, and the Ebola and Marburg viruses that originate in animals.

ATTACKING THE IMMUNE SYSTEM

As with other infections, HIV must evade the immune system, which functions to detect and destroy invaders. To learn how HIV first attacks healthy cells while evading attack by the immune system, it is important to understand the complex structure of HIV and how normal white blood cells work.

Healthy White Blood Cells at Work

White blood cells are major components of the complicated, coordinated system of organs and cells that make up the human immune system. These organs and cells work together to prevent invasion by foreign substances. There are five types of white blood cells: macrophages (scavenger cells of the immune system), T4 or helper T cells, T8 or killer T cells, plasma B cells, and memory B cells. T and B white blood cells are also called lymphocytes. It is these lymphocytes that bear the major responsibility for carrying out immune system activities.

Each type of white blood cell has a specific function. The macrophage, which begins as a smaller monocyte (single cell), readies the T4 cells to respond to particular invaders such as viruses. At the time of a viral attack, the macrophage, which is sometimes referred to as the vacuum cleaner of the immune system, swallows the virus, but leaves a portion displayed so that the T4 cell can make contact. The macrophage also stimulates the production of thousands of T4 cells, which are all programmed to battle the invader. Figure 1.3 shows how the virus attaches to an immune cell and reproduces.

When T4 lymphocytes attack an invading virus, they also send out chemical messages that cause the multiplication of B cells and T8 killer cells. These cells, along with the help of some T4 cells, destroy the infected cell. Other T4 cells, which are not actively involved in destroying the infected cells, send chemical messages to B cells, causing them to reproduce and divide into groups of either plasma cells or memory cells. Plasma cells make antibodies that cripple the invading virus, whereas memory cells increase the immune response if the invader ever attacks again.

HIV's Molecular Structure

HIV has nine genes. Three of these—designated env, gag, and pol code—form the structural components of the virus that surround the genetic material and the outer surface of the virus particle. The remaining genes—tat, nef, rev, vpr, vpu, and vif—are involved in regulating the genetic activities that are necessary to create copies of the infecting virus.

HIV's complement of nine genes is minuscule when compared to the 30,000 genes that are in human DNA. Nevertheless, HIV is more complex than most other retroviruses, which have only three or four genes. Scientists believe these genes direct the production of proteins that make up parts of the virus and regulate its reproduction. The HIV core contains genes that are protected by a protein shell, whereas the entire virus is surrounded by a fatty membrane dotted with glycoproteins (proteins with sugar units attached), adding to its protection. (See Figure 1.2.) Figure 1.4 shows the steps in the replication cycle of HIV.

Once HIV enters the human body, its primary target is a subset of immune cells that contain a molecule called CD4. In particular, the virus attaches itself to CD4+ T cells and, to a lesser extent, to macrophages. Figure 1.5 shows the cell-to-cell spread of HIV through the CD4-mediated fusion of an infected cell with an uninfected cell.

Another Discovery

In November 1995 Ute-Christiane Meier et al. proposed in "Cytotoxic T Lymphocyte Lysis Inhibited by Viable HIV Mutants" (*Science*, vol. 270, no. 5240) that

FIGURE 1.3

How HIV attaches to an immune cell and reproduces

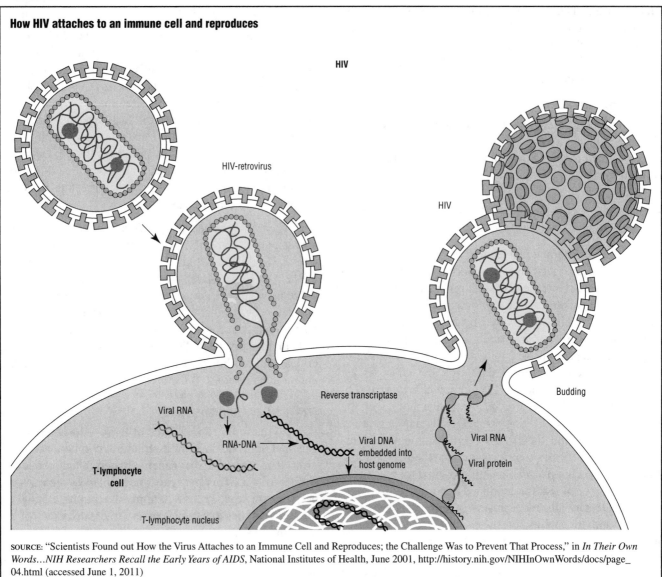

SOURCE: "Scientists Found out How the Virus Attaches to an Immune Cell and Reproduces; the Challenge Was to Prevent That Process," in *In Their Own Words...NIH Researchers Recall the Early Years of AIDS*, National Institutes of Health, June 2001, http://history.nih.gov/NIHInOwnWords/docs/page_04.html (accessed June 1, 2011)

HIV defuses the killer cells that are supposed to destroy virus-stricken cells. The researchers isolated HIV from AIDS patients and demonstrated that the virus had undergone a mutation, or change, in its genetic structure. When killer T cells approached cells infected with the mutated virus, the T cells failed to kill the stricken cells, perhaps because they no longer recognized them. In fact, the T cells were unable to kill even cells infected with the original, unmutated virus. The mutations not only allowed the altered strains to multiply but also allowed unaltered strains to flourish.

AN ALTERNATE THEORY: "FRIENDLY FIRE." Not all researchers agree that the alteration of killer T cells is the underlying basis for the establishment of an HIV infection. Some believe that other cells in the immune system attack and kill CD4-containing cells in what has been called an autoimmune response. The CD4-containing cells that have not been invaded by the virus, but that display fragments of it, become targets for other cells—besides the killer cells—which see the infected cells as a camouflaged virus and kill them. In addition, HIV-infected cells may send out protein signals that weaken or destroy other healthy cells in the immune system.

Whatever the basis of the beginning of an HIV infection, it is agreed that HIV subsequently exhibits various behaviors, depending on the kind of cell it has invaded and how the cell behaves. The virus can remain dormant in T cells for two to 20 years, hidden from the immune system. When the cells are stimulated, however, the viral genes that have been incorporated into the DNA of the T4 cells can be replicated and the gene products assembled into new virus particles that then break free of the T4 cells and attack other cells. Once a T4 cell has been infected, it cannot respond adequately and may reproduce to form as few as 10 cells. An uninfected T4

FIGURE 1.4

HIV replication cycle

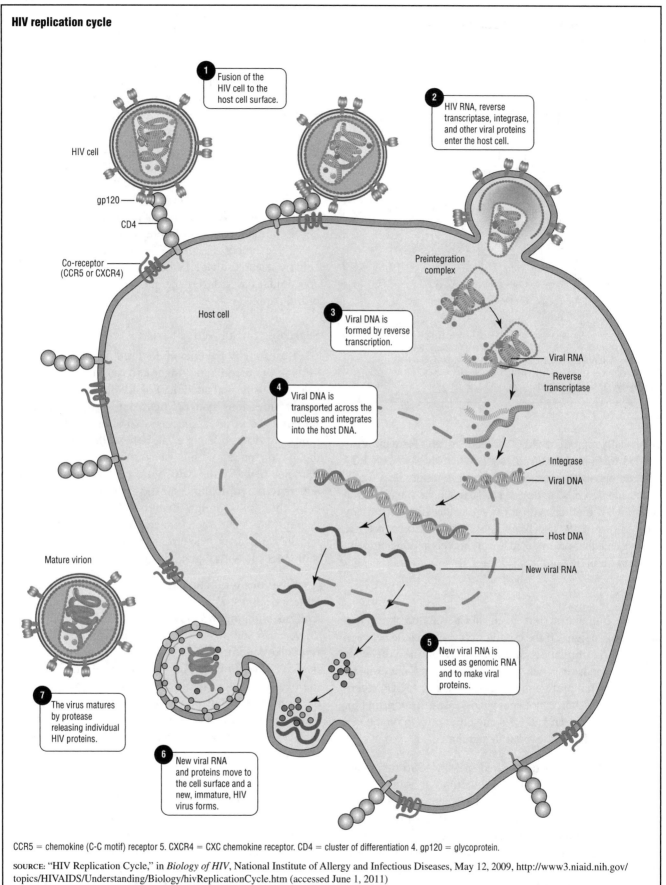

CCR5 = chemokine (C-C motif) receptor 5. CXCR4 = CXC chemokine receptor. CD4 = cluster of differentiation 4. gp120 = glycoprotein.

SOURCE: "HIV Replication Cycle," in *Biology of HIV*, National Institute of Allergy and Infectious Diseases, May 12, 2009, http://www3.niaid.nih.gov/ topics/HIVAIDS/Understanding/Biology/hivReplicationCycle.htm (accessed June 1, 2011)

FIGURE 1.5

Cell-to-cell spread of HIV through the CD4-mediated fusion of an infected cell with an uninfected cell

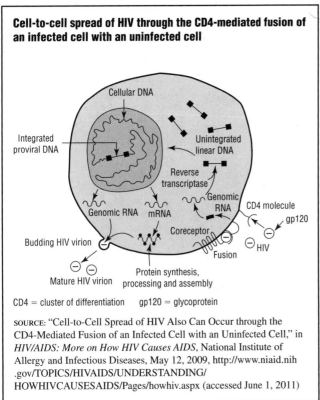

CD4 = cluster of differentiation   gp120 = glycoprotein

SOURCE: "Cell-to-Cell Spread of HIV Also Can Occur through the CD4-Mediated Fusion of an Infected Cell with an Uninfected Cell," in *HIV/AIDS: More on How HIV Causes AIDS*, National Institute of Allergy and Infectious Diseases, May 12, 2009, http://www.niaid.nih .gov/TOPICS/HIVAIDS/UNDERSTANDING/ HOWHIVCAUSESAIDS/Pages/howhiv.aspx (accessed June 1, 2011)

cell usually reproduces 1,000 or more times to form the army needed to fight the HIV invader. When these crippled T4 cells do encounter the invader, the virus inside them reproduces and the cells are destroyed. To make the situation even worse, HIV reproduces itself at a rate far greater than any other known virus. The T4 cells essentially become factories for the invading enemy soldiers, ultimately producing them in overwhelming numbers.

The Attack

The immune system is unable to produce sufficient antibodies to fight off the complex HIV. The battle between HIV and the immune system begins when the virus slips into the bloodstream via a CD4 receptor enzyme on a T4 cell, to which it preferentially attaches itself. A CD4 receptor alone, however, is not enough to cause infection, and for years scientists searched for some other protein on the cell surface that HIV can exploit to gain entry.

This protein was discovered in May 1996 by a team of scientists at the National Institute of Allergy and Infectious Diseases (NIAID). The scientists named the protein fusin because it helps the virus fuse with a healthy cell membrane and inject genetic material into the cell. The CD4-containing cell signals to killer T cells that it is infected by displaying fragments of HIV proteins on its surface. This triggers the killer cells to spring into action, which multiply and seek out the infected CD4-containing cells to pierce them open and destroy them.

CONFIRMING A HIDING PLACE

Typically, an HIV infection begins with a sudden, flu-like illness. Shortly after this first episode, the virus virtually disappears and symptoms may not materialize for as long as 20 years. Over time, the immune system eventually collapses and the virus appears in ever-increasing amounts of CD4-containing cells floating free in the patient's blood. Even though previous studies focused on the presence of the virus in the blood, two independently conducted studies in 1993—Janet Embretson et al.'s "Massive Covert Infection of Helper T Lymphocytes and Macrophages by HIV during the Incubation Period of AIDS" (*Nature*, vol. 362, no. 6418, March 25, 1993) and Anthony S. Fauci et al.'s "Multifactorial Nature of Human Immunodeficiency Virus Disease: Implications for Therapy" (*Science*, vol. 262, no. 5136, November 12, 1993)—confirmed suspicions long held by scientists that HIV hides in a patient's lymph nodes and similar tissue during the quiescent (first or early) stage of infection.

Searching for an Active Virus

Research by Fauci et al. focused on the search for the virus in the blood and lymphoid tissue (the lymph nodes, spleen, tonsils, and adenoids) of 12 HIV-infected patients whose infections had progressed to varying severities. Initially, the virus is concentrated almost entirely in the lymphoid tissues. Fauci et al. believe the virus infiltrates the lymph nodes within weeks of the initial infection. Particles of the virus, which are coated with antibodies, adhere to the follicular dendritic cells, a group of filtering cells that trap foreign material. CD4-containing cells nearby "see" the trapped material and are stimulated to attack the invader. The stronger virus counterattacks and reproduces itself on some of these CD4-containing cells.

After this infiltration, the performance of the immune system declines. This decline, which ultimately is dramatically debilitating, occurs over an extended period—up to 20 years in some AIDS sufferers. During this decline the follicular dendritic cells also begin to deteriorate, and the quantity of HIV in the CD4-containing cells floating free in the blood increases significantly. In the final stage of the disease, there is an almost complete dissolution of the follicular dendritic cell network. At this point the amount of HIV in the blood and in the CD4-containing cells has grown to equal the amount in the lymph nodes.

NOT JUST THE IMMUNE SYSTEM

For some time scientists and researchers believed HIV attacked and affected only the immune system. Many early AIDS cases that provided evidence of the involvement of other regions of the body were not counted due to the narrower definitions of AIDS that existed before 1993. However, after 1993 clear evidence showed that the free virus (not attached to any other cells) could appear in the fluid surrounding the brain and spinal cord and in the bloodstream. HIV can be found not only in T4 lymphocytes but also in other immune system cells, as well as in cells in the nervous system, intestine, and bone marrow.

CDC researchers proposed another reason HIV infections are so difficult to eliminate and why the immune system appears to be so susceptible to them. Their research shows that HIV can infect and grow in immature bone marrow cells, offering no clues about what the mature HIV-infected cells will become. The virus reproduces without revealing itself to the immune system, which under normal circumstances would destroy it. By developing in immature bone marrow cells, a great quantity of the virus can be produced before the body ever attempts to resist it.

As they mature, the cells change, becoming infected monocytes and macrophages that may not only fail to fight infections but may also spread the virus to other immune system cells. Infected marrow cells may seed the virus into other parts of the body, including the brain. The infected cells that develop in the marrow are carried through the bloodstream to the rest of the body.

SEARCHING FOR ANSWERS

Researchers have long been puzzled by the fact that AIDS is virtually always fatal, even though relatively small amounts of the virus are found in patients, compared to other lethal viral infections. How the virus acts to kill the cells has been hotly debated. Certainly, this behavior is inconsistent with other retroviruses, which do not kill all the infected host cells. Even though HIV is considered to be a slow virus (a virus that exerts its effect over a long period), some AIDS activity occurs more quickly and may be associated with the coincidental presence of infectious mycoplasma (bacteria that lack a cell wall).

Restoring Immune Response

In December 1993 the NCI reported that the immune function had been restored to HIV-infected cells grown in a laboratory through the addition of interleukin-12 (IL-12). IL-12 is a member of a group of natural blood proteins called cytokines that were discovered in 1991 by scientists at the Wistar Institute and Hoffmann-La Roche Inc. Despite this promising result, the U.S. Food and Drug Administration (FDA) halted human testing of IL-12 in June 1995, after two patients died. After testing the protein on animals, researchers concluded that the problem was not in IL-12 itself, but in the timing of the doses. Consequently, human testing resumed in November 1995.

In December 1995 a new class of drugs called protease inhibitors received FDA approval. These drugs block the ability of HIV to mature and to infect new cells by suppressing the protein-degrading activity of a viral enzyme. Enzymes with this activity are classified as proteases, hence the designation of the enzyme blocker as a protease inhib-

itor. If protease inhibitors can block the spread of HIV in the immune system, then AIDS will not develop. Though patients may be HIV positive the rest of their life, they may never die from an HIV infection.

Theories of HIV/AIDS Progression

Even after nearly three decades of research, there is still no consensus among HIV experts as to the pathogenesis (the origination and development) of AIDS. Despite this, there is agreement that the latent period between the establishment of an HIV infection and the appearance of the symptoms of AIDS averages from about two to 11 years. However, some people remain symptom free for as long as 20 years. Furthermore, between 5% and 10% of all HIV-infected people do not appear to develop AIDS. Called long-term nonprogressors, these individuals are believed to have genetic and immune response characteristics that slow, or may even halt, the course of disease progression. Much research interest centers on these people, because an understanding of their physiological characteristics that allow them to suppress the infection could be invaluable to the treatment of the disease in other patients.

After the HIV infection is established, the immune system regenerates cells only up to a certain point, which would explain a gradual progression to AIDS. The early regulatory functions of the immune system limit viral replication until a certain threshold is reached. When the number of different viral mutants becomes too large, the regulatory system is overwhelmed and shuts down, opening the door to opportunistic infections and eventual total decline.

When the total CD4+ T cell count falls from the normal 800 to 1,000 per cubic millimeter of blood to 200 per cubic millimeter, the rate of immune decline speeds up and the HIV-positive person becomes prone to the opportunistic infections and other illnesses that are characteristic of AIDS. In searching for an antiretroviral therapy, researchers find that rather than boosting the CD4+ T cell count, interruption of the viral replication may be the way to reverse immune deficiency in an HIV infection, though the nature of a reversing mechanism remains unknown.

SOME INCONSISTENCIES WITH CURRENT THEORIES. Most scientists agree that there are still gaps and inconsistencies in the knowledge of how HIV causes AIDS. One inconsistency concerns the infection and killing of the helper T cells. Initially, researchers thought that the main tactic of HIV was to infect and destroy the T cells. As these cells died, the numerical strength of the helper T cell force was depleted, thus causing the immune deficiency associated with AIDS patients.

Other scientists, however, consider this theory too simplistic, because so few T cells—no more than one infected cell in 500—are infected. Rather, two studies published in 2001 in the *Journal of Experimental Medicine*—Hiroshi

Mohri et al.'s "Increased Turnover of T Lymphocytes in HIV-1 Infection and Its Reduction by Antiretroviral Therapy" (vol. 194, no. 9, November 5, 2001) and Joseph A. Kovacs et al.'s "Identification of Dynamically Distinct Subpopulations of T Lymphocytes That Are Differentially Affected by HIV" (vol. 194, no. 12, December 17, 2001)—support the idea that HIV does not block the production of T cells but instead accelerates the division of existing T cells. This causes the existing T cells to die off more quickly than normal.

Another inconsistency involves the observation that the rapid decline in the number of T cells comes relatively late in the infection, even though there are clear indications that the immune system has been impaired much earlier.

OPPORTUNISTIC INFECTIONS

Once HIV has destroyed the immune system, the body can no longer protect itself against bacterial, fungal, protozoal, and other viral agents that take advantage of the compromised condition and cause infections. These infections, which would not otherwise occur but for an impaired immune system, are known as opportunistic infections (OIs). In the non-AIDS community, OIs are problematic in hospitals, where ill, newborn, or elderly patients may also have less than adequately functioning immune systems. Because the patient is considered to have AIDS if at least one OI appears, OIs are also referred to as "AIDS-defining events," though OIs are not the only AIDS-defining events.

By 1997 the leading OI for Americans suffering from HIV/AIDS was *Pneumocystis carinii* pneumonia (PCP), a lung disease caused by a fungus. Before the discovery of HIV/AIDS, PCP was found almost exclusively in cancer and transplant patients with weakened immune systems. During the 1980s PCP was the AIDS-defining illness for two-thirds of people diagnosed with AIDS in the United States, and it was estimated that 75% of HIV-infected people would develop PCP during their lifetime. According to Laurence Huang et al., in "An Official ATS Workshop Summary: Recent Advances and Future Directions in Pneumocystis Pneumonia (PCP)" (*Proceedings of the American Thoracic Society*, vol. 3, no. 8, November 2006), the incidence of PCP decreased 3.4% per year between 1992 and 1995 and then declined 21.5% annually between 1996 and 1998, when powerful combinations of antiretroviral therapy were beginning to be used. NAM, a charitable organization that produces and distributes information about HIV/AIDS, explains in the fact sheet "PCP" (2011, http://www.aidsmap.com/PCP/page/1044747/) that effective HIV treatment and improved treatment for PCP, including the use of antibiotics to prevent its occurrence, have made PCP infection uncommon among people with HIV in the United States. However, PCP remains the most frequently occurring serious OI among HIV-infected people in developing countries.

Even though prescription drugs such as trimethoprim-sulfamethoxazole were found to be effective at preventing PCP during the late 1980s, and their widespread use along with the addition of antiretroviral therapy a decade later markedly reduced the cases of PCP, researchers find that people who do not adhere to treatment remain at risk of developing the disease. James D. Heffelfinger et al. determine in "Nonadherence to Primary Prophylaxis against *Pneumocystis jirovecii* Pneumonia" (*PLoS ONE*, vol. 4, no. 3, March 2009) that nearly one-fifth of HIV-infected people do not take the drugs prescribed to prevent PCP. The researchers identify illicit drug use and mental health issues including depression and a low CD4 cell count as factors that are associated with nonadherence to treatment prescribed to prevent PCP. Furthermore, NAM indicates that HIV-positive people who smoke are three times more likely to develop PCP than nonsmokers.

Esophageal candidiasis, an infection of the esophagus, and extrapulmonary cryptococcosis, a systemic fungus that enters the body through the lungs and may invade any organ of the body, are also OIs frequently diagnosed in AIDS patients.

Other illnesses such as Burkitt's lymphoma, invasive cervical cancer, and primary brain lymphoma are also considered AIDS-defining events. Wasting syndrome (which is characterized by drastic weight loss and lethargy) is another illness that may be considered an AIDS-defining event. Other examples of AIDS-defining events include diagnosis of *Mycobacterium avium* complex, a serious bacterial infection that may occur in one part of the body such as the liver, bone marrow, and spleen or spread throughout the body; cytomegalovirus disease, a member of the herpesvirus group; Kaposi's sarcoma, a once-rare cancer of the blood vessel walls that causes conspicuous purple lesions on the skin; and toxoplasmic encephalitis, an inflammation of the brain. Patients may experience more than one OI or AIDS-defining event.

In 2006 NIAID researchers identified a critical human cell surface molecule—protein xCT—as the receptor that can make cells vulnerable to infection with Kaposi's sarcoma herpesvirus (KSHV). At the close of the first decade of the 21st century, Kaposi's sarcoma was less common in the United States than it had been during the early years of the AIDS pandemic; however, it remained the most common cancer that was associated with HIV infection. Figure 1.6 shows how KSHV fuses to and enters a human cell after binding to the protein xCT.

HIV and Tuberculosis

Tuberculosis (TB) is a communicable infection that is caused by the bacterium *Mycobacterium tuberculosis*. TB was a widespread pandemic in North America during the late 19th and early 20th centuries. Subsequently, it faded from prominence. However, TB regained a foothold during

FIGURE 1.6

How the Kaposi's sarcoma herpesvirus enters cells

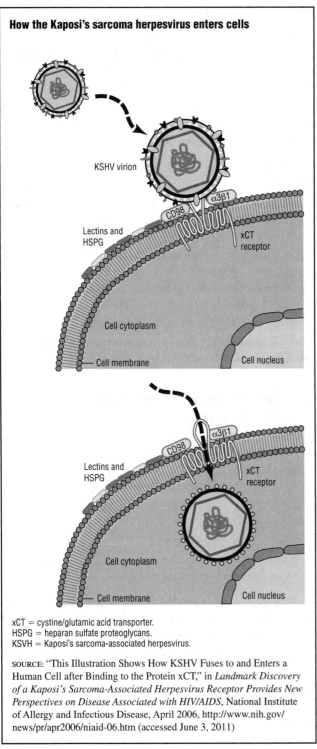

xCT = cystine/glutamic acid transporter.
HSPG = heparan sulfate proteoglycans.
KSVH = Kaposi's sarcoma-associated herpesvirus.

SOURCE: "This Illustration Shows How KSHV Fuses to and Enters a Human Cell after Binding to the Protein xCT," in *Landmark Discovery of a Kaposi's Sarcoma-Associated Herpesvirus Receptor Provides New Perspectives on Disease Associated with HIV/AIDS*, National Institute of Allergy and Infectious Disease, April 2006, http://www.nih.gov/news/pr/apr2006/niaid-06.htm (accessed June 3, 2011)

Activation Induced Apoptosis in CD4 Lymphocytes from HIV Seropositive Patients" (January 28–February 1, 1996)—first concluded that the decline in CD4+ T cells is greater in HIV-infected patients who develop TB than in those who remain free of TB. In some geographic areas up to 58% of those diagnosed with TB were also HIV positive. Of the many diseases that are associated with HIV infection, TB is one of the few that is transmissible (capable of being transmitted), treatable, and preventable.

TB is spread from person to person through the inhalation of airborne particles containing *M. tuberculosis*. The particles, called droplet nuclei, are produced when a person with infectious TB of the lung or larynx forcefully exhales, such as when coughing, sneezing, speaking, or singing. These infectious particles remain suspended in the air and may be inhaled by someone sharing the same air. The risk of transmission is increased when ventilation is poor and when susceptible people share air for prolonged periods with a person who has untreated pulmonary TB.

Approximately 85% of TB infections occur in the lungs. This infection is called pulmonary TB. However, TB may occur at any site of the body, such as the larynx, the lymph nodes, the brain, the kidneys, or the bones. These cases are called extrapulmonary TB. Except for laryngeal TB, people with extrapulmonary TB are usually not considered infectious to others. It is important to note that, as mentioned earlier, HIV is a bloodborne infection and cannot be spread through the air. An HIV-positive person who has TB can spread TB nuclei through the air, but not HIV.

According to the CDC, in "Tuberculosis (TB)" (June 1, 2011, http://www.cdc.gov/tb/statistics/default.htm), the number of TB cases in the United States declined by 10.5% from 2008 to 2009; however, TB remains one of the leading causes of death of people who are HIV infected. This is because people who are not HIV infected usually can defend themselves successfully against TB infection. The risk that TB will develop in people infected only with *M. tuberculosis* is 10% within their lifetime. People with HIV, who may have weakened immune systems, are less able to resist infection and are more likely to develop active TB. HIV-infected people with either latent TB infection or active TB disease can be effectively treated with prescription drugs that kill the bacteria.

Extensively drug-resistant TB (XDR-TB), which does not respond to the conventional drugs that are used to combat the disease, poses a new threat to public health initiatives aimed at reducing the numbers of TB infections. In "Extensively Drug-Resistant Tuberculosis: New Strains, New Challenges" (*Expert Review of Anti-infective Therapy*, vol. 6, no. 5, October 2008), Ritu Banerjee et al. observe that high HIV coinfection rates in many parts of the world have contributed to the emergence of XDR-TB. Jason R. Andrews et al. report in "Predictors of Multidrug- and Extensively Drug-Resistant

the 1990s, with the number of cases increasing in the United States. Part of this increase is the parallel increase in the occurrence of the infection in HIV-positive individuals. Indeed, HIV infection has become one of the strongest known risk factors for the progression of TB from infection to disease.

A landmark report from the 1996 Conference on Retroviruses and Opportunistic Infections—Andrew D. Badley et al.'s "Enhanced Fas/Fas Ligand Dependent

Tuberculosis in a High HIV Prevalence Community" (*PLoS One*, vol. 5, no. 12, December 29, 2010) that multidrug-resistant TB and XDR-TB continue to appear in places with high HIV prevalence, where the death rate for HIV-coinfected patients remains high. In the developing world, where many cases are undetected, delays in diagnosis and treatment serve to increase the death rate.

HIV and Cancer

People with AIDS are susceptible to cancer. Some malignant tumors, such as Kaposi's sarcoma and cancers of the lymph system, have been common among AIDS patients since the disease was first discovered in 1981. More recently, however, physicians and researchers have found that certain forms of cancer are more prevalent among HIV/AIDS patients who are living longer.

Most AIDS-related cancers are believed to be caused by viruses. These cancers are more common among HIV-infected people because HIV suppresses the immune system, enabling cancer-causing viruses to attack more successfully. These cancers include non-Hodgkin's lymphoma (found in lymph tissues) and primary lymphoma of the brain. People infected with HIV are also at greater risk of oral, lung, anal, liver, and skin cancers as well as myeloma (malignant tumors of the bone marrow), brain tumors, testicular cancers, and leukemia (cancer of the blood cells).

Because anti-HIV-combination drug therapies, such as highly active antiretroviral therapy (HAART), have become widely used, researchers report a decline in Kaposi's sarcoma and primary lymphoma of the brain. One possible explanation for the decline may be that the combination drug therapies enable the body to recover partial immunity, which in turn helps prevent the development of cancer.

Lung cancer is the third most commonly diagnosed cancer among people with HIV, after non-Hodgkin's lymphoma and Kaposi's sarcoma. Until recently it was assumed that the high rate of lung cancer in HIV-infected people was solely attributable to smoking, but recent research questions this assumption. In "HIV Infection Is Associated with an Increased Risk for Lung Cancer, Independent of Smoking" (*Clinical Infectious Diseases*, vol. 45, no. 1, July 1, 2007), Gregory D. Kirk et al. examine the relationship between HIV infection and lung cancer death and smoking. The researchers find strong evidence that HIV infection contributes to lung cancer, independent of smoking, and conclude that HIV infection alone increases the risk of developing lung cancer. They also find that HIV increased the lung cancer risk among smokers. Even though it is not known how HIV influences the development of lung cancer, Kirk et al. speculate that it might be directly involved in promoting the development of cancer or might increase susceptibility by

compromising immune function. HIV might also increase susceptibility to the cancer-causing effects of tobacco.

Other researchers also report an association between HIV and lung cancer, independent of smoking. Alexandra Bazoes, Mark Bower, and Thomas Powles speculate in "Smoke and Mirrors: HIV-Related Lung Cancer" (*Current Opinions in Oncology*, vol. 20, no. 5, September 2008) that lung cancer in HIV-positive patients is a more aggressive and extensive disease.

Meredith S. Shiels et al. explain in "Cancer Burden in the HIV-Infected Population in the United States" (*Journal of the National Cancer Institute*, vol. 103, no. 9, May 4, 2011) that since the introduction of combination antiretroviral therapy, the incidence of AIDS-defining infections and cancers, including Kaposi's sarcoma, non-Hodgkin lymphoma, and invasive cervical carcinoma, have decreased significantly. However, the incidence and numbers of deaths that are attributable to non-AIDS-related malignancies and other diseases have increased among patients with HIV-1 infection. This shift is the result of increased life expectancy and the reduction of competing causes of death.

TOWARD A VACCINE: THE HOPE AND THE REALITIES

The different routes of attack of HIV on the immune system and the ability of the virus to mutate has prompted the suggestion by some researchers that the development of an effective vaccine will be difficult to achieve. This admission is contrary to what Margaret M. Heckler (1931–), the U.S. secretary of the Department of Health and Human Services under President Ronald Reagan (1911–2004), announced in 1984 that the identification of HIV would lead to a vaccine within two years.

The intervening years have made many AIDS researchers realize that the chances of developing a vaccine that will prevent AIDS (confer immunity on the person receiving the vaccine) are remote. Testing the effectiveness of an AIDS vaccine is also difficult, because the deliberate contamination of people with HIV is both unethical and illegal. As a result, the focus of research has shifted to vaccines that do not prevent infections but lessen their effects and delay the progress of the disease. For example, recent studies, including one that was conducted in Thailand in 2009, overcome ethical concerns by offering vaccine trials in regions such as Thailand provinces that have some of the highest prevalence rates of HIV infection. These studies also advise their subjects to practice safe sex and supply condoms to help prevent infection.

According to Margaret I. Johnston and Anthony S. Fauci, in "An HIV Vaccine—Evolving Concepts" (*New England Journal of Medicine*, vol. 356, no. 20, May 17, 2007), such vaccine efforts continue. The huge genetic diversity and other unique features of the HIV envelope protein have frustrated attempts to identify an effective vaccine of the traditional type—one that imitates the effects of natural exposure and confers a high level of long-lasting protection against infection in the vast majority of recipients. As a result, most research focuses on harnessing T cells to stimulate cellular immunity to HIV. Research demonstrates the importance of cellular immunity during the early and later stages of HIV infection, and even though T cell vaccines have not completely eliminated the virus, they can produce cellular immune responses that may act to reduce virus levels or help people remain disease free for longer periods following infection. In animal studies, T cell vaccines decreased the amount of virus produced during early infection, prompted a reduction in virus levels after the acute stage of infection, delayed disease progression, or generated a combination of these beneficial effects.

In "HIV-1 Vaccines and Adaptive Trial Designs" (*Science Translational Research*, vol. 3, no. 79, April 2011), Lawrence Corey et al. describe the challenges of vaccine development. The researchers explain that even though animal models provide valuable information, they do not accurately predict HIV vaccine efficacy (the ability of an intervention to produce the intended diagnostic or therapeutic effect in optimal circumstances) in humans. The lack of an ideal animal model with a predictive value for humans and the fact that there are no universally accepted standardized measures of immune protection against HIV suggests that human vaccine trials are the only accurate way to assess promising vaccine candidates.

As of August 2011, the best human clinical trial results came from a 2009 study involving more than 16,000 people in Thailand. The study involved the use of two vaccines. When these vaccines were combined, they reduced the risk of infection by 30%. Leia Wren and Stephen J. Kent observe in "HIV Vaccine Efficacy Trial: Glimmers of Hope and the Potential Role of Antibody-Dependent Cellular Cytotoxicity" (*Human Vaccines*, vol. 7, no. 4, April 1, 2011) that the modest success of the vaccine trial in Thailand has reinvigorated vaccine research efforts and focused research on the role of antibody-dependent cellular cytotoxicity (the extent to which something can harm or kill cells).

Despite the challenges that HIV provides, clinical trials of HIV vaccines continue. In "Search for HIV/AIDS Clinical Trials" (August 16, 2011, http://www.aidsinfo.nih.gov/clinicaltrials/), AIDSinfo, a service of the U.S. Department of Health and Human Services, notes that 142 clinical trials of HIV preventive vaccines were planned, underway, or completed in 2011.

Promise and Progress

Even though human trials have not yet produced favorable results and animal study findings are not necessarily applicable to humans, several animal studies have yielded promising findings. Jennifer D. Watkins et al. report in "An Anti-HIV-1 V3 Loop Antibody Fully Protects Cross-Clade and Elicits T-Cell Immunity in Macaques Mucosally Challenged with an R5 Clade C SHIV" (*PLoS One*, vol. 6, no. 3, March 31, 2011) that neutralizing antibodies may prove effective as a vaccine. The neutralizing antibodies act by binding to the surface of HIV and prevent it from attaching itself to a cell and infecting it. The researchers tested this theory on Asian monkeys. When they injected the monkeys with the neutralizing antibodies and then exposed the monkeys to HIV, the HIV was unable to attach and as a result the monkeys did not become HIV infected.

Another auspicious finding was reported by Scott G. Hansen et al. in "Profound Early Control of Highly Pathogenic SIV by an Effector Memory T-cell Vaccine" (*Nature*, vol. 473, no. 7348, May 2011). The researchers theorize that because most people become infected with cytomegalovirus (CMV) early in life and because the virus lives in them without causing disease, it might be a vehicle for carrying some HIV genes into the body to evoke an immune response. To test this theory, Hansen et al. injected 24 monkeys with a strain of CMV that infects rhesus monkeys loaded with a vaccine candidate aimed at SIV. In more than half of the monkeys, the vaccine quickly eliminated SIV infections, and the protection lasted for at least one year.

HAART Treatment Is Effective but Adherence May Be Difficult

During the mid-1990s a "hit-hard-early" strategy gained favor. In this strategy a cocktail of anti-HIV drugs was given to patients shortly after they had been diagnosed with having HIV. The idea of HAART is to suppress the reproduction of the virus as much as possible. Some of the drugs target the virus's reverse transcriptase. By inhibiting the enzyme's activity, the ability of HIV to reproduce is thwarted. However, HAART has a downside. Even though it is able to suppress the viral load, it is unable to eradicate it, and once HAART is initiated, treatment must be continued over a lifetime. The therapy is expensive and hard to maintain, and its long-term use is associated with a number of serious side effects. If patients do not adhere to the treatment, then they may not adequately suppress the virus.

Historically, HAART treatment was initiated when CD4 cell counts fell below 350 cells per cubic millimeter and in many countries with limited resources, treatment was deferred until CD4 counts dropped below 200 cells per cubic millimeter. However, Emma Hitt reports in "Starting HAART at Higher T-Cell Counts Improves Survival in Early-Stage HIV" (*Medscape Medical News*, June 10, 2009) that early HAART treatment, when CD4 cell counts are between 200 and 350 cells per cubic millimeter, improves survival. Early treatment may also improve tolerability of antiviral drugs and reduce HIV transmission to other uninfected people.

CHAPTER 2
DEFINITION, SYMPTOMS, AND TRANSMITTAL

A DEFINITION OF AIDS

The Centers for Disease Control and Prevention (CDC) is the federal government's clearinghouse, research center, and monitoring agency for all infectious diseases, including HIV/AIDS. The CDC tracks the diseases in the United States and notifies health officials of their occurrence via *Morbidity and Mortality Weekly Report* notices and a website that is updated frequently.

The CDC defines AIDS as a specific group of diseases or conditions that are indicative of severe immunosuppression related to infection with HIV. The health agency first outlined a surveillance (a constant observation of a process) case definition in 1982, and then revised it in 1983, 1985, 1987, 1993, 2000, and again in 2008 as knowledge about HIV infection increased and additional severe and common symptoms were included in the definitions. The 1993 definition emphasized the clinical importance of the CD4+ T cell count and included the addition of three clinical conditions.

THE 1993 AND 2008 CLASSIFICATION REVISIONS AND EXPANDED SURVEILLANCE CASE DEFINITIONS

In 1991 the CDC released a draft of the document that eventually became the "1993 Revised Classification System for HIV Infection and Expanded Surveillance Case Definition for AIDS among Adolescents and Adults" (*Morbidity and Mortality Weekly Report*, vol. 41, RR-17, December 18, 1992), by Kenneth G. Castro et al. of the CDC. This classification scheme was slightly revised in 2008 and published as "Revised Surveillance Case Definitions for HIV Infection among Adults, Adolescents, and Children Aged <18 Months and for HIV Infection and AIDS among Children Aged 18 Months to <13 Years—United States, 2008" (*Morbidity and Mortality Weekly Report*, vol. 57, RR-10, December 5, 2008), by Eileen Schneider et al. of the CDC. As of August 2011, it was the standard surveillance case definition.

The 1993 revision addressed the concerns of many women, their attorneys, and physicians, who had strongly advocated the inclusion of diseases such as pelvic inflammatory disease (inflammation of the female reproductive organs by microorganisms) and vaginal candidiasis (a fungal infection, commonly called a yeast infection or thrush) as conditions that could precede the development of AIDS, so that women infected with HIV would be included in the revised definition. Advocates cautioned that if the CDC omitted such inclusive criteria, many women would be denied access to disability benefits, necessary treatment, and education.

The 2008 revision combined surveillance case definitions for adults and adolescents by offering a single definition for people aged 13 years and older. It also revised the HIV infection case definition for children under the age of 13 years and the AIDS case definition for children aged 18 months to 13 years old. The case definition for HIV infection includes AIDS and incorporates the HIV infection classification system in which AIDS is called stage 3 infection. Laboratory-confirmed evidence of HIV infection, as opposed to simply the diagnosis of an AIDS-defining condition without confirmation from laboratory tests, is now required to meet the surveillance case definition for HIV infection.

Even though reporting criteria include recommendations for diagnosing HIV infection, the primary purpose of the original and updated case definitions for HIV and AIDS is public health surveillance as opposed to the diagnosis of individual patients.

The 2008 Revised Definition and Classification: Tied to CD4+ Cells

The 2008 surveillance case definition emphasizes the central role of the CD4+ T cell counts and percentages, which are objective measures of immunosuppression that are routinely used in the care of HIV-infected people and

TABLE 2.1

Surveillance case definition for HIV infection among adults and adolescents, 2008

[Aged >13 years. United States.]

Stage	Laboratory evidence[a]	Clinical evidence
Stage 1	Laboratory confirmation of HIV infection and CD4+ T-lymphocyte count of ≥500 cells/μL or CD4+ T-lymphocyte percentage of ≥29	None required (but no AIDS-defining condition)
Stage 2	Laboratory confirmation of HIV infection and CD4+ T-lymphocyte count of 200–499 cells/μL or CD4+ T-lymphocyte percentage of 14–28	None required (but no AIDS-defining condition)
Stage 3 (AIDS)	Laboratory confirmation of HIV infection and CD4+ T-lymphocyte count of <200 cells/μL or CD4+ T-lymphocyte percentage of <14[b]	Or documentation of an AIDS-defining condition (with laboratory confirmation of HIV infection)[b]
Stage unknown[c]	Laboratory confirmation of HIV infection and no information on CD4+ T-lymphocyte count or percentage	And no information on presence of AIDS-defining conditions

μL = Microliter.

[a]The CD4+ T-lymphocyte percentage is the percentage of total lymphocytes. If the CD4+ T-lymphocyte count and percentage do not correspond to the same HIV infection stage, select the more severe stage.

[b]Documentation of an AIDS-defining condition supersedes a CD4= T-lymphocyte count of ≥200 cells/μL and a CD4+ T-lymphocyte percentage of total lymphocytes of ≥14.

[c]Although cases with no information on CD4+ T-lymphocyte count or percentage or on the presence of AIDS-defining conditions can be classified as stage unknown, every effort should be made to report CD4+ T-lymphocyte counts or percentages and the presence of AIDS-defining conditions at the time of diagnosis. Additional CD4+ T-lymphocyte counts or percentages and any identified AIDS-defining conditions can be reported as recommended.

SOURCE: Eileen Schneider et al., "Table. Surveillance Case Definition for Human Immunodeficiency Virus (HIV) Infection among Adults and Adolescents (Aged >13 years)—United States, 2008," in "Revised Surveillance Case Definitions for HIV Infection among Adults, Adolescents, and Children Aged <18 Months and for HIV Infection and AIDS among Children Aged 18 Months to <13 Years—United States, 2008," *Morbidity and Mortality Weekly Report*, vol. 57, no. RR-10, December 5, 2008, http://www.cdc.gov/mmwr/pdf/rr/rr5710.pdf (accessed June 3, 2011)

are available to surveillance programs. As shown in Table 2.1, the 2008 classification system is based on three ranges of CD4+ T-lymphocyte counts and does not require the presence of an AIDS-defining condition. Table 2.2 lists a number of AIDS-defining conditions.

Historically, one of the difficulties that researchers faced when making international comparisons were varying case definitions and reporting practices. The World Health Organization (WHO) and CDC surveillance case definitions both require laboratory confirmation to establish HIV infection; however, their staging systems are slightly different from one another. In addition, because there is no universal method for measuring CD4+ T-lymphocyte counts and percentages, the WHO advises using clinical and immunologic criteria for staging. Table 2.3 compares the WHO and the CDC case definitions.

The Impact of the 1993 Definition on Case Reporting

CDC data indicate that expansion of the AIDS surveillance criteria changed both the process of AIDS surveillance and the number of reported cases. In "Current Trends Update: Impact of the Expanded AIDS Surveillance Case Definition for Adolescents and Adults on Case Reporting—United States, 1993" (*Morbidity and Mortality Weekly Report*, vol. 43, no. 9, March 11, 1994), the CDC reports that in 1993, 103,500 AIDS cases were reported in the United States among adults and adolescents aged 13 years and older. This number was just over twice the 49,016 cases reported in 1992 and likely represented a one-time effect of the 1993 expansion of the AIDS definition. The steep increase probably represented the reporting of people who

were diagnosed with the newly added conditions before 1993. Newly reported AIDS cases declined again beginning in 1996 in response to treatments, such as highly active antiretroviral therapy (HAART), that slowed the progression from HIV infection to AIDS. Between 1998 and 1999 the decline in the incidence of AIDS began to level. (See Figure 2.1.) Between 1999 and 2008 the numbers of diagnoses and deaths remained fairly stable.

Table 2.4 shows the estimated numbers and rates of people living with HIV infection in 2008, the most recent year for which data were available as of August 2011. It also indicates that 20.1% of people were undiagnosed with having an HIV infection.

DIAGNOSIS AND SYMPTOMS OF AIDS

Only a qualified health professional can diagnose AIDS. To evaluate a patient with a positive HIV test, the health care practitioner performs a complete physical examination and collects the patient's social and family history. Diagnostic laboratory tests are also performed. These tests typically include complete blood count and routine chemistry; CD4+ T cell count; assays (analyses) that measure the amount of HIV-1 ribonucleic acid (RNA) in plasma; tuberculin skin tests to detect the presence of the bacterium that causes tuberculosis; and assays for the microbial agents that cause syphilis, toxoplasmosis, and hepatitis B and C. Female patients are screened for cervical cancer using the *Papanicolaou* smear.

HIV infection progresses through a range of stages. Following the establishment of the infection (primary

TABLE 2.2

AIDS-defining conditions

- Bacterial infections, multiple or recurrent[a]
- Candidiasis of bronchi, trachea, or lungs
- Candidiasis of esophagus[b]
- Cervical cancer, invasive[c]
- Coccidioidomycosis, disseminated or extrapulmonary
- Cryptococcosis, extrapulmonary
- Cryptosporidiosis, chronic intestinal (>1 month's duration)
- Cytomegalovirus disease (other than liver, spleen, or nodes), onset at age >1 month
- Cytomegalovirus retinitis (with loss of vision)[b]
- Encephalopathy, HIV related
- Herpes simplex: chronic ulcers (>1 month's duration) or bronchitis, pneumonitis, or esophagitis (onset at age >1 month)
- Histoplasmosis, disseminated or extrapulmonary
- Isosporiasis, chronic intestinal (>1 month's duration)
- Kaposi sarcoma[b]
- Lymphoid interstitial pneumonia or pulmonary lymphoid hyperplasia complex[a, b]
- Lymphoma, Burkitt (or equivalent term)
- Lymphoma, immunoblastic (or equivalent term)
- Lymphoma, primary, of brain
- *Mycobacterium avium* complex or *Mycobacterium kansasii*, disseminated or extrapulmonary[b]
- *Mycobacterium tuberculosis* of any site, pulmonary,[b, c] disseminated,[b] or extrapulmonary[b]
- *Mycobacterium*, other species or unidentified species, disseminated[b] or extrapulmonary[b]
- *Pneumocystis jirovecii* pneumonia[b]
- Pneumonia, recurrent[b, c]
- Progressive multifocal leukoencephalopathy
- *Salmonella* septicemia, recurrent
- Toxoplasmosis of brain, onset at age >1 month[b]
- Wasting syndrome attributed to HIV

HIV = Human immunodeficiency virus.
[a]Only among children aged <13 years.
[b]Condition that might be diagnosed presumptively.
[c]Only among adults and adolescents aged >13 years.

SOURCE: Eileen Schneider et al., "Appendix A. AIDS-Defining Conditions," in "Revised Surveillance Case Definitions for HIV Infection among Adults, Adolescents, and Children Aged <18 Months and for HIV Infection and AIDS among Children Aged 18 Months to <13 Years—United States, 2008," *Morbidity and Mortality Weekly Report*, vol. 57, no. RR-10, December 5, 2008, http://www.cdc.gov/mmwr/pdf/rr/rr5710.pdf (accessed June 3, 2011)

infection), there follows a typically prolonged asymptomatic (symptom free) period before the appearance of symptoms and the deterioration of the patient's health. Among the symptoms that develop are weight loss; profound, unexplained fatigue; nausea; fever; night sweats; swollen lymph glands; a heavy, persistent, dry cough; easy bruising or unexplained bleeding; watery diarrhea; loss of memory; balance problems; mood changes; blurring or loss of vision; and oral lesions, such as thrush (a fungal infection caused by *Candida albicans*, which appears as a white coating on the tongue and throat). The infecting virus is basically the same in all infected people in terms of its structure and genetic makeup, but individual reactions to the virus vary greatly. Death is usually the result of the opportunistic infections (OIs) and cancers that arise due to the impaired immune system—not HIV.

Dementia

Before the 1987 case definition many researchers were reluctant to include dementia as a symptom indicative of AIDS. Lawrence K. Altman notes in "New Study Is Easing Fears on AIDS and Mental Illness" (*New York Times*, June 3, 1989) that some observers cited early studies that showed as many as 40% to 70% of people infected with the virus developed neurological and psychological complications several years before other clinical symptoms, such as weight loss and fever, appeared. This fear led the military and civilian authorities to bar infected people from certain jobs involving public safety, including commercial pilots and bus drivers.

Altman reports that officials of the WHO and the National Institutes of Health (NIH) jointly found these estimates to be false. They reported that even though neurological

TABLE 2.3

Comparison of World Health Organization (WHO) and Centers for Disease Control and Prevention (CDC) stages of HIV infection

[For reporting purposes only. By CD4+ T-lymphocyte count and percentage of total lymphocytes.]

WHO stage[a]	WHO T-lymphocyte count and percentage[b]	CDC stage[c]	CDC T-lymphocyte count and percentage
Stage 1 (HIV infection)	CD4+ T-lymphocyte count of ≥500 cells/μL	Stage 1 (HIV infection)	CD4+ T-lymphocyte count of ≥500 cells/μL or CD4+ T-lymphocyte percentage of ≥29
Stage 2 (HIV infection)	CD4+ T-lymphocyte count of 350–499 cells/μL	Stage 2 (HIV infection)	CD4+ T-lymphocyte count of 200–499 cells/μL or CD4+ T-lymphocyte percentage of 14–28
Stage 3 (advanced HIV disease [AHD])	CD4+ T-lymphocyte count of 200–349 cells/μL	Stage 2 (HIV infection)	CD4+ T-lymphocyte count of 200–499 cells/μL or CD4+ T-lymphocyte percentage of 14–28
Stage 4 (acquired immunodeficiency syndrome [AIDS])	CD4+ T-lymphocyte count of <200 cells/μL or CD4+ T-lymphocyte percentage of <15	Stage 3 (AIDS)	CD4+ T-lymphocyte count of <200 cells/μL or CD4+ T-lymphocyte percentage of <14

HIV = Human immunodeficiency virus.
μL = Microliter.
[a]Among adults and children aged ≥5 years.
[b]Percentage applicable for stage 4 only.
[c]Among adults and adolescents (aged ≥13 years). CDC also includes a fourth stage, stage unknown: laboratory confirmation of HIV infection but no information on CD4+ T-lymphocyte count or percentage and no information on AIDS-defining conditions.

SOURCE: Eileen Schneider et al., "Table. Comparison of World Health Organization (WHO) and CDC Stages of Human Immunodeficiency Virus (HIV) Infection, by CD4+ T-Lymphocyte Count and Percentage of Total Lymphocytes," in "Revised Surveillance Case Definitions for HIV Infection among Adults, Adolescents, and Children Aged <18 Months and for HIV Infection and AIDS among Children Aged 18 Months to <13 Years—United States, 2008," *Morbidity and Mortality Weekly Report*, vol. 57, no. RR-10, December 5, 2008, http://www.cdc.gov/mmwr/pdf/rr/rr5710.pdf (accessed June 3, 2011)

FIGURE 2.1

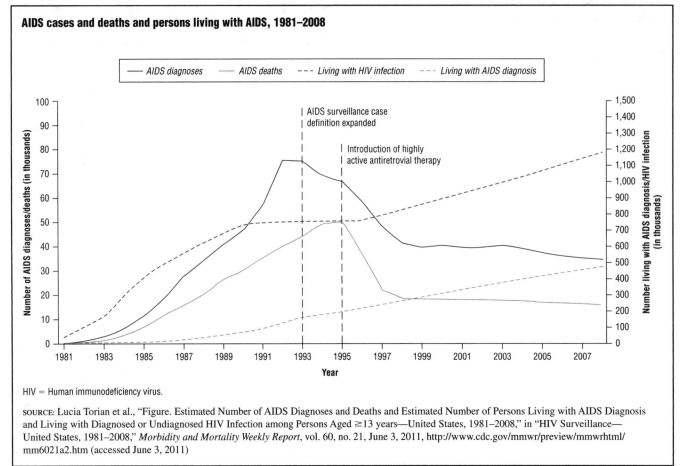

AIDS cases and deaths and persons living with AIDS, 1981–2008

— AIDS diagnoses   — AIDS deaths   --- Living with HIV infection   --- Living with AIDS diagnosis

AIDS surveillance case definition expanded

Introduction of highly active antiretroviral therapy

HIV = Human immunodeficiency virus.

SOURCE: Lucia Torian et al., "Figure. Estimated Number of AIDS Diagnoses and Deaths and Estimated Number of Persons Living with AIDS Diagnosis and Living with Diagnosed or Undiagnosed HIV Infection among Persons Aged ≥13 years—United States, 1981–2008," in "HIV Surveillance—United States, 1981–2008," *Morbidity and Mortality Weekly Report*, vol. 60, no. 21, June 3, 2011, http://www.cdc.gov/mmwr/preview/mmwrhtml/mm6021a2.htm (accessed June 3, 2011)

complications are common in the later stages of AIDS, dementia is rarely diagnosed in asymptomatic HIV-infected people, affecting fewer than 1% of those infected with HIV who have not yet developed AIDS.

A number of research studies were initiated during the 1990s to determine conclusively if there was any link between dementia and the subsequent diagnosis of AIDS. The data from studies conducted by the U.S. Air Force; a joint effort by the CDC and the San Francisco Health Department; and the Multicenter AIDS Cohort Study of men who have sex with other men in Baltimore, Maryland; Chicago, Illinois; Los Angeles, California; and Pittsburgh, Pennsylvania (sponsored by the National Institute of Allergy and Infectious Diseases and the National Cancer Institute), confirmed that the 40% to 70% frequency rate of dementia for HIV-infected people was far higher than the actual rate. One explanation for the higher figures reported during the 1980s is that the data came from centers to which AIDS patients with dementia had been referred for treatment. Put another way, the sample population was skewed toward the increased prevalence of dementia.

HIV-associated dementia (also called AIDS dementia complex) is now recognized as a declining cognitive (thinking) function that generally occurs during the late stages of HIV infection. The dementia is caused directly by HIV infection of the central nervous system, which includes the brain, and is different from the forgetfulness and difficulty in concentrating that can be the by-products of depression and fatigue. Christopher Power et al. estimate in "NeuroAIDS: An Evolving Epidemic" (*Canadian Journal of Neurological Sciences*, vol. 36, no. 3, May 2009) that more than 50% of people infected with HIV will develop a neurological disorder, such as dementia, despite the availability of HAART.

Selected Cancers

Historically, the frequent diagnosis of specific AIDS-defining cancers—non-Hodgkin's lymphoma, Kaposi's sarcoma, and cervical cancer—was attributed to compromised immune systems, and the occurrence of other cancers was thought to result from the fact that people with HIV/AIDS were living longer because of the widespread use of HAART.

In "Incidence of Non-AIDS-Defining Malignancies in HIV-Infected versus Noninfected Patients in the HAART Era: Impact of Immunosuppression" (*Journal of Acquired Immune Deficiency Syndromes*, vol. 52, no. 2, October 1, 2009), Roger J. Bedimo et al. discuss the results of their

TABLE 2.4

Estimated number and rate of persons with HIV infection, and number and percentage with undiagnosed HIV infection by selected characteristics, 2008

Characteristic	Total persons living with HIV infection		Persons whose HIV infection was undiagnosed	
	No.	Rate[a]	No.	%
Total	1,178,350	469.4	236,400	20.1
Sex				
Male	883,450	719.5	182,450	20.6
Female	294,900	230.0	53,950	18.3
Age group (yrs)				
13–24	68,600	134.1	40,400	58.9
25–34	180,600	440.9	56,800	31.5
35–44	357,500	846.3	64,300	18.0
45–54	385,400	871.3	53,200	13.8
55–64	147,700	439.3	17,600	11.9
≥65	38,400	99.0	4,100	10.7
Race				
American Indian/Alaska Native	5,000	268.8	1,250	25.0
Asian/Pacific Islander	16,750	147.0	4,350	26.0
Black/African American	545,000	1,819.0	116,750	21.4
White	406,000	238.4	75,200	18.5
Ethnicity				
Hispanic/Latino	205,400	592.9	38,900	18.9
Transmission category				
MSM	580,000	NC	128,400	22.1
IDU (male)	131,600	NC	18,900	14.4
IDU (female)	73,900	NC	10,400	14.1
MSM and IDU	55,200	NC	6,200	11.2
Heterosexual contact[b] (male)	110,900	NC	27,700	25.0
Heterosexual contact[b] (female)	217,400	NC	42,900	19.7
Other[c]	9,350	NC	1,900	20.3

HIV = Human immunodeficiency virus. MSM = Men who have sex with men. NC = Not calculated because population denominators for transmission category subgroups were unavailable. IDU = Injection drug users.

Notes: Estimates derived using extended back-calculation on HIV and acquired immunodeficiency syndrome (AIDS) data for persons aged ≥13 years at diagnosis from 40 states that have had confidential name-based HIV infection reporting since at least January 2006, and AIDS data from 10 states (California, Delaware, Hawaii, Maryland, Massachusetts, Montana, Oregon, Rhode Island, Vermont, and Washington) and the District of Columbia.

[a]Per 100,000 population.

[b]Heterosexual contact with a person known to have, or to be at high risk for, HIV infection.

[c]Includes hemophilia, blood transfusion, perinatal exposure, and risk factors not reported or not identfied.

SOURCE: Lucia Torian et al., "Table. Estimated Number and Rate of Persons Aged ≥13 Years Living with HIV Infection, and Number and Percentage Whose HIV infection Was Undiagnosed, by Selected Characteristics—United States, 2008," in "HIV Surveillance—United States, 1981–2008," *Morbidity and Mortality Weekly Report*, vol. 60, no. 21, June 3, 2011, http://www.cdc.gov/mmwr/pdf/wk/mm6021.pdf (accessed June 3, 2011)

study, which considered 33,420 HIV-infected and 66,840 HIV-uninfected patients. They find that other cancers, called non-AIDS-defining malignancies, appear to occur more frequently among people with HIV/AIDS. People with HIV/AIDS were found to be at 60% greater risk for anal, lung, and liver cancer as well as Hodgkin's lymphoma and melanoma than people who were not HIV infected.

Even though investigators do not yet know exactly why the rates of the cancers are higher among people with HIV infection, they hypothesize that:

- HIV or another as yet undetected virus may increase the risk of developing cancer.

- HAART may increase the risk of developing cancer.

- People with HIV may have lifestyle or other environmental exposures that increase their risk for cancer, such as smoking or excessive alcohol consumption.

Anouk Kesselring et al. opine in "Immunodeficiency as a Risk Factor for Non-AIDS-Defining Malignancies in HIV-1-Infected Patients Receiving Combination Antiretroviral Therapy" (*Clinical Infectious Diseases*, vol. 52, no. 12, June 15, 2011) that HIV itself may play a role in the development of cancer, either by a direct effect or as an effect of immune suppression.

From HIV to AIDS

Through 2011, among people who were not treated with antiretroviral therapy, the average amount of time from initial HIV infection to the development of AIDS was about 10 years. However, medical developments such as the use of HAART have significantly increased the life expectancy of AIDS patients.

In "The Lifetime Cost of Current Human Immunodeficiency Virus Care in the United States" (*Medical Care*, vol. 44, no. 11, November 2006), Bruce R. Schackman et al. note that a 1993 estimate of life expectancy for an asymptomatic person infected with HIV was less than seven years. During the 1990s life expectancy for HIV-infected people was about 10 years. A decade later, in 2006, life expectancy after HIV diagnosis averaged 24.2 years.

According to the Antiretroviral Therapy Cohort Collaboration, in "Life Expectancy of Individuals on Combination Antiretroviral Therapy in High-Income Countries: A Collaborative Analysis of 14 Cohort Studies" (*Lancet*, vol. 372, no. 9635, July 26, 2008), a 20-year-old HIV-positive person starting antiretroviral therapy in 2008 could expect to live to age 69. The collaboration observes that this projection represents a 37% increase in life expectancy from the late 1990s, when a 20-year-old HIV-positive person starting antiretroviral therapy could be expected to live an additional 36 years (to age 56).

Ard I. van Sighem et al. indicate in "Life Expectancy of Recently Diagnosed Asymptomatic HIV-Infected Patients Approaches That of Uninfected Individuals" (*AIDS*, vol. 24, no. 10, June 19, 2010) that many people who are diagnosed with HIV infection in the 21st century will have normal life expectancies. Research involving more than 80,000 HIV-infected people from 30 European countries confirms that people who maintain CD4 counts of over 500 per cubic millimeter of blood for three years or more and who abstain from illicit drug use can anticipate a lifespan that is comparable in length to their uninfected peers.

THE EARLY STAGE. Even though the timing and progression of HIV infection vary among people, the disease follows a basic pattern. In the beginning of the early stage, shortly after the virus has entered the bloodstream, the T4 cell count is normal (around 1,000 per cubic millimeter). The virus is undetectable at this stage using assays that are geared to detect the presence of anti-HIV antibodies. The antibody assays can remain negative for up to six weeks. In unusual cases antibodies may remain undetectable for a year or more. Even after testing positive for the virus, or for the presence of the antiviral antibodies, many people remain asymptomatic for years. These people may develop a disorder that is similar to infectious mononucleosis with fatigue, fever, swollen glands, and possibly a rash. Often, these symptoms disappear within a few weeks, and a connection with an HIV infection is not made. Throughout this stage, however, the virus is multiplying and destroying healthy cells. Most people continue to feel fine, though some may have chronically swollen lymph nodes. This stage usually lasts about five years.

THE MIDDLE STAGE. By the middle stage of infection, the CD4+ T cell count is reduced by half, to around 500 per cubic millimeter. Even with this physiological change, many people may still be asymptomatic. As the infection advances, skin tests will likely show that cell-mediated immunity, a form of immunological defense, is disintegrat-

ing. The deterioration of the immune system has begun. This stage can also last up to five years.

During the 1980s a drug called azidothymidine (AZT; now called zidovudine), which had failed to fulfill its early potential as an anticancer compound, garnered a lot of publicity when it was shown to help slow the attachment of HIV to host cells. AZT delayed the onset of symptoms and extended this middle stage of the infection. However, AZT's benefits proved to be temporary, as HIV mutated to counteract the effect of the drug. The drug is still used today in conjunction with other medicines, and some studies suggest that people who receive AZT may develop AIDS later than those who do not take it.

Newer and more promising drugs have since been developed, in particular protease inhibitors, which prevent the virus from destructively degrading cell protein. Protease inhibitors were licensed for use by the U.S. Food and Drug Administration (FDA) in December 1995. In 2011 there were 10 FDA-approved protease inhibitors available. However, because HIV mutates, it can become resistant to these drugs. In "Novel Antiretroviral Combinations in Treatment-Experienced Patients with HIV Infection: Rationale and Results" (*Drugs*, vol. 70, no. 13, September 10, 2010), Babafemi Taiwo, Robert Murphy, and Christine Katlama explain that combinations of newer antiretroviral drugs may be effective in patients who have developed drug-resistant HIV.

Structured treatment interruptions (STIs), initially proposed during the late 1990s, in which the multiple drug therapy that patients receive is stopped for short periods of time, have also shown promise. However, the disastrous consequences that have resulted from patients taking self-initiated "drug holidays" underscore the importance of receiving a physician's approval before embarking on an STI program.

Considerable research indicates that STI may be associated with worse health outcomes in terms of immune function and viral load than continuous antiretroviral therapy. Nonetheless, some investigators believe there is a role for STI, especially as a short-term strategy to help patients who are experiencing severe side effects of treatment such as drug toxicity. Calvin J. Cohen et al. report in "Pilot Study of a Novel Short-Cycle Antiretroviral Treatment Interruption Strategy: 48-Week Results of the Five-Days-On, Two-Days-Off (FOTO) Study" (*HIV Clinical Trials*, vol. 8, no. 1, January–February 2007), a study of STI that treated 30 patients on a five-day-on antiretroviral therapy and a two-day-off cycle, that after eight weeks on this schedule 90% of the patients maintained adequate suppression of the virus. In "Virologic Determinants of Success after Structured Treatment Interruptions of Antiretrovirals in Acute HIV-1 Infection" (*Journal of Acquired Immune Deficiency Syndromes*, vol. 47, no. 2, February 1, 2008), Sharon R. Lewin et al. hypothesize that the total pool of infected cells and the degree of persistent viral replication would determine the likelihood of successful control of the virus after STIs. The researchers also posit that starting antiretroviral therapy early—during primary HIV infection—might help limit viral replication during STIs.

THE LATE STAGE. The third and final stage of HIV infection is reached when the CD4+ T cell count drops to 200 per cubic millimeter or below. Though many patients are still asymptomatic at this point, the functioning of the immune system has by now been markedly weakened. The body is far less able to defend itself from invasion. As a consequence, the risk of infection due to opportunistic bacteria, viruses, fungi, and parasites and the possibility of cancer increase dramatically. To prevent *Pneumocystis carinii* pneumonia, a lung disease caused by a fungus and one of the most common OIs, patients are usually treated with antibiotics during this stage.

At the onset of the late stage, patients may experience weight loss, diarrhea, lethargy, and recurring fever. Skin and mucous membrane infections increase. Oral fungal infections such as thrush and chronic infection caused by the herpes simplex virus are also common.

As the late stage progresses, the immune system collapses. OIs move deeper into the body. It is not uncommon for a parasitic infection called toxoplasmosis to attack the brain, while the cryptococcosis fungus attacks the nervous system, liver, bones, and skin. Cytomegalovirus can cause pneumonia, encephalitis, and retinitis. The latter, an inflammation of the retina, can cause blindness. Many other infections can occur. The consequences and complications of compromised immune function are many, and death becomes a matter of time. The average survival rate, once the late stage has been reached, is two years.

THE TRANSMISSION OF HIV

When AIDS was first identified, it was often compared to the Black Death of the 14th century, in terms of the public panic surrounding the disease and its possible spread. The comparison has not proved to be valid. The bacterium that caused the Black Death (and that still causes bubonic plague) is highly contagious, largely because it is readily transmitted via food, water, and air. HIV is not nearly as contagious. Moreover, by observing precautions that prevent the sharing of bodily fluids, the transmission of HIV can be almost entirely prevented.

The accumulated knowledge of 30 years of research has definitively established that HIV can only be transmitted by the following routes:

- Oral, anal, or vaginal sex with an infected person. Sexual intercourse—particularly heterosexual sex—is the most common mode of HIV transmission worldwide.

- Sharing drug needles or syringes with an infected person.

- Maternal transmission to a baby at the time of birth and through breast milk. Paul J. Weidle and Steven Nesheim report in "HIV Drug Resistance and Mother-to-Child Transmission of HIV" (*Clinics in Perinatology*, vol. 37, no. 4, December 2010) that pregnant women who develop HIV drug resistance may transmit this resistance to their infants via breastfeeding. Even though breastfeeding is a known source of HIV transmission, in many developing countries where alternative sources of nutrition are unavailable, the benefits of breastfeeding outweigh the risks. For this reason, the WHO recommends in *HIV Transmission through Breastfeeding: A Review of Available Evidence, 2007 Update* (2008, http://whqlibdoc .who.int/publications/2008/9789241596596_eng.pdf) that HIV-infected women "breastfeed their infants exclusively for the first six months of life, unless replacement feeding is acceptable, feasible, affordable, sustainable and safe for them and their infants before that time. When those conditions are met, WHO recommends avoidance of all breastfeeding by HIV-infected women."

- Transplantation of HIV-infected organs or transfusion of infected bodily fluids, such as blood or blood products. During the mid-1980s the transfusion of HIV-infected blood caused thousands of cases of AIDS and led to many deaths in separate incidents in Europe, the United States, and Canada. The blood agencies of the affected countries have revamped their blood-testing policies so that molecular assay techniques, which detect HIV genetic material, are used to screen every donated blood sample.

Confirming the involvement of bodily fluids in HIV transmission, high concentrations of HIV have been found in blood, semen, and cerebrospinal fluid. Not all body fluids seem to be involved, because HIV concentrations 1,000 times less have been found in saliva, tears, vaginal secretions, breast milk, and feces. However, there have been no reports of HIV transmission from saliva, tears, or human bites. In fact, Altman reports in "Protein in Saliva Found to Block AIDS Virus in Test Tube Study" (*New York Times*, February 7, 1995) that a small protein found in human saliva actually blocks the virus from entering the system. Table 2.5 shows the estimated distribution of HIV/AIDS diagnoses in adolescents and adults by sex and transmission category in the United States in 2009 and the cumulative totals from the beginning of the epidemic through 2009.

Casual Contact

Even though HIV is an infectious, contagious disease, it is not spread in the same manner as a common cold or chicken pox. It is not spread by sneezing or coughing, as are airborne illnesses. HIV is not spread by sharing a bathroom,

TABLE 2.5

AIDS cases by transmission category, 2009 and cumulative through 2009

Transmission category	Estimated number of AIDS diagnoses, 2009		
	Adult and adolescent males	Adult and adolescent females	Total
Male-to-male sexual contact	17,005	—	17,005
Injection drug use	3,012	1,930	4,942
Male-to-male sexual contact and injection drug use	1,580	—	1,580
Heterosexual contact[a]	3,832	6,561	10,393
Other[b]	158	155	313
	Cumulative estimated number of AIDS diagnoses, through 2009[c]		
Male-to-male sexual contact	529,908	—	529,908
Injection drug use	186,318	87,126	273,444
Male-to-male sexual contact and injection drug use	77,213	—	77,213
Heterosexual contact[a]	72,183	126,637	198,820
Other[b]	12,744	7,032	19,776

[a]Heterosexual contact with a person known to have, or to be at high risk for, HIV infection.
[b]Includes hemophilia, blood transfusion, perinatal exposure, and risk not reported or not identified.
[c]From the beginning of the epidemic through 2009.

SOURCE: "AIDS Cases by Transmission Category," in *HIV Surveillance Report: Diagnoses of HIV infection and AIDS in the United States and Dependent Areas, 2009*, Centers for Disease Control and Prevention, Divisions of HIV/AIDS Prevention, February 28, 2011, http://www.cdc.gov/hiv/topics/surveillance/basic.htm#exposure (accessed June 3, 2011)

by swimming in a pool, or by hugging or shaking hands. Studies of family members who lived with and cared for AIDS patients have not found definitive evidence that anyone has become infected through casual contact. Still, myths abound. To combat misinformation, the U.S. surgeon general and public health education initiatives continue to stress that HIV is not spread by:

- Bites from mosquitoes or other insects.

- Bites from animals.

- Food handled, prepared, or served by HIV-infected people.

- Forks, spoons, knives, or drinking glasses used by HIV-infected people.

- Chairs previously occupied by HIV-infected people.

- Casual contact such as touching, hugging, or kissing a person who is HIV positive (open-mouth kissing with a person who is HIV positive is not recommended because of potential exposure to blood).

Donating Blood

Health officials agree that donating blood poses no danger of HIV infection for the donors. The needles used to draw blood from donors are new and are thrown away after one use. Therefore, contact with HIV from donating blood is impossible.

SAFETY OF BLOOD AND TRANSPLANT PROCEDURES

To safeguard the nation's transplant recipients, the CDC suggests that all donors of blood products, tissue, and organs be screened and tested. The recommendations include screening for behaviors—risk factors—that are associated with the acquisition of HIV infection, a physical examination for signs and symptoms that are related to HIV infection, and laboratory screening for antibodies to HIV. It is important to remember that the CDC does not regulate medical protocol; its main function is to offer health care guidelines and information to the nation and its health care providers.

The U.S. Blood Supply

Before HIV-antibody testing began in 1985, it is estimated that 70% of hemophiliacs (people with inherited bleeding disorders) who received blood products were given tainted blood-clotting factor (a concentrate of blood used to stem bleeding) and were therefore infected with HIV. According to Steve Sternberg, in "A Legacy of Tainted Blood" (*USA Today*, July 11, 2006), approximately 10,000 of these patients developed AIDS and approximately 5,000 have died.

The widespread use of two blood-screening tests, both of which are also used on plasma and other blood products, has strengthened the safety of the U.S. blood and plasma supply. Since 1992 the U.S. Public Health Service, an arm of the U.S. Department of Health and Human Services, has required that all blood and plasma donations be screened for the rare HIV-2 antibody, as well as for the more common HIV-1 antibody.

In 2001 the FDA approved the first nucleic acid test (NAT) system to screen plasma donors for HIV. Rather than relying on the identification of antigens or antibodies, the new test provides extremely sensitive detection of RNA from HIV-1. Even with the new test, however, there is still some risk due to the "window period," during which a person who has acquired the HIV-1 infection may still test negative. For HIV-1 antigen and antibody detection, the window period is 16 and 21 days, respectively, following infection. NAT systems reduce the window period to 12 days. Put another way, anyone who is infected with HIV and who donates blood more than 12 days after exposure to the virus will register HIV positive.

Barbee I. Whitaker et al. indicate in *The 2007 National Blood Collection and Utilization Survey Report* (October 2008, http://www.hhs.gov/ash/bloodsafety/2007nbcus_survey.pdf) that 16.2 million units of blood were donated in the United States in 2006. There are many measures in place to ensure the safety of the U.S. blood supply; however, the FDA admits that it is impossible to ensure zero risk of transmitting infectious disease. So even though the U.S. blood supply is considered safe, blood banks across the country nonetheless encourage individuals concerned about tainted blood to bank their own blood for possible future use.

In "New Technologies Promise to Improve Blood Supply Safety" (*Nature Medicine*, vol. 17, no. 5, May 5, 2011), Michelle Pflumm explains that to further improve the safety of the blood supply, U.S. blood banks have introduced new technologies that use deoxyribonucleic acid–based screening to detect previously undetectable levels of HIV and other pathogens in blood. Even though officials assert that the U.S. blood supply is "safer than it's ever been," they concede that "transfusion is still associated with [a] risk of transmission."

Foreign Blood Supplies

Historically, HIV infection from contaminated blood has been much more common in other countries. According to Craig R. Whitney, in "Top French Officials Cleared over Blood with AIDS Virus" (*New York Times*, March 10, 1999), a French court ruled in 1998 that a former prime minister and two former cabinet members would be tried on charges that they allowed HIV-contaminated blood to be used for transfusions during 1984 and 1985. Relatives of the patients argued that the French government had refused U.S. technology that would have detected antibodies in the tainted blood in favor of a French procedure that was in development. Approximately 4,400 people acquired HIV as a result of this action. Many of the victims were hemophiliacs, and about 40% of the total number infected had died of AIDS. The former French officials, Prime Minister Laurent Fabius (1946–), Minister of Social Affairs Georgina Dufoix (1943–), and Minister of Health Edmond Herve (1942–), faced charges of involuntary homicide and went to trial in 1999. Herve was convicted without a penalty and Dufoix and Fabius were acquitted. The tragedy resulted in the overhaul of the blood supply and donation networks in France.

Jane Perlez notes in "Parents Sue Romania over Child's H.I.V. Infection" (*New York Times*, August 31, 1995) that the WHO reported in 1995 that 3,000 children in Romania—home to thousands of abandoned babies left in squalid institutions after the fall of the Romanian dictator Nicolae Ceausescu (1918–1989)—were infected by contaminated blood and syringes during the late 1980s. The WHO estimated that 1,000 of those children had died. According to Perlez, "Romania has more than half of the juvenile AIDS cases in Europe. More than 90 percent of the country's reported AIDS cases are among children, most of whom were infected by contaminated needles and syringes." The Romanian Health Ministry faced litigation for causing the spread of HIV.

According to the article "Another German Trial for H.I.V.-Tainted Blood" (Reuters, November 30, 1995), Gunter Kurt Eckert, the owner of a German drug laboratory, was charged in 1995 with nearly 6,000 counts of murder or attempted murder for selling HIV-tainted blood products to German hospitals in 1987. Nearly 90% of the 6,000 batches had not been tested for HIV. Testing has been mandatory in Germany since 1986. Eckert was found guilty and sentenced to six and a half years in prison.

The article "Canada's Tainted Blood Scandal: A Timeline" (CBC News, October 1, 2007) notes that the Canadian blood collection, testing, and distribution system was completely overhauled in the wake of the distribution of blood that was contaminated with HIV and the hepatitis C virus. In 1989 Ottawa established a $150 million fund to compensate the 1,250 Canadians who were infected with HIV as a result of contact with infected blood. It was discovered that 95% of hemophiliacs who received blood products prior to 1990 had been infected with hepatitis C. In 2001 the Canadian supreme court ruled that the negligence of the blood agency during the early years of the AIDS crisis entitled several thousand affected Canadians to a $1.2 billion federal-provincial government compensation offer. Legal wrangling in the intervening years delayed the implementation of the court's ruling.

Even though blood safety has been examined by the WHO and all developed countries have strengthened their screening efforts, problems persist in developing countries. The WHO notes in the fact sheet "Blood Safety and Availability" (November 2009, http://www.who.int/mediacentre/factsheets/fs279/en/index.html) that 41 of the 162 countries reporting blood screening data in 2007 were unable to screen all donated blood for transmissible infections, including HIV. The article "Blood Racket: Contaminated Blood Could Have Caused Hepatitis" (ProKerala.com, August 30, 2009) reports the use of outdated blood screening kits in India and alleges that contaminated blood was sold for transfusions in Uttar Pradesh in 2009.

Organ and Tissue Transplants

There are cases that HIV has been transmitted through organ (kidney, liver, heart, lung, and pancreas) and other tissue transplants. However, the risk of such transmission is low simply because there are far fewer transplant cases than blood transfusions.

In 1994 the FDA began regulating the sale of bone, skin, corneas, cartilage, tendons, and similar nonblood vessel–bearing tissues that are used for transplants. The FDA requires that all procurement agencies conduct behavioral screening and infectious-disease (HIV-1, HIV-2, hepatitis B virus, and hepatitis C virus) testing of donors.

TESTING PEOPLE FOR HIV

A person who is infected with HIV produces antibodies specific to the virus as part of the body's immune response to the invader. Even though the antibodies are not enough to successfully fight HIV, they are of diagnostic value, as they can indicate the presence of the virus.

Antibody-based HIV testing is done, rather than a direct test for the virus itself, because it is too difficult to isolate the virus from the blood. Testing serves to determine if there is a viral infection in donated blood, tissues, or organs. This protects the recipients of the donated material and can be used to identify HIV-infected donors.

An antibody-based test cannot detect all HIV-positive blood. It can typically take between four and 12 weeks following HIV infection for antibodies to appear, although in rare cases this period can be up to one year. The introduction of tests that detect the viral nucleic acid rather than the HIV antibodies has markedly increased the detection sensitivity of blood screening. Still, even nucleic acid detection has a window period, albeit a shorter one, of about 12 days.

The fact that detection is not absolute from the moment of HIV infection means that the possibility exists that some HIV-infected donors may not be diagnosed and their blood may enter the nation's blood supply. However, the number of predicted contaminated blood samples is extremely small. To further reduce the chances of contaminated blood entering the blood supply, blood banks routinely question potential donors about high-risk behaviors. Any donor whose behavior might indicate an increased risk of HIV infection (such as injection drug use or unsafe sex) is automatically excluded from donating blood.

Diagnostic Tools for HIV Antibodies

Two tests commonly used to detect HIV antibodies are believed to be about 99% reliable. These tests are the enzyme-linked immunosorbent assay (ELISA) and the Western blot.

Introduced in 1985, ELISA is a test that was designed for screening rather than for diagnosing. The assay uses purified HIV antigens to probe for the presence of complimentary antibodies in a sample such as blood. If anti-HIV antibodies are present in the sample, they attach themselves to the viral proteins that have been immobilized on a plastic surface. A second antibody that has been raised against the anti-HIV antibody (antibodies are proteins, too, so they can function as antigens, stimulating the formation of antibodies) is bound to the anti-HIV antibodies. The second antibody contains a chemical that can be made to change color. The color change reveals the presence of the anti-HIV antibody. If no color change appears, no anti-HIV antibody is present in the blood sample. This test is reliable, simple to conduct, and inexpensive.

The Western blot, introduced in 1987, is a confirmatory test. This means the test is commonly used to verify the results of the less-specific assays. The Western blot technique separates the various HIV proteins from one another, based on their speed of movement through a gel under the influence of electricity. The separated proteins are transferred from the gel to a membrane made of a material such as nitrocellulose. When the nitrocellulose is exposed to a blood sample, antibodies that recognize one of the proteins on the nitrocellulose will bind to the particular protein. As with ELISA, a color reaction can be induced to indicate the site of the bound antibodies. The Western blot provides a positive, negative, or intermediate result. The presence of three or more of the color bands confirms an HIV infection. If fewer—one or two—bands appear, the test is considered intermediate and retesting is performed six months later. If no color bands appear, the test is considered negative with no HIV present, though many people who test negative also repeat the test six months later.

Body Fluid Tests

In June 1998 the FDA approved a urine-based diagnostic kit for HIV marketed by Calypte Biomedical Corporation that does not require confirmation by a blood test. Urine tests are easier to use and cost less than blood tests for health care providers. According to the NIH, there is no evidence that HIV is spread through urine. Therefore, the chances of accidental infection through needle sticks or the handling of samples are lessened. The urine test and its urine-based confirmation test, like most blood tests, recognize the existence of antibodies, not the actual virus.

The test is marketed to life insurance companies, clinical laboratories, public health agencies, the military, immigration authorities, and the criminal justice system. In the press release "Calypte Appoints Distributor for Its HIV-1 Urine Test in People's Republic of China" (Business Wire, June 12, 2000), Calypte announced its partnership with the Chinese National Center for AIDS Prevention and Control to distribute the first HIV-1 antibody urine test in China. In 2002 the company completed clinical trials involving more than 10,000 subjects in China and reported in the press release "Calypte Completes China Clinical Trials" (October 8, 2002, http://www.prnewswire.com/news-releases/calypte-completes-china-clinical-trials-72424722.html) excellent results in terms of the sensitivity (the ability of the test to accurately detect disease in people who have the disease) and specificity (the ability of the test to accurately identify people who do not have the disease) of the urine test. The WHO observes in *Towards Universal Access: Scaling up Priority HIV/AIDS Interventions in the Health Sector* (October 2010, http://whqlibdoc.who.int/publications/2010/9789241500395_eng.pdf) that between 2007 and the close of 2009 the number of facilities offering HIV testing in China grew from 4,293 to 7,335.

In July 2005 Calypte began marketing its products in developing countries; however, as of August 2011, Calypte rapid test products, which detect HIV-1 and HIV-2 antibodies in the blood, oral fluids, and urine, were not yet available in the United States. In 2011 Calypte (http://www.calypte.com/products.asp) was developing a rapid test for professional use at its Portland, Oregon, facility. An over-the-counter version for consumers was slated to follow. In September 2007 the U.S. Agency for International Development (USAID) placed the Calypte oral test on its rapid HIV test waiver list, which, under the U.S. Acquisition and Assistance Policy Directive, permits the test to be used in USAID-funded projects. The USAID decision allows countries whose governments have approved the test to purchase it with funds from the President's Emergency Plan for AIDS Relief (this program was launched in 2003 to combat global HIV/AIDS).

According to the article "Calypte Biomedical Announces Successful Conclusion of Internal Trials" (Reuters, March 2, 2011), in March 2011 Calypte announced the successful completion of internal studies of its oral fluid rapid test, which was performed in South Africa and the United States. The company indicated that the test is 100% accurate.

Home Testing

As of 2011, the FDA had approved only one method of home testing for HIV-1, the Home Access Express HIV-1 Test System, which is produced by the Home Access Health Corporation. The FDA warned that the more than one dozen nonapproved home HIV tests advertised could produce inaccurate results. Users mail an anonymous blood sample to a laboratory and receive results seven days after the sample arrives at the laboratory, or if they choose the "express" option, results are available the same day the sample arrives at the laboratory. Proponents of home testing state that it offers the advantages of privacy and ease of use. Critics of home testing point out that it is expensive; a kit costs as much as $65 and may be prohibitively expensive for poorer populations—for whom such a test is most needed. Critics also question the impersonal practice of relaying HIV-positive results and follow-up counseling by telephone.

A. David Paltiel and Harold A. Pollack maintain in "Price, Performance, and the FDA Approval Process: The Example of Home HIV Testing" (*Medical Decision Making*, vol. 30, no. 2, March–April 2010) that in addition to evidence of the test's performance and its sensitivity and specificity when administered by untrained users, the FDA should consider the population of end-users. Paltiel and Pollack assert that the performance of the home HIV test, which is measured in terms of its ability to correctly detect the presence and absence of HIV infection among the people who purchase it, depends on market factors such as its retail price. For example, their analysis suggests that a cheaper test may work better when marketed at a lower price because there is a greater chance that it will be used by people likely to be infected, rather than by the uninfected "worried well" who can afford to purchase it.

Rapid-Response Tests

According to Bernard M. Branson of the CDC, in "Point-of-Care Rapid Tests for HIV Antibody" (September 12, 2006, http://www.cdc.gov/hiv/topics/testing/resources/journal_article/J_Lab_Med_20031.htm), during the mid- to late 1990s the CDC recommended the development of a new HIV test that would give results instantly. The CDC hoped that this would encourage people to learn the results of their tests. Currently, about half of the people who are tested at voluntary counseling and testing clinics and at perinatal screening do not return to collect their results, so the benefit of testing is lost. The CDC stresses the importance of obtaining results quickly. It contends that people are not only more likely to take a test that gives results instantly but also will benefit from the opportunity to learn they are infected before their immune system has been seriously damaged. Furthermore, rapid results may lead to earlier, more effective treatment and might reduce transmission of the virus.

The FDA has approved a number of rapid-response tests that are designed for use in clinics in the United States. The first test to be approved is manufactured by Murex Diagnostics Inc. This test detects the presence of HIV antibody in about 10 minutes. The test is as accurate as the standard Western blot test. However, because the Western blot test also looks for protein bands, this test remains the absolute antibody-based indicator of HIV.

In late 2002 the FDA announced approval of another blood-based antibody test (OraQuick Rapid HIV-1 by OraSure Technologies Inc.) for use. As of 2011 the test, which produces results within about 10 minutes, was not licensed for home use and could only be performed in a clinical setting. However, the fact that the test does not require any specialized equipment or refrigeration offers the possibility of home use in the future.

Another similar rapid-response test kit, developed and manufactured by the Canadian-based MedMira Inc., was granted FDA approval in April 2003 for sale in the United States. The kit is also approved in China, where HIV infection rates dramatically increased during the first decade of the 21st century.

Table 2.6 lists the rapid HIV tests that had been approved by the FDA as of 2008. It also shows the body fluids that could be used and the sensitivity and specificity of each of the rapid HIV tests. Sensitivity is the ability or extent to which a diagnostic test detects a disease when it is truly present. Specificity is the ability or extent to which a diagnostic test excludes the presence of a disease when it is truly not present. In other words, a sensitive test will produce a positive test result when the patient has the disease, whereas a specific test will give a negative result when the patient does not have the disease.

TABLE 2.6

FDA-approved rapid HIV tests, 2008

	FDA approval received	Specimen type	CLIA category[a]	Sensitivity[b]	Specificity[b]	Manufacturer	Approved for HIV-2 detection?	List price per device[c]	External controls
OraQuick Advance Rapid HIV-1/2 Antibody Test	Nov 2002	Oral fluid Whole blood (finger stick or venipuncture) Plasma	Waived Waived	99.3% 99.6%	99.8% 100%	OraSure Technologies, Inc. www.orasure.com	Yes	$17.50	Sold separately ($25 each)
Uni-Gold Recombigen HIV	Dec 2003	Whole blood (finger stick or venipuncture) Serum & plasma	Moderate complexity Waived Moderate complexity	99.6% 100% 100%	99.9% 99.7% 99.8%	Trinity Biotech www.unigoldhiv.com	No	$15.75 $8.00[d]	Sold separately ($26.25 each)
Reveal G-3 Rapid HIV-1	Apr 2003	Serum Plasma	Moderate complexity Moderate complexity	99.8% 99.8%	99.1% 98.6%	MedMira, Inc. www.medmira.com	No	$14.00	Included
MultiSpot HIV-1/HIV-2 Rapid Test	Nov 2004	Serum Plasma	Moderate complexity Moderate complexity	100% 100%	99.93% 99.91%	BioRad Laboratories www.biorad.com	Yes - differentiates HIV-1 from HIV-2	$25.00	Included
Clearview HIV 1/2 STAT-PAK	May 2006	Whole blood (finger stick or venipuncture) Serum & plasma	Waived Non-waived	99.7% 99.7%	99.9% 99.9%	Inverness Medical Professional Diagnostics www.invernessmedicalpd.com	Yes	$17.50 $8.00[d]	Sold separately ($50/set)
Clearview COMPLETE HIV 1/2	May 2006	Whole blood (finger stick or venipuncture) Serum & plasma	Waived Non-waived	99.7% 99.7%	99.90% 99.9%	Inverness Medical Professional Diagnostics www.invernessmedicalpd.com	Yes	$18.50 $9.00[d]	Sold separately ($50/set)

[a]Clinical Laboratory Improvement Amendments: CLIA regulations identify three categories of tests: waived, moderate complexity, or high complexity.
[b]Sensitivity is the probability that the test result will be reactive if the specimen is a true positive; specificity is the probability that the test result will be nonreactive if the specimen is a true negative. Data are from the FDA summary basis of approval, for HIV-1 only.
[c]Actual price may vary by purchasing agreements with manufacturers.
[d]"Public health" price for public health programs that are recipients of CDC funds for expanded HIV testing.
Note: Trade names are for identification purposes only and do not imply endorsement. This information was compiled from package inserts and direct calls to manufacturers.

SOURCE: "FDA-Approved Rapid HIV Antibody Screening Tests, February 4, 2008," in *Rapid HIV Testing*, Centers for Disease Control and Prevention, February 15, 2008, http://www.cdc.gov/hiv/topics/testing/rapid/pdf/RT_Comparison-Chart_2-4-08.pdf (accessed June 3, 2011)

Rapid HIV tests are used more frequently in other countries, such as China. In developing countries quick-response tests are used to screen blood before transfusions and to screen pregnant women so medical interventions can be given to prevent mother-to-child transmission of the virus. They are also used in rural clinics.

Revised Recommendations for HIV Testing

In 2006 the CDC revised its recommendations for HIV testing, which were published by Bernard M. Branson et al. in "Revised Recommendations for HIV Testing of Adults, Adolescents, and Pregnant Women in Health-Care Settings" (*Morbidity and Mortality Weekly Report*, vol. 55, RR-14, September 22, 2006). The new recommendations updated and replaced guidelines issued in 1993. The major revisions from the 1993 guidelines are to advise routine HIV screening of adults, adolescents, and pregnant women in health care settings in the United States; to screen people at high risk for HIV infection at least annually; to eliminate the requirement for separate written consent for HIV testing, making general consent sufficient to permit HIV testing; and to remove the requirement to provide prevention counseling as part of HIV screening and testing in health care settings. The 2006 guidelines also advise that HIV screening be part of routine prenatal screening for all pregnant women and that repeat screening during the third trimester of pregnancy be performed in areas where there are high levels of HIV infection among pregnant women.

Test Tracks HIV/AIDS Progression

In June 1996 the FDA approved a test to help determine how fast an HIV infection will progress to full-blown AIDS. Developed by Roche Diagnostic Systems Inc., the Amplicor HIV-1 monitor test is not intended to screen for HIV or to confirm an HIV diagnosis. Instead, the test detects the amount of HIV in the blood (the viral load) by measuring HIV genetic material. An increased viral load indicates the advancement of the infection toward AIDS and an increasing predisposition to the development of OIs. The test is based on a technique developed in 1984 called the polymerase chain reaction (PCR). PCR uses a heat-resistant bacterial enzyme to amplify the copies of target stretches of genetic material to detectable amounts. The process can be completed in less than one hour. This test was the first PCR-based test to be approved.

FDA approval was granted in 1997 to expand the use of the test as an aid in managing HIV in patients undergoing antiretroviral therapy. In 1999 a more sensitive version of the test became available, and this test has been widely used since then—to help evaluate and track the progression of HIV infection and disease and to predict the risk of complications and debilitating infections.

David March reports in "Viral Load Testing: Way to Predict Anti-HIV Failures in Africa" (*JHU Gazette*, March 23, 2009) that in February 2009 a research team led by Steven Reynolds presented its findings about how to track the progress of HIV and predict treatment failures at the 2009 Conference on Retroviruses and Opportunistic Infections in Montreal, Canada. According to March, Reynolds and his colleagues asserted that "counting the number of HIV viruses in the blood rather than relying solely on counting the number of circulating HIV-fighting CD4 immune system cells" is a more effective way to detect early signs that antiretroviral drugs are no longer working. March quoted Reynolds, who observed that "detecting antiretroviral drug failures accurately and early is essential to avoiding HIV drug resistance, which could result in HIV disease progressing to AIDS and leading to illness and death."

In "Detection of Drug Resistance Mutations at Low Plasma HIV-1 RNA Load in a European Multicentre Cohort Study" (*Journal of Antimicrobial Chemotherapy*, vol. 66, no. 8, August 2011), Mattia C. F. Prosperi et al. report that even though there are not yet conclusive data to support the clinical utility of this approach, "testing at low viral load may identify emerging antiretroviral drug resistance at an early stage," when prompt treatment changes may most effectively reduce the accumulation of resistance and viral adaptive changes.

CHAPTER 3
PATTERNS AND TRENDS IN HIV/AIDS SURVEILLANCE

DETERMINING THE NUMBER OF PEOPLE INFECTED WITH HIV

The Centers for Disease Control and Prevention (CDC) keeps track of the number of people in the United States who are infected with HIV, the virus that causes AIDS.

These CDC figures, which have always been acknowledged as estimates, have been criticized as being inaccurate—either too high or too low. Nonetheless, the historical continuity of CDC data permits trend analyses. Therefore, when viewed over a number of years, the figures provide a reasonable indication of the progress of the disease in the United States.

Estimates of HIV infection are important because they directly influence public health and medical resource allocation as well as political and economic decisions. Definitive figures are difficult to obtain because laws prevent testing for HIV without consent and permission. Furthermore, many people are understandably reluctant to participate in community or household surveys because of confidentiality concerns and fear of losing or failing to obtain insurance coverage.

Health officials contend that knowing the prevalence of HIV infections (prevalence is a measure of all cases of illness existing at a given point in time) is not as crucial as knowing whether the number of HIV infections is rising or falling. The rate at which people develop HIV/AIDS during a specified period is known as the incidence rate. Because there are no national studies to collect these data (not all states require reporting of new HIV cases), estimates are based on reports from states that mandate confidential reporting of HIV cases, along with other small studies and surveys. CDC officials explain that a major problem is the lack of knowledge about how many people were infected before the beginning of the agency's regular collection of data. This would help determine how the current incidence of HIV compares to previous years. The comparison of incidence rates is important because they are

a direct measure of the rate at which individuals become ill and provide data to help estimate the risk or probability of illness.

CDC data through 2008 from states and U.S.-dependent areas with confidential HIV reporting indicate that 679,590 adults and adolescents were living with HIV infection. (See Figure 3.1.) During this same period, 3,079 children under the age of 13 years were living with HIV infection. (See Figure 3.2.)

In the 40 states and five U.S. dependent areas (American Samoa, Guam, the Northern Mariana Islands, Puerto Rico, and the U.S. Virgin Islands) with confidential name-based HIV infection reporting since at least 2003, the prevalence rate of HIV infection among adults and adolescents was estimated at 337.5 per 100,000 population at the end of 2008. Figure 3.1 shows that the rates of HIV infection varied widely from state to state, from a low of 46.5 per 100,000 in Wyoming to 826.7 per 100,000 in New York.

The CDC also compiles figures on the numbers of people living with AIDS. Figure 3.3 shows that 489,976 adults and adolescents were living with AIDS at the end of 2008. According to the CDC, in *Epidemiology of HIV Infection through 2009* (April 22, 2011, http://www.cdc.gov/hiv/topics/surveillance/resources/slides/general/slides/general.pdf), the number of children under the age of 13 years living with AIDS through 2008 was 720.

AIDS CASE NUMBERS

The first cases of what came to be recognized as AIDS were reported in the United States in June 1981. Five young, homosexual males in Los Angeles, California, were diagnosed with *Pneumocystis carinii* pneumonia and other opportunistic infections. The CDC notes in *HIV/AIDS Surveillance Report, 1997* (December 1997, http://www.cdc.gov/hiv/topics/surveillance/resources/reports/pdf/hivsur92.pdf) that by August 1989 approximately 100,000 cases of AIDS had

FIGURE 3.1

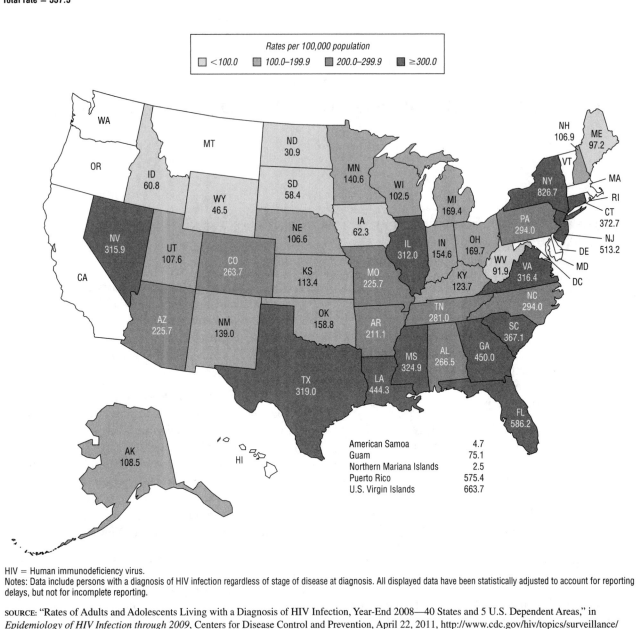

Adults and adolescents living with diagnosed HIV infection, 2008

[40 states and 5 U.S. dependent areas. Population = 679,590.]

Total rate = 337.5

Rates per 100,000 population

☐ < 100.0   ☐ 100.0–199.9   ☐ 200.0–299.9   ☐ ≥ 300.0

American Samoa	4.7
Guam	75.1
Northern Mariana Islands	2.5
Puerto Rico	575.4
U.S. Virgin Islands	663.7

HIV = Human immunodeficiency virus.
Notes: Data include persons with a diagnosis of HIV infection regardless of stage of disease at diagnosis. All displayed data have been statistically adjusted to account for reporting delays, but not for incomplete reporting.

SOURCE: "Rates of Adults and Adolescents Living with a Diagnosis of HIV Infection, Year-End 2008—40 States and 5 U.S. Dependent Areas," in *Epidemiology of HIV Infection through 2009*, Centers for Disease Control and Prevention, April 22, 2011, http://www.cdc.gov/hiv/topics/surveillance/resources/slides/general/slides/general.pdf (accessed June 4, 2011)

been reported to the agency. By December 1997 that number had risen to 641,086; of these, 390,692 people had died. Cumulatively, through 2009 there were 1,108,611 reported cases of AIDS in the United States—1,099,163 among adults and adolescents and 9,448 among children under the age of 13 years. (See Table 3.1.) According to the CDC, in *HIV Surveillance Report: Diagnoses of HIV Infection and AIDS in the United States and Dependent Areas, 2009* (February 2011, http://www.cdc.gov/hiv/surveillance/resources/reports/2009report/pdf/2009SurveillanceReport.pdf), as of 2009, 617,025 people had died of the disease.

During the mid-1990s the number of AIDS cases rose dramatically. This surge was not an actual numerical increase, but was due to the expanded 1993 AIDS surveillance definition, which added diseases and conditions that had not been part of the previous definition of AIDS. By the late 1990s the number of AIDS cases leveled off and began to decline, probably as a result of the increasing use of effective antiretroviral drugs that delay the progression of AIDS. Between 2006 and 2009 the number of cases diagnosed each year decreased, from 41,237 in 2006 to 35,825 in 2009, and the rate decreased slightly from 17.5 in 2006

FIGURE 3.2

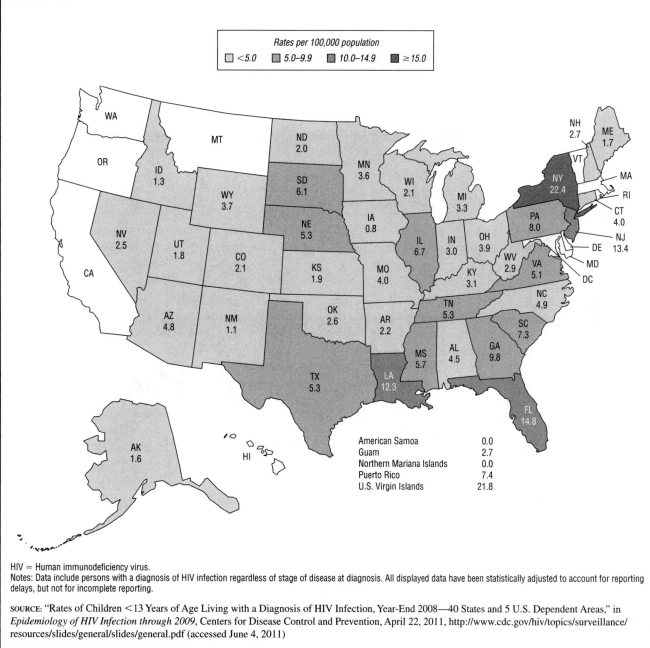

Children under 13 years of age living with diagnosed HIV infection, 2008

[40 states and 5 U.S. dependent areas. Population = 3,079.]

Total rate = 7.2

Rates per 100,000 population

☐ <5.0   ▨ 5.0–9.9   ▨ 10.0–14.9   ■ ≥15.0

American Samoa	0.0
Guam	2.7
Northern Mariana Islands	0.0
Puerto Rico	7.4
U.S. Virgin Islands	21.8

HIV = Human immunodeficiency virus.
Notes: Data include persons with a diagnosis of HIV infection regardless of stage of disease at diagnosis. All displayed data have been statistically adjusted to account for reporting delays, but not for incomplete reporting.

SOURCE: "Rates of Children <13 Years of Age Living with a Diagnosis of HIV Infection, Year-End 2008—40 States and 5 U.S. Dependent Areas," in *Epidemiology of HIV Infection through 2009*, Centers for Disease Control and Prevention, April 22, 2011, http://www.cdc.gov/hiv/topics/surveillance/resources/slides/general/slides/general.pdf (accessed June 4, 2011)

to 17.4 per 100,000 in 2009. (See Table 3.2.). The numbers of AIDS diagnoses also decreased during this same period, with the rate per 100,000 population falling from 12.1 in 2006 to 11.2 in 2009. (See Table 3.3.)

THE NATURE OF THE EPIDEMIC

Changes in the distribution of HIV infection illustrate the increasing diversity of those affected by the epidemic in the 30 years since AIDS was first diagnosed. The CDC notes in "Current Trends Update: Acquired Immunode-ficiency Syndrome—United States, 1981–1990" (*Morbidity and Mortality Weekly Report*, vol. 40, no. 22, June 7, 1991) that all the 189 AIDS cases reported in 1981 in the United States were males. Three-fourths (76%) of them were men who had sex with men (MSM) living in New York and California. In 1990, of the 43,339 AIDS cases reported by all states, approximately 30% were from New York and California, 11.5% were women, and about 2% were children. In 1999 the proportions of reported cases among women, African-Americans, Hispanics, and people exposed through heterosexual contact all increased.

FIGURE 3.3

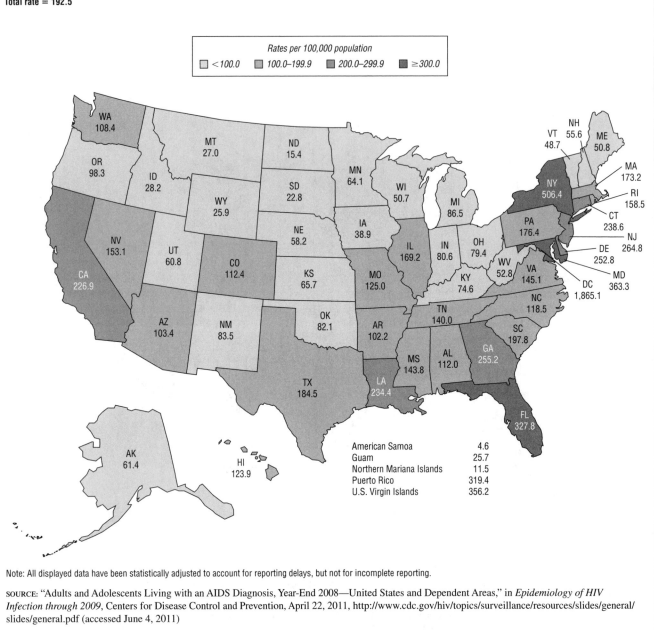

Adults and adolescents living with diagnosed AIDS, 2008

[United States and dependent areas. Population = 489,976.]

Total rate = 192.5

Rates per 100,000 population

☐ <100.0   ▨ 100.0–199.9   ▨ 200.0–299.9   ■ ≥300.0

WA 108.4
OR 98.3
ID 28.2
MT 27.0
ND 15.4
MN 64.1
WI 50.7
MI 86.5
NY 506.4
VT 48.7
NH 55.6
ME 50.8
MA 173.2
RI 158.5
CT 238.6
NJ 264.8
DE 252.8
MD 363.3
DC 1,865.1
PA 176.4
OH 79.4
IN 80.6
IL 169.2
IA 38.9
NE 58.2
SD 22.8
WY 25.9
NV 153.1
UT 60.8
CO 112.4
KS 65.7
CA 226.9
AZ 103.4
NM 83.5
OK 82.1
MO 125.0
AR 102.2
TX 184.5
LA 234.4
MS 143.8
AL 112.0
GA 255.2
TN 140.0
KY 74.6
WV 52.8
VA 145.1
NC 118.5
SC 197.8
FL 327.8
AK 61.4
HI 123.9

American Samoa   4.6
Guam   25.7
Northern Mariana Islands 11.5
Puerto Rico   319.4
U.S. Virgin Islands   356.2

Note: All displayed data have been statistically adjusted to account for reporting delays, but not for incomplete reporting.

SOURCE: "Adults and Adolescents Living with an AIDS Diagnosis, Year-End 2008—United States and Dependent Areas," in *Epidemiology of HIV Infection through 2009*, Centers for Disease Control and Prevention, April 22, 2011, http://www.cdc.gov/hiv/topics/surveillance/resources/slides/general/slides/general.pdf (accessed June 4, 2011)

By contrast, the percentage of reported cases among whites and MSM declined somewhat.

Table 3.2 and Table 3.3 show that between 2006 and 2009 MSM sexual contact continued to account for the largest proportion of diagnosed cases; however, there were still substantial numbers of HIV and AIDS diagnoses attributable to injection drug use, and high-risk heterosexual contact also grew among males and females. By contrast, the number of cases diagnosed in children under the age of 13 years declined during this period.

Regional Differences

AIDS cases have been reported in all 50 states, the District of Columbia, and dependent areas. However, the distribution of cases is far from even. (See Figure 3.3.) At the end of 2008, the highest rate by far was in the District of Columbia, where the rate was 1,865.1 per 100,000 population. There was a concentration in the states on the East Coast (particularly in New York, Maryland, New Jersey, Delaware, and Connecticut, with respective rates of 506.4, 363.3, 264.8, 252.8, and 238.6, and in Florida, with a rate of 327.8). Also prominent were Puerto Rico

TABLE 3.1

AIDS diagnoses by age, 2009 and cumulative

Age (years)	Estimated number of AIDS diagnoses, 2009	Cumulative estimated number of AIDS diagnoses, through 2009*
Under 13	13	9,448
Ages 13–14	58	1,321
Ages 15–19	484	7,214
Ages 20–24	2,095	42,920
Ages 25–29	3,476	129,639
Ages 30–34	4,043	214,149
Ages 35–39	4,893	234,575
Ages 40–44	5,689	193,237
Ages 45–49	5,466	126,380
Ages 50–54	3,983	72,327
Ages 55–59	2,191	39,025
Ages 60-64	1,010	20,633
Ages 65 or older	846	17,743

*From the beginning of the epidemic through 2009.

SOURCE: "AIDS Diagnoses by Age," in *HIV Surveillance Report: Diagnoses of HIV infection and AIDS in the United States and Dependent Areas, 2009*, Centers for Disease Control and Prevention, Divisions of HIV/AIDS Prevention, February 28, 2011, http://www.cdc.gov/hiv/topics/surveillance/basic.htm (accessed June 4, 2011)

(319.4) and the U.S. Virgin Islands (356.2). Figure 3.4 shows the corresponding AIDS rates for children under the age of 13 years at the end of 2008. The estimated rates for children living with AIDS ranged from 0 per 100,000 population in Idaho, Montana, Wyoming, Utah, Vermont, Maine, American Samoa, Guam, and the Northern Mariana Islands to 24.4 per 100,000 population in the District of Columbia.

RATES IN MAJOR METROPOLITAN AREAS. Most AIDS cases are concentrated in larger metropolitan regions (the city and surrounding suburbs). In 2009 the annual metropolitan AIDS diagnosis rates per 100,000 people were highest on the coasts, such as in the Fort Lauderdale, Florida, division (45.7); the Miami, Florida, division (37.1); the New York–White Plains–Wayne, New York, division (35.3); the Washington division (29.8); the San Francisco, California, division (24.3); and in Baltimore–Towson, Maryland (22.8). (See Table 3.4.) By contrast, the midwestern metropolitan areas displayed some of the lowest rates: Akron, Ohio (4.4), Grand Rapids, Michigan (5.3), and Youngstown–Warren–Boardman, Ohio (6.7). Provo–Orem, Utah, had the lowest overall rate (1), followed by Boise City–Nampa, Idaho (1.9), Colorado Springs, Colorado (3), and Honolulu, Hawaii (3).

There are several reasons for the higher rates in urban areas. First, metropolitan areas are more cosmopolitan and, by definition, more tolerant of alternative lifestyles such as those of MSM, a group with high-risk sexual behaviors. Second, large metropolitan areas have greater numbers of people who use injection drugs, which is another major risk factor for HIV infection. Third, even though HIV infection and transmission are not restricted to more populated areas, those who need and seek treat-

ment may migrate to these areas for access to medical care and social services. In many smaller communities medical care may be unavailable and financial and/or social barriers may limit access to health care services.

AIDS Transmission Categories Have Changed

The distribution of AIDS diagnoses by transmission category has changed since the beginning of the epidemic. In 1985 MSM accounted for about two-thirds of all AIDS diagnoses, but in 1999 MSM accounted for 40% of diagnoses. (See Figure 3.5.) Beginning in 2001 the percentage of AIDS diagnoses attributable to MSM began to increase and by 2009 it accounted for about half (49%) of all AIDS diagnoses.

AIDS diagnoses attributable to injection drug use grew from 20% to 32% between 1985 and 1993 and subsequently decreased to 15% in 2009. AIDS diagnoses attributable to MSM and injection drug use declined from 9% in 1985 to 5% in 2009. In contrast, the percentage of AIDS diagnoses attributable to heterosexual contact skyrocketed from 3% in 1985 to nearly 31% in 2009.

Rates among Women

In 2009 reported AIDS cases among women that were attributable to injection drug use (1,930) accounted for 22% of the total number of cases (8,647). (See Table 3.3.) The number of AIDS cases among women that were attributable to injection drug use declined between 2006 and 2009, from an estimated 2,469 cases in 2006 to 1,930 in 2009.

When considering the role of heterosexual contact in the acquisition of AIDS, the proportion was far higher for women in 2009 (an estimated 6,561 cases, representing 76% of the total of 8,647) than for men (an estimated 3,832, representing 15% of the total of 25,587). (See Table 3.3.)

Decline in AIDS Due to Blood Transfusions

As a result of screening procedures for blood and blood products that began in 1985, the CDC indicates that the number of AIDS cases among adult and adolescent transfusion recipients decreased between 1995 (664 cases) and 1997 (409 cases). A pronounced decrease in 1999 (256 cases) was followed by a steady decline after an initial slight increase to 282 cases in 2000: 218 cases in 2001, 219 in 2003, 160 in 2005, and 109 in 2007. By 2008 the numbers had dropped so low that the CDC began reporting cases attributable to blood transfusion along with hemophilia, perinatal exposure, and other unidentified risk factors in a category called "Other." This category has declined steadily among men, from an estimated 194 cases in 2006 to 158 in 2009. (See Table 3.3.)

Current Age and Sex Distribution

Of the 1,108,611 estimated cumulative total reported cases of AIDS in 2009, 1,099,163 (99% of the cumulative

TABLE 3.2

HIV diagnoses by year of diagnosis and selected characteristics, 2006–09

[40 states with confidential name-based HIV infection reporting.]

| | 2006 | | | 2007 | | | 2008 | | | 2009 | | |
	No.	Estimated[a] No.	Rate	No.	Estimated[a] No.	Rate	No.	Estimated[a] No.	Rate	No.	Estimated[a] No.	Rate
Age at diagnosis (year)												
<13	204	215	0.5	190	204	0.5	194	215	0.5	141	166	0.4
13–14	55	57	0.9	37	40	0.6	34	37	0.6	19	21	0.3
15–19	1,530	1,605	9.6	1,742	1,861	11.0	1,817	1,996	11.8	1,752	2,036	12.0
20–24	4,481	4,695	28.2	4,700	5,020	30.1	5,156	5,662	33.8	5,327	6,237	36.9
25–29	5,117	5,370	33.7	5,351	5,723	34.9	5,239	5,743	34.4	5,078	5,951	35.2
30–34	4,917	5,155	34.1	4,732	5,056	33.6	4,685	5,160	34.0	4,294	5,020	32.5
35–39	5,995	6,287	38.5	5,562	5,944	36.3	4,961	5,450	33.5	4,448	5,232	32.6
40–44	6,281	6,590	37.7	5,833	6,238	36.4	5,244	5,752	34.3	4,704	5,519	33.6
45–49	4,677	4,899	27.4	4,734	5,059	28.2	4,630	5,093	28.4	4,141	4,865	27.1
50–54	3,029	3,176	19.7	3,185	3,412	20.6	2,977	3,271	19.3	2,834	3,323	19.3
55–59	1,629	1,705	11.9	1,715	1,827	12.7	1,761	1,926	13.1	1,691	2,004	13.4
60–64	749	786	7.4	829	884	7.7	872	953	7.9	772	900	7.2
Over 65	665	696	2.3	731	780	2.6	679	747	2.4	624	736	2.3
Race/ethnicity												
American Indian/Alaska Native	156	163	8.8	175	185	9.9	175	193	10.2	163	189	9.8
Asian	345	366	5.5	434	473	6.9	418	466	6.6	395	470	6.4
Black/African American	19,701	20,672	65.7	19,542	20,922	65.7	19,667	21,709	67.4	18,320	21,652	66.6
Hispanic/Latino[b]	6,931	7,285	25.1	6,977	7,463	24.8	6,568	7,177	23.0	6,318	7,347	22.8
Native Hawaiian/other Pacific Islander	44	46	31.4	39	41	27.1	29	31	20.0	29	34	21.0
White	11,576	12,099	7.4	11,592	12,332	7.5	10,873	11,860	7.2	10,160	11,803	7.2
Multiple races	576	606	21.8	582	631	21.9	519	567	19.0	440	516	16.7
Transmission category												
Male adult or adolescent												
Male-to-male sexual contact	15,979	20,877	—	16,292	22,177	—	16,030	22,849	—	15,488	23,846	—
Injection drug use	2,040	3,245	—	1,676	2,907	—	1,269	2,540	—	1,018	2,449	—
Male-to-male sexual contact and injection drug use	1,040	1,407	—	904	1,318	—	744	1,188	—	632	1,131	—
Heterosexual contact[c]	2,971	4,541	—	2,893	4,680	—	2,705	4,634	—	2,266	4,399	—
Other[d]	6,745	101	—	7,342	55	—	7,729	72	—	7,749	47	—
Subtotal	28,775	30,171	31.9	29,107	31,137	32.6	28,477	31,283	32.4	27,153	31,872	32.7
Female adult or adolescent												
Injection drug use	1,067	1,954	—	887	1,756	—	791	1,654	—	591	1,483	—
Heterosexual contact[c]	4,896	8,826	—	4,674	8,894	—	4,268	8,813	—	3,453	8,461	—
Other[d]	4,387	71	—	4,482	55	—	4,519	40	—	4,487	29	—
Subtotal	10,350	10,851	10.9	10,043	10,705	10.7	9,578	10,506	10.4	8,531	9,973	9.8

TABLE 3.2

HIV diagnoses by year of diagnosis and selected characteristics, 2006–09 [CONTINUED]

[40 states with confidential name-based HIV infection reporting.]

	2006			2007			2008			2009		
		Estimated[a]			Estimated[a]			Estimated[a]			Estimated[a]	
	No.	No.	Rate	No.	No.	Rate	No.	No.	Rate	No.	No.	Rate
Child (<13 years at diagnosis)												
Perinatal	173	182	—	161	173	—	156	171	—	112	131	—
Other[e]	31	34	—	29	32	—	38	44	—	29	35	—
Subtotal	**204**	**215**	**0.5**	**190**	**204**	**0.5**	**194**	**215**	**0.5**	**141**	**166**	**0.4**
Total[f]	**39,329**	**41,237**	**17.5**	**39,341**	**42,047**	**17.7**	**38,249**	**42,005**	**17.5**	**35,825**	**42,011**	**17.4**

Note: Data include persons with a diagnosis of HIV infection regardless of stage of disease at diagnosis.
[a]Estimated numbers resulted from statistical adjustment that accounted for reporting delays and missing risk-factor information, but not for incomplete reporting. Rates are per 100,000 population. Rates are not calculated by transmission category because of the lack of denominator data.
[b]Hispanics/Latinos can be of any race.
[c]Heterosexual contact with a person known to have, or to be at high risk for, HIV infection.
[d]Includes hemophilia, blood transfusion, perinatal exposure, and risk factor not reported or not identified.
[e]Includes hemophilia, blood transfusion, and risk factor not reported or not identified.
[f]Because column totals for estimated numbers were calculated independently of the values for the subpopulations, the values in each column may not sum to the column total.

source: "Table 1a. Diagnoses of HIV infection, by Year of Diagnosis and Selected Characteristics, 2006–2009—40 States with Confidential Name-Based HIV Infection Reporting," in "Diagnoses of HIV Infection and AIDS in the United States and Dependent Areas, 2009," *HIV Surveillance Report, 2009,* vol. 21, Centers for Disease Control and Prevention, February 2011, http://www.cdc.gov/hiv/surveillance/resources/reports/2009report/pdf/table1a.pdf (accessed June 4, 2011)

TABLE 3.3

AIDS diagnoses by year of diagnosis and selected characteristics, 2006–09

[United States]

	2006 No.	2006 Estimated[a] No.	2006 Estimated[a] Rate	2007 No.	2007 Estimated[a] No.	2007 Estimated[a] Rate	2008 No.	2008 Estimated[a] No.	2008 Estimated[a] Rate	2009 No.	2009 Estimated[a] No.	2009 Estimated[a] Rate	Cumulative[b] No.	Cumulative[b] Est. No.[a]
Age at diagnosis (year)														
<13	37	39	0.1	29	31	0.1	35	40	0.1	10	13	0.0	9,369	9,448
13–14	73	78	0.9	74	80	1.0	51	58	0.7	39	58	0.7	1,262	1,321
15–19	376	398	1.9	416	449	2.1	429	480	2.2	376	484	2.2	6,910	7,214
20–24	1,548	1,637	7.7	1,750	1,880	8.9	1,675	1,869	8.8	1,667	2,095	9.7	41,628	42,920
25–29	3,176	3,353	16.3	3,135	3,378	16.1	3,064	3,428	16.0	2,753	3,476	16.0	126,954	129,639
30–34	4,048	4,279	22.0	3,805	4,096	21.2	3,716	4,147	21.2	3,227	4,043	20.3	210,270	214,149
35–39	5,911	6,254	29.8	5,317	5,741	27.3	4,776	5,367	25.7	3,888	4,893	23.8	229,584	234,575
40–44	6,760	7,159	32.1	6,181	6,680	30.6	5,540	6,222	29.1	4,502	5,689	27.1	188,102	193,237
45–49	5,236	5,543	24.4	5,307	5,731	25.2	4,885	5,518	24.2	4,303	5,466	23.9	122,228	126,380
50–54	3,405	3,608	17.7	3,340	3,599	17.2	3,274	3,660	17.1	3,138	3,983	18.3	69,691	72,327
55–59	1,901	2,013	11.1	1,855	1,998	11.0	1,877	2,091	11.3	1,723	2,991	11.5	37,604	39,025
60–64	900	954	7.2	909	979	6.8	965	1,075	7.1	805	1,010	6.4	19,947	20,633
≥65	788	836	2.2	732	791	2.1	721	800	2.1	669	846	2.1	17,165	17,743
Race/ethnicity														
American Indian/Alaska Native	138	145	6.4	132	141	6.1	161	177	7.6	127	155	6.6	3,599	3,700
Asian[c]	395	422	3.3	416	454	3.5	434	489	3.7	329	429	3.1	7,995	8,324
Black/African American	16,357	17,300	47.4	15,926	17,171	46.5	15,226	17,065	45.7	13,196	16,741	44.4	452,985	466,351
Hispanic/Latino[d]	6,652	7,065	16.1	6,390	6,912	15.2	5,962	6,701	14.3	5,285	6,719	13.9	184,719	190,263
Native Hawaiian/other Pacific Islander	47	49	11.7	48	51	12.0	37	41	9.2	40	50	11.2	810	839
White	9,924	10,484	5.3	9,331	10,050	5.0	8,640	9,668	4.8	7,595	9,467	4.7	418,074	426,102
Multiple races	646	686	16.5	607	656	15.3	548	616	13.9	528	686	15.1	12,229	12,726
Transmission category														
Male adult or adolescent														
Male-to-male sexual contact	13,006	16,517	—	12,621	16,521	—	11,871	16,469	—	10,773	17,005	—	473,724	529,908
Injection drug use	2,743	3,853	—	2,361	3,505	—	2,061	3,303	—	1,523	3,012	—	160,614	186,318
Male-to-male sexual contact and injection drug use	1,595	1,957	—	1,394	1,798	—	1,264	1,706	—	1,000	1,580	—	70,586	77,213
Heterosexual contact[e]	2,829	3,952	—	2,607	3,882	—	2,552	3,949	—	2,148	3,832	—	56,074	72,183
Other[f]	4,827	194	—	4,964	165	—	5,072	185	—	4,741	158	—	96,383	12,744
Subtotal	25,000	26,473	22.0	23,947	25,871	21.3	22,820	25,612	20.9	20,185	25,587	20.6	857,381	878,366
Female adult or adolescent														
Injection drug use	1,599	2,469	—	1,491	2,392	—	1,221	2,141	—	900	1,930	—	70,856	87,126
Heterosexual contact[e]	4,580	6,980	—	4,355	6,955	—	3,965	6,824	—	3,241	6,561	—	96,111	126,637
Other[f]	2,943	190	—	3,027	184	—	2,967	137	—	2,764	155	—	46,995	7,032
Subtotal	9,122	9,639	7.7	8,873	9,531	7.5	8,153	9,102	7.1	6,905	8,647	6.7	213,962	220,795

TABLE 3.3

AIDS diagnoses by year of diagnosis and selected characteristics, 2006–09 [CONTINUED]

[United States]

| | 2006 | | | 2007 | | | 2008 | | | 2009 | | | Cumulative[b] | |
| | | Estimated[a] | | | Estimated[a] | | | Estimated[a] | | | Estimated[a] | | | |
	No.	No.	Rate	No.	No.	Rate	No.	No.	Rate	No.	No.	Rate	No.	Est. No.[a]
Child (<13 years at diagnosis)														
Perinatal	34	36	—	28	30	—	31	35	—	9	12	—	8,568	8,640
Other[c]	3	3	—	1	1	—	4	5	—	1	1	—	801	807
Subtotal	**37**	**39**	**0.1**	**29**	**31**	**0.1**	**35**	**40**	**0.1**	**10**	**13**	**0.0**	**9,369**	**9,448**
Region of residence														
Northeast	8,742	9,369	17.1	8,298	9,082	16.5	6,986	8,064	14.6	5,807	8,171	14.8	330,979	340,357
Midwest	3,903	4,154	6.3	3,675	4,006	6.0	3,687	4,218	6.3	3,435	4,394	6.6	112,560	116,029
South	15,718	16,453	15.1	15,371	16,383	14.8	15,003	16,506	14.7	13,188	15,806	13.9	419,910	430,141
West	5,796	6,174	9.0	5,506	5,964	8.5	5,332	5,967	8.4	4,670	5,875	8.2	217,265	222,083
Total[b]	**34,159**	**36,151**	**12.1**	**32,850**	**35,434**	**11.7**	**31,008**	**34,755**	**11.4**	**27,100**	**34,247**	**11.2**	**1,080,714[i]**	**1,108,611**

[a]Estimated numbers resulted from statistical adjustment that accounted for reporting delays and missing risk-factor information, but not for incomplete reporting. Rates are per 100,000 population. Rates are not calculated by transmission category because of the lack of denominator data.

[b]From the beginning of the epidemic through 2009.

[c]Includes Asian/Pacific Islander legacy cases.

[d]Hispanics/Latinos can be of any race.

[e]Heterosexual contact with a person known to have or to be at high risk for, HIV infection.

[f]Includes hemophilia, blood transfusion, perinatal exposure, and risk factor not reported or not identified.

[g]Includes hemophilia, blood transfusion, and risk factor not reported or not identified.

[h]Because column totals for estimated numbers were calculated independently of the values for the subpopulations, the values in each column may not sum to the column total.

[i]Includes persons of unknown race/ethnicity.

SOURCE: "Table 2a. AIDS Diagnoses, by Year of Diagnosis and Selected Characteristics, 2006–2009 and Cumulative—United States," in "Diagnoses of HIV Infection and AIDS in the United States and Dependent Areas, 2009," *HIV Surveillance Report, 2009*, vol. 21, Centers for Disease Control and Prevention, February 2011, http://www.cdc.gov/hiv/surveillance/resources/reports/2009report/pdf/table2a.pdf (accessed June 4, 2011)

FIGURE 3.4

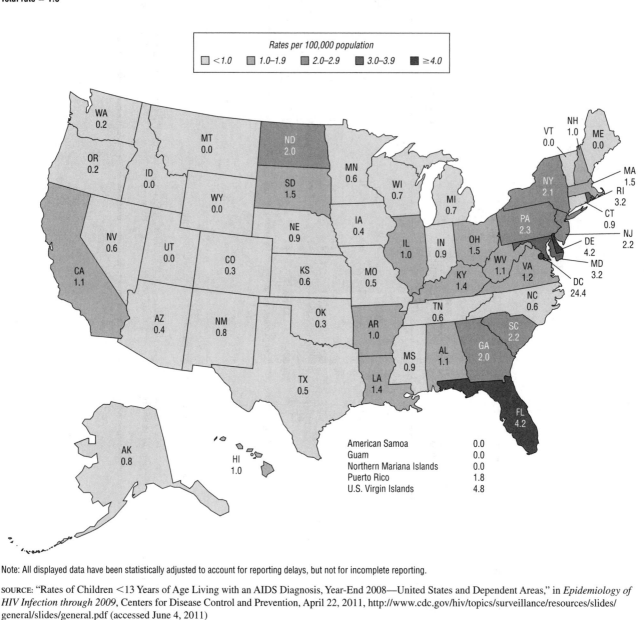

Children under 13 years of age living with diagnosed AIDS, 2008

[United States and dependent areas. Population = 720.]

Total rate = 1.3

Rates per 100,000 population

□ <1.0 ▨ 1.0–1.9 ▨ 2.0–2.9 ▨ 3.0–3.9 ■ ≥4.0

WA 0.2
MT 0.0
ND 2.0
MN 0.6
VT 0.0
NH 1.0
ME 0.0
OR 0.2
ID 0.0
SD 1.5
WI 0.7
NY 2.1
MA 1.5
RI 3.2
CT 0.9
WY 0.0
MI 0.7
PA 2.3
NJ 2.2
NV 0.6
UT 0.0
NE 0.9
IA 0.4
IL 1.0
IN 0.9
OH 1.5
DE 4.2
MD 3.2
CA 1.1
CO 0.3
KS 0.6
MO 0.5
WV 1.1
VA 1.2
DC 24.4
AZ 0.4
NM 0.8
OK 0.3
AR 1.0
KY 1.4
TN 0.6
NC 0.6
SC 2.2
MS 0.9
AL 1.1
GA 2.0
TX 0.5
LA 1.4
FL 4.2
AK 0.8
HI 1.0

American Samoa	0.0
Guam	0.0
Northern Mariana Islands	0.0
Puerto Rico	1.8
U.S. Virgin Islands	4.8

Note: All displayed data have been statistically adjusted to account for reporting delays, but not for incomplete reporting.

SOURCE: "Rates of Children <13 Years of Age Living with an AIDS Diagnosis, Year-End 2008—United States and Dependent Areas," in *Epidemiology of HIV Infection through 2009*, Centers for Disease Control and Prevention, April 22, 2011, http://www.cdc.gov/hiv/topics/surveillance/resources/slides/general/slides/general.pdf (accessed June 4, 2011)

total) were among adults and adolescents. (See Table 3.3.) The remaining 9,448 cases (1%) were children under the age of 13 years. According to the CDC, in 2008 more people between the ages of 45 to 49 years (104,575) and 40 to 44 years (91,237) were living with AIDS (195,812, or 41% of all cases) than in any other age category. (See Table 3.5.)

Cumulatively, the total number of AIDS cases that were reported in adults and adolescents at the end of 2009 occurred predominantly in males (878,366 cases, or 79% of the cumulative total). (See Table 3.3.) Adult and adolescent females accounted for 220,795 cumulative cases (20% of the cumulative total).

Race and Ethnicity Influence Risk

The changing racial and ethnic profile and characteristics of Americans with HIV/AIDS from 1993 through 2009 reflect a shift in the population at risk for HIV/AIDS. In *HIV/AIDS Surveillance Report, 2001* (December 2001, http://www.cdc.gov/hiv/topics/surveillance/resources/reports/2001report/pdf/2001surveillance-report_year-end.pdf), the CDC indicates that in 1993 there were 60,587 cases reported

TABLE 3.4

Reported AIDS cases and annual rates, by metropolitan area of residence and age category, 2009, and cumulative

[United States and Puerto Rico]

Area of residence	Diagnosis, 2009				Diagnosis, cumulative[a]			Living with AIDS, year-end 2008		
	No.	Estimated[b] No.	Rate	Rank[c]	Adults or adolescents No.	Children Estimated[b] No.	Total No.	No.	Estimated[b] No.	Rate
Akron, OH	20	31	4.4	93	878	1	880	382	382	54.5
Albany—Schenectady—Troy, NY	42	58	6.8	71	2,575	27	2,602	1,202	1,215	142.2
Albuquerque, NM	48	56	6.6	75	1,627	3	1,630	698	691	81.6
Allentown—Bethlehem—Easton, PA—NJ	44	52	6.4	80	1,610	19	1,629	830	827	101.9
Atlanta—Sandy Springs—Marietta, GA	735	1,023	18.7	14	27,170	143	27,313	13,148	13,678	254.0
Augusta—Richmond County, GA—SC	42	53	9.8	45	2,165	24	2,189	1,036	1,066	199.3
Austin—Round Rock, TX	162	180	10.5	35	5,479	26	5,505	2,535	2,547	154.0
Bakersfield, CA	39	51	6.3	81	1,921	9	1,930	1,163	1,185	148.7
Baltimore—Towson, MD	457	614	22.8	10	23,651	224	23,875	10,321	10,543	393.7
Baton Rouge, LA	221	241	30.6	2	4,545	20	4,565	1,947	1,944	249.5
Birmingham—Hoover, AL	36	39	3.5	98	2,920	25	2,945	1,228	1,220	108.7
Boise City—Nampa, ID	8	12	1.9	101	328	0	328	160	162	27.1
Boston, Mass—NH[d]	206	286	6.2	82	15,207	156	15,363	6,681	6,696	147.3
Boston division	118	168	8.8	—	9,494	96	9,589	3,999	3,996	210.5
Cambridge division	53	73	4.8	—	3,561	36	3,597	1,680	1,697	114.1
Essex division	27	35	4.7	—	1,789	23	1,812	836	837	113.5
Bradenton—Sarasota—Venice, FL	60	68	10.0	41	2,278	29	2,307	998	988	144.0
Bridgeport—Stamford—Norwalk, CT	85	114	12.7	28	4,170	57	4,228	1,835	1,834	205.1
Buffalo—Niagara Falls, NY	67	93	8.3	60	2,886	22	2,908	1,235	1,247	110.9
Cape Coral—Fort Myers, FL	70	78	13.2	24	2,009	25	2,034	866	861	146.2
Charleston—North Charleston, SC	83	95	14.4	20	2,403	20	2,423	1,092	1,060	163.8
Charlotte—Gastonia—Concord, NC—SC	236	275	15.7	18	4,101	22	4,123	1,904	1,876	110.0
Chattanooga, TN—GA	34	44	8.3	59	1,152	3	1,155	561	564	108.5
Chicago, IL—IN—WI	782	1,068	11.2	32	34,807	268	35,074	15,513	15,824	166.3
Chicago division	700	962	12.0	—	32,622	255	32,876	14,498	14,809	186.5
Gary division	47	61	8.6	—	1,256	8	1,264	538	528	75.2
Lake division	35	46	5.2	—	929	5	934	477	487	55.8
Cincinnati—Middletown, OH—KY—IN	162	214	9.8	44	3,363	20	3,383	1,451	1,465	67.9
Cleveland—Elyria—Mentor, OH	146	198	9.5	48	4,871	50	4,921	2,111	2,103	100.4
Colorado Springs, CO	17	19	3.0	99	646	5	651	291	290	47.0
Columbia, SC	153	175	23.5	6	3,925	24	3,949	2,067	2,031	277.3
Columbus, OH	176	232	12.9	25	3,944	22	3,966	1,559	1,564	87.9
Dallas, TX	726	828	12.8	26	23,022	62	23,084	10,631	10,690	169.7
Dallas division	602	680	15.7	—	18,290	37	18,327	8,472	8,527	201.8
Fort Worth division	124	149	7.0	—	4,732	25	4,757	2,159	2,163	104.3
Dayton, OH	46	61	7.3	68	1,461	15	1,476	649	656	78.3
Denver—Aurora, CO	212	237	9.3	50	7,823	22	7,845	3,472	3,473	138.9
Des Moines, IA	33	36	6.4	79	632	4	636	292	294	53.0
Detroit, MI	332	382	8.7	57	11,861	75	11,936	4,965	4,811	108.7
Detroit division	256	293	15.2	—	9,378	58	9,436	3,789	3,656	187.6
Warren division	76	89	3.6	—	2,483	17	2,500	1,176	1,155	46.7
Durham—Chapel Hill, NC	43	48	9.5	47	1,410	10	1,420	580	564	114.9

TABLE 3.4

Reported AIDS cases and annual rates, by metropolitan area of residence and age category, 2009, and cumulative [CONTINUED]

[United States and Puerto Rico]

Area of residence	Diagnosis, 2009 Estimated[b] No.	Rate	Rank[c]	Diagnosis, cumulative[a] Adults or adolescents No.	Children Estimated[b] No.	Total No.	Living with AIDS, year-end 2008 No.	Estimated[b] No.	Rate
El Paso, TX	51	56	7.4	67	1,765	10	1,775	952	963	130.3
Fresno, CA	94	124	13.5	23	1,818	11	1,829	777	785	86.9
Grand Rapids—Wyoming, MI	37	41	5.3	86	948	6	954	454	448	57.7
Greensboro—High Point, NC	65	72	10.1	39	1,536	19	1,555	659	645	91.2
Greenville, SC	53	60	9.4	49	1,501	4	1,505	679	662	105.1
Harrisburg—Carlisle, PA	49	56	10.4	36	1,457	9	1,466	717	715	134.0
Hartford—West Hartford—East Hartford, CT	88	118	9.9	43	5,678	47	5,726	2,405	2,376	199.5
Honolulu, HI	24	27	3.0	100	2,348	14	2,362	916	910	100.8
Houston—Baytown—Sugar Land, TX	797	885	15.1	19	29,381	175	29,556	11,978	12,022	209.9
Indianapolis, IN	160	178	10.2	38	4,415	25	4,440	2,060	2,008	116.7
Jackson, MS	103	120	22.2	11	2,851	30	2,881	1,295	1,281	238.5
Jacksonville, FL	346	387	29.1	3	7,212	79	7,292	3,158	3,116	236.7
Kansas City, MO—KS	147	201	9.7	46	5,670	16	5,686	2,569	2,628	128.5
Knoxville, TN	45	50	7.2	69	1,055	5	1,060	503	503	72.7
Lakeland, FL	98	110	18.9	13	2,189	21	2,210	946	935	161.2
Lancaster, PA	22	24	4.7	90	841	21	862	400	402	79.7
Las Vegas—Paradise, NV	199	236	12.4	29	5,547	28	5,575	2,688	2,670	142.1
Little Rock—North Little Rock, AR	46	52	7.6	63	1,588	14	1,602	864	880	130.2
Los Angeles, CA	993	1,328	10.3	37	65,647	300	65,947	27,824	28,438	222.7
Los Angeles division	812	1,084	11.0	—	57,846	256	58,102	24,268	24,864	254.3
Santa Ana division	181	244	8.1	—	7,800	45	7,845	3,556	3,574	119.6
Louisville, KY—IN	79	98	7.8	62	2,770	27	2,797	1,312	1,297	103.8
Madison, WI	22	24	4.3	94	601	5	606	291	285	50.8
McAllen—Edinburg—Pharr, TX	26	29	3.9	95	766	12	778	460	460	63.7
Memphis, TN—MS—AR	267	305	23.3	7	5,998	20	6,018	2,806	2,801	215.7
Miami, FL	1,831	2,061	37.2	1	63,557	1,016	64,573	26,152	25,819	469.3
Fort Lauderdale division	712	807	45.7	—	19,334	267	19,601	8,289	8,214	468.5
Miami division	827	927	37.1	—	33,333	522	33,855	13,301	13,111	528.9
West Palm Beach division	292	327	25.5	—	10,890	226	11,116	4,562	4,494	354.0
Milwaukee—Waukesha—West Allis, WI	79	87	5.6	85	2,859	18	2,877	1,334	1,306	84.2
Minneapolis—St. Paul—Bloomington, MN—WI	173	193	5.9	83	5,038	23	5,061	2,447	2,454	75.8
Modesto, CA	25	33	6.6	77	799	6	805	379	384	75.6
Nashville—Davidson—Murfreesboro, TN	194	217	13.7	22	4,550	20	4,570	2,355	2,356	151.4
New Haven—Milford, CT	58	78	9.2	52	4,994	77	5,071	2,195	2,175	257.3
New Orleans—Metairie—Kenner, LA	262	274	23.0	9	9,871	70	9,941	3,973	3,956	338.5
New York, NY—NJ—PA	3,531	5,153	27.0	4	220,499	3,009	223,508	82,812	87,026	458.8
Edison division	127	208	8.9	—	7,453	143	7,597	2,679	2,718	117.1
Nassau division	176	244	8.5	—	9,267	119	9,386	3,657	3,662	127.7
New York—White Plains—Wayne division	2,873	4,145	35.3	—	181,653	2,394	184,047	69,286	73,333	628.7
Newark division	355	557	26.2	—	22,125	352	22,477	7,190	7,312	345.4
Ogden—Clearfield, UT	7	8	1.5	102	293	4	297	139	138	26.0
Oklahoma City, OK	72	80	6.5	78	2,615	5	2,620	1,127	1,147	95.0
Omaha—Council Bluffs, NE—IA	49	56	6.6	76	1,217	4	1,221	591	592	70.5
Orlando, FL	433	485	23.3	8	10,360	97	10,457	4,800	4,759	230.9
Oxnard—Thousand Oaks—Ventura, CA	22	30	3.8	96	1,135	3	1,138	490	491	61.8

TABLE 3.4

Reported AIDS cases and annual rates, by metropolitan area of residence and age category, 2009, and cumulative [CONTINUED]

[United States and Puerto Rico]

Area of residence	Diagnosis, 2009 No.	Estimated[b] No.	Estimated[b] Rate	Rank[c]	Cumulative[a] Adults or adolescents No.	Children Estimated[b] No.	Total No.	Living with AIDS, year-end 2008 No.	Estimated[b] No.	Estimated[b] Rate
Palm Bay—Melbourne—Titusville, FL	36	40	7.4	66	1,696	11	1,707	771	764	142.5
Philadelphia, PA—NJ—DE—MD	544	676	11.3	31	32,156	320	32,477	15,500	15,416	259.5
Camden division	78	118	9.4	—	3,578	42	3,620	1,467	1,495	119.5
Philadelphia division	382	444	11.1	—	25,104	256	25,360	12,548	12,436	311.5
Wilmington division	84	114	16.2	—	3,474	22	3,497	1,485	1,485	213.0
Phoenix—Mesa—Scottsdale, AZ	394	441	10.1	40	8,905	32	8,937	3,986	3,973	92.7
Pittsburgh, PA	111	122	5.2	87	3,634	20	3,655	1,567	1,548	65.7
Portland—South Portland, ME	23	34	6.6	73	676	1	677	297	300	58.1
Portland—Vancouver—Beaverton, OR—WA	154	177	7.9	61	5,450	10	5,460	2,457	2,456	111.4
Poughkeepsie—Newburgh—Middletown, NY	52	72	10.7	34	3,538	25	3,564	1,455	1,457	216.8
Providence—New Bedford—Fall River, RI—MA	101	139	8.7	56	4,430	44	4,475	2,043	2,056	128.5
Provo-Orem, UT	5	5	1.0	103	141	3	144	73	72	13.4
Raleigh—Cary, NC	141	161	14.3	21	2,618	14	2,632	1,369	1,354	124.1
Richmond, VA	91	123	9.9	42	3,974	36	4,010	1,765	1,771	144.4
Riverside—San Bernardino—Ontario, CA	274	364	8.8	55	10,070	63	10,133	4,898	4,939	120.7
Rochester, NY	82	114	11.0	33	3,648	15	3,663	1,734	1,751	169.5
Sacramento—Arden-Arcade—Roseville, CA	78	105	4.9	88	4,485	28	4,514	1,914	1,918	91.3
St. Louis, MO—IL	265	365	12.8	27	7,042	40	7,083	3,389	3,301	119.2
Salt Lake City, UT	44	50	4.4	92	1,931	10	1,941	955	955	85.9
San Antonio, TX	220	255	12.3	30	5,861	31	5,892	2,743	2,729	135.1
San Diego—Carlsbad—San Marcos, CA	366	489	16.0	17	14,655	68	14,723	6,724	6,676	222.7
San Francisco, CA	592	792	18.3	15	44,319	103	44,422	15,504	15,586	365.8
Oakland division	271	359	14.2	—	11,198	53	11,250	4,591	4,616	184.9
San Francisco division	321	433	24.3	—	33,122	50	33,172	10,913	10,970	621.7
San Jose—Sunnyvale—Santa Clara, CA	124	166	9.0	53	4,402	15	4,417	2,015	2,039	112.6
San Juan—Caguas—Guaynabo, PR	395	524	20.0	12	23,842	285	24,126	7,728	7,451	285.6
Scranton—Wilkes-Barre, PA	23	26	4.7	91	648	6	654	318	320	58.3
Seattle, WA	273	306	9.0	54	10,233	29	10,262	4,503	4,495	133.9
Seattle division	245	275	10.5	—	9,091	19	9,111	4,013	4,010	156.1
Tacoma division	28	31	3.9	—	1,141	10	1,151	490	485	61.6
Springfield, MA	25	34	4.9	89	2,375	28	2,404	988	985	141.4
Stockton, CA	44	56	8.4	58	1,304	15	1,319	626	630	94.2
Syracuse, NY	36	49	7.5	64	1,519	9	1,528	674	679	105.2
Tampa—St. Petersburg—Clearwater, FL	426	477	17.4	16	13,014	121	13,135	5,554	5,491	201.1
Toledo, OH	33	44	6.6	74	991	14	1,005	425	428	63.6
Tucson, AZ	83	94	9.2	51	2,270	10	2,280	925	914	90.6
Tulsa, OK	62	70	7.5	65	1,745	10	1,755	779	793	86.6
Virginia Beach—Norfolk—Newport News, VA—NC	88	117	7.0	70	5,511	63	5,575	2,533	2,538	152.0

TABLE 3.4

Reported AIDS cases and annual rates, by metropolitan area of residence and age category, 2009, and cumulative [CONTINUED]

[United States and Puerto Rico]

Area of residence	Diagnosis, 2009				Diagnosis, cumulative[a]				Living with AIDS, year-end 2008	
		Estimated[b]			Adults or adolescents	Children Estimated[b]	Total		Estimated[b]	
	No.	No.	Rate	Rank[c]	No.	No.	No.		No.	Rate
Washington, DC—VA—MD—WV	939	1,455	26.6	5	37,593	323	37,916		17,836	341.4
Bethesda division	109	181	15.1	—	3,548	24	3,572		1,886	166.2
Washington division	830	1,273	29.8	—	34,045	298	34,344		15,950	390.7
Wichita, KS	32	36	5.8	84	955	2	957		424	69.5
Worcester, MA	23	29	3.7	97	2,031	21	2,053		974	122.3
Youngstown—Warren—Boardman, OH—PA	29	38	6.7	72	656	0	656		267	47.2
Subtotal for MSAs (population ≥500,000)	22,278	28,342	13.8	—	956,528	8,516	965,044		404,473	202.0
Metropolitan areas (population of 50,000–499,999)	3,142	3,805	6.8	—	107,430	835	108,265		48,142	86.5
Nonmetropolitan areas	2,016	2,438	4.9	—	63,921	467	64,388		29,737	59.8
Total[e]	**27,653**	**34,981**	**11.2**	**—**	**1,132,030**	**9,858**	**1,141,888**		**484,532**	**159.0**

Note: Because of the lack of U.S. census information for all U.S. dependent areas, includes data for only the 50 states, the District of Columbia, and Puerto Rico. MSA = Metropolitan statistical area.

[a]From the beginning of the epidemic through 2009.

[b]Estimated numbers resulted from statistical adjustment that accounted for reporting delays, but not for incomplete reporting. Rates are per 100,000 population.

[c]Based on estimated rate.

[d]Counts of AIDS diagnoses for the metropolitan divisions do not sum to the MSA total. MSA total includes data from 1 metropolitan division with population of <500,000.

[e]Includes persons whose county of residence is unknown. Because column totals for estimated numbers were calculated independently of the values for the subpopulations, the values in each column may not sum to the column total.

SOURCE: "Table 24. AIDS Diagnoses, 2009 and Cumulative, and Persons Living with an AIDS Diagnosis, Year-End 2008, by Metropolitan Statistical Area of Residence—United States and Puerto Rico," in "Diagnoses of HIV Infection and AIDS in the United States and Dependent Areas, 2009," HIV Surveillance Report, 2009, vol. 21, Centers for Disease Control and Prevention, February 2011, http://www.cdc.gov/hiv/surveillance/resources/reports/2009report/pdf/table24.pdf (accessed June 4, 2011)

FIGURE 3.5

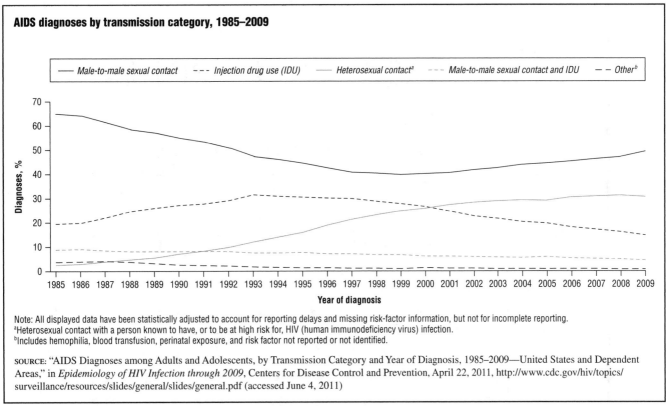

AIDS diagnoses by transmission category, 1985–2009

Note: All displayed data have been statistically adjusted to account for reporting delays and missing risk-factor information, but not for incomplete reporting.
aHeterosexual contact with a person known to have, or to be at high risk for, HIV (human immunodeficiency virus) infection.
bIncludes hemophilia, blood transfusion, perinatal exposure, and risk factor not reported or not identified.

SOURCE: "AIDS Diagnoses among Adults and Adolescents, by Transmission Category and Year of Diagnosis, 1985–2009—United States and Dependent Areas," in *Epidemiology of HIV Infection through 2009*, Centers for Disease Control and Prevention, April 22, 2011, http://www.cdc.gov/hiv/topics/surveillance/resources/slides/general/slides/general.pdf (accessed June 4, 2011)

among African-Americans. By 2009 the number of cases had reached 466,351. (See Table 3.3.) As Table 3.5 shows, the number of African-Americans living with HIV/AIDS continued to outpace the number of whites living with HIV/AIDS between 2006 and 2008.

In 1999 African-Americans accounted for 41% (127,169) of people estimated to be living with HIV/AIDS. By 2008 this figure had risen to 44% (208,983). (See Table 3.5.) In contrast, the proportion of whites living with HIV/AIDS in 1999 was 38% (120,731), and by 2009 it was 34% (163,238).

In 2009 Hispanics accounted for an estimated 6,719 new reported AIDS cases. (See Table 3.3.) The corresponding figures for whites and African-Americans were 9,467 and 16,741, respectively. The total number of male and female adult and adolescent reported AIDS cases in native Hawaiians/Other Pacific Islanders (50) and Asian-Americans (429) were the lowest of all the racial and ethnic groups in the United States.

In 2009 the total (male and female) estimated AIDS incidence rate per 100,000 adults and adolescents among African-Americans (44.4) was nine times higher than that among whites (4.7), about four times higher than that of native Hawaiians/Other Pacific Islanders (11.2), and three times higher than that of Hispanics (13.9). (See Table 3.3.) The rates were lowest among Asian-Americans (3.1).

The racial and ethnic difference is particularly alarming among children under the age of 13 years. As shown in Table 3.6, in 2009 the rate of HIV infection per 100,000 population for African-American children (2) was nearly seven times the rate for Hispanic and Asian-American children (both at 0.3). The other racial and ethnic categories were negligible.

The racial disparity is also reflected in the acquisition of HIV infection by infants born to HIV-infected mothers. From 1994 through 2009 the number of reported cases of HIV/AIDS among African-American infants was significantly greater than the reported cases for white and Hispanic infants born to HIV-infected mothers. In 2009 more than 10 times as many African-American infants were HIV-infected (96) through perinatal exposure (before, during, or immediately after birth) than were white infants (9). (See Table 3.7.)

Causes of Racial Disparities

In "Disparities in Diagnoses of HIV Infection between Blacks/African Americans and Other Racial/Ethnic Populations—37 States, 2005–2008" (*Morbidity and Mortality Weekly Report*, vol. 60, no. 4, February 4, 2011), the CDC notes that between 2005 and 2008 African-Americans were diagnosed with HIV infection more frequently than any other racial/ethnic population. This disparity is attributed to factors such as disproportion-

TABLE 3.5

Numbers of persons living with AIDS, by year and selected characteristics, 2006–08

[United States]

	2006			2007			2008		
	No.	Estimated[a] No.	Rate	No.	Estimated[a] No.	Rate	No.	Estimated[a] No.	Rate
Age at end of year									
<13	1,163	1,181	2.2	903	920	1.7	688	707	1.3
13–14	735	743	8.8	674	684	8.2	595	607	7.4
15–19	2,517	2,565	12.0	2,675	2,737	12.7	2,697	2,781	12.9
20–24	5,296	5,488	25.9	5,663	5,908	27.8	6,154	6,501	30.5
25–29	14,193	14,678	71.6	14,679	15,286	72.7	15,095	15,878	74.1
30–34	28,710	29,470	151.7	27,845	28,724	148.4	27,691	28,768	147.4
35–39	59,768	60,943	290.8	56,520	57,819	275.4	53,263	54,742	262.6
40–44	95,710	96,997	434.6	93,598	95,055	434.9	89,657	91,237	426.5
45–49	91,208	91,970	405.2	97,377	98,292	431.4	103,530	104,575	458.6
50–54	66,543	66,891	327.8	73,289	73,633	351.3	79,925	80,193	374.2
55–59	38,835	38,942	214.3	44,276	44,344	243.5	49,815	49,732	268.2
60–64	17,896	17,926	134.4	21,135	21,131	146.1	25,032	24,905	165.1
Over 65	14,268	14,197	38.2	16,795	16,668	44.0	19,541	19,242	49.6
Race/ethnicity									
American Indian/Alaska Native	1,562	1,569	69.1	1,629	1,633	70.9	1,727	1,731	74.2
Asian[b]	3,986	4,073	32.2	4,339	4,453	34.2	4,709	4,861	36.4
Black/African American	188,986	191,446	524.2	197,429	200,094	541.8	206,148	208,983	560.0
Hispanic/Latino[c]	83,835	85,552	194.4	88,058	90,070	197.9	91,959	94,247	200.6
Native Hawaiian/other Pacific Islander	365	371	87.9	405	413	95.8	432	441	100.4
White	152,272	153,008	77.1	157,514	158,337	79.5	162,470	163,238	81.8
Multiple races	5,682	5,822	139.9	5,901	6,046	140.8	6,086	6,214	140.3
Transmission category									
Male adult or adolescent									
Male-to-male sexual contact	183,053	205,653	—	191,238	216,154	—	199,299	226,739	—
Injection drug use	52,487	62,833	—	52,695	63,481	—	52,850	63,973	—
Male-to-male sexual contact and injection drug use	27,610	30,186	—	27,984	30,713	—	28,372	31,185	—
Heterosexual contact[d]	28,720	35,579	—	30,237	37,838	—	31,725	40,039	—
Other[a]	41,944	3,058	—	45,187	3,103	—	48,606	3,172	—
Subtotal	333,814	337,309	280.7	347,341	351,289	289.1	360,852	365,107	297.3
Female adult or adolescent									
Injection drug use	26,468	33,951	—	26,713	34,626	—	26,804	35,052	—
Heterosexual contact[d]	49,935	64,689	—	52,657	69,154	—	55,210	73,536	—
Other[a]	22,715	2,110	—	24,822	2,217	—	26,935	2,277	—
Subtotal	99,118	100,751	80.1	104,192	105,997	83.4	108,949	110,864	86.5

TABLE 3.5

Numbers of persons living with AIDS, by year and selected characteristics, 2006–08 [CONTINUED]

[United States]

| | 2006 | | | 2007 | | | 2008 | | |
| | No. | Estimated[a] | | No. | Estimated[a] | | No. | Estimated[a] | |
		No.	Rate		No.	Rate		No.	Rate
Child (<13 years at diagnosis)									
Perinatal	3,701	3,724	—	3,691	3,710	—	3,677	3,691	—
Other[f]	208	209	—	203	203	—	203	203	—
Subtotal	**3,909**	**3,932**	**7.5**	**3,894**	**3,913**	**7.4**	**3,880**	**3,894**	**7.3**
Region of residence									
Northeast	127,887	131,191	239.8	132,298	136,076	248.0	135,812	140,136	254.5
Midwest	46,818	46,948	71.0	49,182	49,340	74.4	51,668	51,902	77.9
South	175,202	176,418	162.0	183,442	184,653	167.0	192,021	192,827	172.1
West	86,935	87,435	127.0	90,507	91,132	130.6	94,182	95,003	134.4
Total[g]	**436,842**	**441,993**	**148.0**	**455,429**	**461,201**	**152.9**	**473,683**	**479,868**	**157.7**

[a]Estimated numbers resulted from statistical adjustment that accounted for reporting delays and missing risk-factor information, but not for incomplete reporting. Rates are per 100,000 population. Rates are not calculated by transmission category because of the lack of denominator data.

[b]Includes Asian/Pacific Islander legacy cases.

[c]Hispanics/Latinos can be of any race.

[d]Heterosexual contact with a person known to have, or to be at high risk for, HIV infection.

[e]Includes hemophilia, blood transfusion, perinatal exposure, and risk factor not reported or not identified.

[f]Includes hemophilia, blood transfusion, and risk factor not reported or not identified.

[g]Includes persons of unknown race/ethnicity. Because column totals for estimated numbers were calculated independently of the values for the subpopulations, the values in each column may not sum to the column total.

SOURCE: "Table 16a. Persons Living With an AIDS Diagnosis, by Year and Selected Characteristics, 2006–2008—United States," in "Diagnoses of HIV Infection and AIDS in the United States and Dependent Areas, 2009," *HIV Surveillance Report, 2009*, vol. 21, Centers for Disease Control and Prevention, February 2011, http://www.cdc.gov/hiv/surveillance/resources/reports/2009report/pdf/table16a.pdf (accessed June 4, 2011)

TABLE 3.6

Diagnosed HIV infection, by age, race/ethnicity, and transmission category, 2009

[40 states with confidential name-based HIV infection reporting]

	American Indian/ Alaska Native			Asian			Black/African American			Hispanic/Latino[a]			Native Hawaiian/other Pacific Islander			White			Multiple races			Total		
	No.	Estimated[b] No.	Rate	No.	Estimated[b] No.	Rate	No.	Estimated[b] No.	Rate	No.	Estimated[b] No.	Rate	No.	Estimated[b] No.	Rate	No.	Estimated[b] No.	Rate	No.	Estimated[b] No.	Rate	No.[c]	Estimated[b] No.	Rate
Age at diagnosis (year)																								
<13	0	0	0.0	3	4	0.3	107	127	2.0	20	23	0.3	0	0	0.0	10	11	0.0	1	1	0.1	141	166	0.4
13–14	0	0	0.0	1	1	0.6	13	14	1.4	3	3	0.3	0	0	0.0	2	2	0.1	0	0	0.0	19	21	0.3
15–19	4	4	2.6	8	10	2.3	1,274	1,482	51.9	224	264	10.3	1	1	11.3	219	248	2.4	22	26	8.5	1,752	2,036	12.0
20–24	19	23	13.5	44	52	10.5	3,313	3,895	144.7	830	970	38.3	4	5	35.3	1,047	1,208	11.2	70	85	34.3	5,327	6,237	36.9
25–29	27	31	19.9	64	76	12.7	2,525	2,987	117.0	1,053	1,225	44.5	3	3	21.9	1,334	1,546	14.6	72	84	40.0	5,078	5,951	35.2
30–34	29	33	25.7	76	87	13.1	2,009	2,370	107.1	977	1,145	42.3	5	6	41.7	1,150	1,323	13.8	48	56	34.8	4,294	5,020	32.5
35–39	20	23	18.8	82	97	13.9	1,959	2,335	105.1	923	1,059	42.2	3	4	28.4	1,397	1,638	15.9	64	75	52.8	4,448	5,232	32.6
40–44	25	28	22.9	49	61	10.2	2,124	2,524	114.3	855	984	44.9	5	5	49.5	1,605	1,868	16.7	41	47	38.1	4,704	5,519	33.6
45–49	20	24	17.4	30	35	6.6	1,936	2,293	98.9	635	740	38.4	3	4	36.3	1,463	1,704	13.2	54	65	50.0	4,141	4,865	27.1
50–54	7	8	6.6	18	22	4.8	1,482	1,753	82.5	361	421	27.8	3	4	41.3	934	1,083	8.4	29	33	27.8	2,834	3,323	19.3
55–59	10	12	11.8	9	11	2.8	863	1,023	58.9	206	242	20.8	0	0	0.0	574	683	5.9	29	34	34.0	1,691	2,004	13.4
60–64	0	0	0.0	3	4	1.2	387	455	35.7	117	140	15.9	1	1	20.5	263	299	3.0	1	1	1.3	772	900	7.2
≥65	2	3	1.7	8	10	1.7	328	393	13.9	114	131	6.8	1	1	11.7	162	188	0.7	9	10	6.0	624	736	2.3
Transmission category																								
Male adult or adolescent																								
Male-to-male sexual contact	60	91	—	171	293	—	6,212	10,128	—	2,894	4,418	—	14	22	—	5,928	8,608	—	209	287	—	15,488	23,846	—
Injection drug use	11	16	—	8	16	—	410	1,333	—	269	592	—	1	1	—	304	462	—	15	29	—	1,018	2,449	—
Male-to-male sexual contact and injection drug use	9	16	—	5	7	—	128	389	—	115	199	—	0	0	—	362	501	—	13	18	—	632	1,131	—
Heterosexual contact[d]	9	13	—	26	44	—	1,411	3,029	—	466	755	—	2	2	—	318	505	—	34	49	—	2,266	4,399	—
Other[e]	29	1	—	95	3	—	4,405	19	—	1,401	7	—	5	0	—	1,761	17	—	53	0	—	7,749	47	—
Subtotal	**118**	**137**	**18.4**	**305**	**363**	**12.7**	**12,566**	**14,898**	**122.2**	**5,145**	**5,972**	**48.3**	**22**	**26**	**41.2**	**8,673**	**10,093**	**14.8**	**324**	**383**	**41.3**	**27,153**	**31,872**	**32.7**
Female adult or adolescent																								
Injection drug use	4	9	—	2	6	—	248	826	—	108	234	—	0	0	—	219	387	—	10	22	—	591	1,483	—
Heterosexual contact[d]	16	43	—	45	96	—	2,231	5,787	—	514	1,113	—	6	8	—	587	1,304	—	54	111	—	3,453	8,461	—
Other[e]	25	0	—	40	1	—	3,168	14	—	531	6	—	1	0	—	671	8	—	51	0	—	4,487	29	—
Subtotal	**45**	**51**	**6.6**	**87**	**103**	**3.4**	**5,647**	**6,627**	**47.8**	**1,153**	**1,352**	**11.9**	**7**	**8**	**13.3**	**1,477**	**1,699**	**2.4**	**115**	**132**	**13.4**	**8,531**	**9,973**	**9.8**

TABLE 3.6

Diagnosed HIV infection, by age, race/ethnicity, and transmission category, 2009 [CONTINUED]

[40 states with confidential name-based HIV infection reporting]

	American Indian/ Alaska Native			Asian			Black/African American			Hispanic/Latino[a]			Native Hawaiian/other Pacific Islander			White			Multiple races			Total		
		Estimated[b]			Estimated[b]			Estimated[b]			Estimated[b]			Estimated[b]			Estimated[b]			Estimated[b]			Estimated[b]	
	No.	No.	Rate	No.	No.	Rate	No.	No.	Rate	No.	No.	Rate	No.	No.	Rate	No.	No.	Rate	No.	No.	Rate	No.[c]	No.[c]	Rate
Child (<13 years at diagnosis)																								
Perinatal	0	0	—	3	4	—	82	96	—	18	20	—	0	0	—	8	9	—	1	1	—	112	131	—
Other[f]	0	0	—	0	0	—	25	31	—	2	2	—	0	0	—	2	2	—	0	0	—	29	35	—
Subtotal	0	0	0.0	3	4	0.3	107	127	2.0	20	23	0.3	0	0	0.0	10	11	0.0	1	1	0.1	141	166	0.4
Total[g]	163	189	9.8	395	470	6.4	18,320	21,652	66.6	6,318	7,347	22.8	29	34	21.0	10,160	11,803	7.2	440	516	16.7	35,825	42,011	17.4

Note: Data include persons with a diagnosis of HIV infection regardless of stage of disease at diagnosis. HIV = Human immunodeficiency virus.

[a]Hispanics/Latinos can be of any race.

[b]Estimated numbers resulted from statistical adjustment that accounted for reporting delays and missing risk-factor information, but not for incomplete reporting. Rates are per 100,000 population. Rates are not calculated by transmission category because of the lack of denominator data.

[c]Because the estimated totals were calculated independently of the corresponding values for each subpopulation, the subpopulation values may not sum to the totals shown here.

[d]Heterosexual contact with a person known to have, or to be at high risk for, HIV infection.

[e]Includes hemophilia, blood transfusion, perinatal exposure, and risk factor not reported or not identified.

[f]Includes hemophilia, blood transfusion, and risk factor not reported or not identified.

[g]Because column totals for estimated numbers were calculated independently of the values for the subpopulations, the values in each column may not sum to the column total.

SOURCE: "Table 3a. Diagnoses of HIV Infection, by Race/Ethnicity and Selected Characteristics, 2009—40 States with Confidential Name-Based HIV Infection Reporting," in "Diagnoses of HIV Infection and AIDS in the United States and Dependent Areas, 2009," *HIV Surveillance Report, 2009*, vol. 21, Centers for Disease Control and Prevention, February 2011, http://www.cdc.gov/hiv/surveillance/resources/reports/2009report/pdf/table3a.pdf (accessed June 4, 2011)

TABLE 3.7

Diagnosed HIV infection, by race/ethnicity and selected characteristics, 2009

[40 states and 5 U.S. dependent areas with confidential name-based HIV infection reporting]

	American Indian/ Alaska Native		Asian		Black/African American		Hispanic/Latino[a]		Native Hawaiian/ other Pacific Islander		White		Multiple races		Total	
	No.	Est. No.[b]	No.	Est. No.[b]	No.	Est. No.[b]	No.	Est. No.[b]	No.	Est. No.[b]	No.	Est. No.[b]	No.	Est. No.[b]	No.	Est. No.[b,c]
Age at diagnosis (yr)																
<13	0	0	3	4	107	127	20	23	0	0	10	11	1	1	141	166
13–14	0	0	1	1	13	14	3	3	0	0	2	2	0	0	19	21
15–19	4	4	8	10	1,274	1,482	239	284	1	1	220	249	22	26	1,768	2,057
20–24	19	23	44	52	3,314	3,897	886	1,045	4	5	1,047	1,208	70	85	5,384	6,314
25–29	28	31	64	76	2,527	2,990	1,135	1,335	4	4	1,335	1,548	72	84	5,165	6,068
30–34	29	33	76	87	2,011	2,373	1,076	1,278	5	6	1,150	1,323	48	56	4,395	5,156
35–39	20	23	82	97	1,960	2,336	1,011	1,177	3	4	1,397	1,638	64	75	4,537	5,351
40–44	25	28	51	64	2,127	2,528	957	1,123	3	5	1,605	1,868	41	47	4,811	5,665
45–49	20	24	30	35	1,940	2,300	725	862	3	4	1,463	1,704	54	65	4,235	4,993
50–54	7	8	18	22	1,483	1,754	424	506	3	4	936	1,086	29	33	2,900	3,413
55–59	10	12	9	11	863	1,023	238	285	0	0	574	683	29	34	1,723	2,047
60–64	3	0	3	4	388	457	138	169	1	1	264	301	1	1	795	932
≥65	2	3	8	10	328	393	142	171	1	1	162	188	9	10	652	776
Transmission category																
Male adult or adolescent																
Male-to-male sexual contact	60	91	171	293	6,215	10,135	3,069	4,692	14	22	5,931	8,613	209	287	15,669	24,132
Injection drug use	11	16	8	17	410	1,336	388	790	1	1	304	462	15	29	1,137	2,652
Male-to-male sexual contact and injection drug use	9	16	5	7	128	389	130	225	0	0	362	501	13	18	647	1,157
Heterosexual contact[d]	9	13	26	44	1,411	3,035	557	901	2	2	318	505	34	49	2,357	4,551
Other[e]	29	1	96	3	4,413	19	1,475	7	5	0	1,762	17	53	0	7,833	47
Subtotal	118	137	306	365	12,577	14,914	5,619	6,615	22	26	8,677	10,098	324	383	27,643	32,538
Female adult or adolescent																
Injection drug use	4	9	2	6	248	827	128	269	0	0	220	388	10	22	612	1,520
Heterosexual contact[d]	16	43	46	97	2,232	5,792	656	1,350	6	9	587	1,304	54	111	3,597	8,706
Other[e]	26	0	40	1	3,171	14	571	6	2	0	671	8	51	0	4,532	29
Subtotal	46	51	88	105	5,651	6,632	1,355	1,625	8	10	1,478	1,700	115	132	8,741	10,255
Child (<13 yrs at diagnosis)																
Perinatal	0	0	3	4	82	96	18	20	0	0	8	9	1	1	112	131
Other[f]	0	0	0	0	25	31	2	2	0	0	2	2	0	0	29	35
Subtotal	0	0	3	4	107	127	20	23	0	0	10	11	1	1	141	166
Total[g]	164	189	397	473	18,335	21,673	6,994	8,263	30	36	10,165	11,810	440	516	36,525	42,959

Note: Data include persons with a diagnosis of HIV infection regardless of stage of disease at diagnosis.

[a] Hispanics/Latinos can be of any race.

[b] Estimated numbers resulted from statistical adjustment that accounted for reporting delays and missing risk-factor information, but not for incomplete reporting.

[c] Because the estimated totals were calculated independently of the corresponding values for each subpopulation, the subpopulation values may not sum to the totals shown here.

[d] Heterosexual contact with a person known to have, or to be at high risk for, HIV infection.

[e] Includes hemophilia, blood transfusion, perinatal exposure, and risk factor not reported or not identified.

[f] Includes hemophilia, blood transfusion, and risk factor not reported or not identified.

[g] Because column totals for estimated numbers were calculated independently of the values for the subpopulations, the values in each column may not sum to the column total.

SOURCE: "Table 3b. Diagnoses of HIV infection, by Race/Ethnicity and Selected Characteristics, 2009—40 States and 5 U.S. Dependent Areas with Confidential Name-Based HIV Infection Reporting," in "Diagnoses of HIV Infection and AIDS in the United States and Dependent Areas, 2009," HIV Surveillance Report, 2009, vol. 21, Centers for Disease Control and Prevention, February 2011, http://www.cdc.gov/hiv/surveillance/resources/reports/2009report/pdf/table3b.pdf (accessed June 4, 2011)

FIGURE 3.6

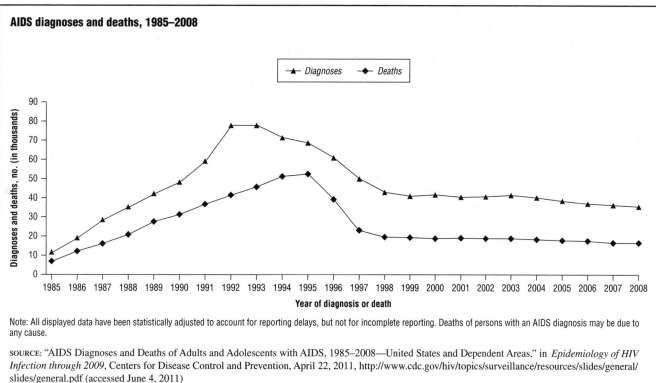

AIDS diagnoses and deaths, 1985–2008

Note: All displayed data have been statistically adjusted to account for reporting delays, but not for incomplete reporting. Deaths of persons with an AIDS diagnosis may be due to any cause.

SOURCE: "AIDS Diagnoses and Deaths of Adults and Adolescents with AIDS, 1985–2008—United States and Dependent Areas," in *Epidemiology of HIV Infection through 2009*, Centers for Disease Control and Prevention, April 22, 2011, http://www.cdc.gov/hiv/topics/surveillance/resources/slides/general/slides/general.pdf (accessed June 4, 2011)

ately higher prevalence rates of other sexually transmitted infections, housing conditions, lack of education and social support, and poverty. To reduce these disparities, the CDC recommends addressing patient-specific behavioral risk factors, such as having multiple sex partners and unprotected sex, as well as social and environmental factors, such as access to testing and health care services, incarceration, stigma, homophobia, sexism, and racism.

To reduce disparities in the incidence and prevalence of HIV infection, the CDC supports prevention and intervention programs for African-Americans, such as the Act against AIDS campaign (2011, http://www.cdc.gov/hiv/aaa/), which aims to improve knowledge and dispel misperceptions about HIV in the United States. In 2010 the CDC launched an expanded HIV testing program to increase the rate of HIV testing among African-Americans.

HOW HIV IS TRANSMITTED

HIV can be transmitted by sexual contact with an infected person; by needle sharing among infected injection drug users; through the receipt of infected blood, blood products, or tissue; and directly from an infected mother to her infant during pregnancy, delivery, or breastfeeding.

In the United States MSM remain the majority of HIV carriers, although prevalence among heterosexuals is on the rise. The CDC reports in *HIV/AIDS Surveillance Report, 1988* (January 1989, http://www.cdc.gov/hiv/topics/surveillance/resources/reports/pdf/surveillance88.pdf) that

70% of adult and adolescent males with AIDS had a single risk factor of a history of high-risk sexual activity in 1987. Even though 50% of reported cases of AIDS among male adults and adolescents were attributable to MSM in 2009, cumulatively the percentage of affected MSM was 48%. (See Table 3.3.) Adult and adolescent males with a history of injection drug use as their only risk factor made up 14% of all cases in 1987. This proportion has remained relatively constant in the intervening years, and even though a cumulative of 21% of AIDS cases in adult and adolescent males were attributable to injection drug use, they accounted for 12% of cases in 2009. (See Table 2.5 in Chapter 2.)

The proportion of adult and adolescent females with AIDS whose only risk factor was injection drug use had dropped from 49% in 1987 to 22% in 2009. (See Table 2.5 in Chapter 2.) Adult and adolescent females with a history of heterosexual contact as their only risk factor made up 31% of all female cases in 1987. By 2009 this percentage had increased to 76%. Researchers suggest that one reason for steadily increasing HIV infection and AIDS among heterosexuals is that an increased proportion report multiple sex partners, which is a risk factor for HIV infection.

MORTALITY FROM AIDS

In "Deaths: Preliminary Data for 2009" (*National Vital Statistics Reports*, vol. 59, no. 4, March 16, 2011),

Kenneth D. Kochanek et al. of the CDC note that in 2009 the average life expectancy for Americans was 78.2 years, an all-time high. This figure would have been higher were it not for heart diseases (the leading cause of death for all age categories), malignant neoplasms (cancers, which were the leading cause of death for those aged 45 to 64 years), and accidents (the leading cause of death for those aged 1 to 44 years). (See Table 1.1 in Chapter 1.) AIDS was also among the leading causes of death among those aged 25 to 44 years. The CDC indicates in *HIV Surveillance Report: Diagnoses of HIV Infection and AIDS in the United States and Dependent Areas, 2009* that through 2008 there were an estimated 406,725 reported AIDS deaths among Americans aged 15 to 44 years, representing two-thirds (66%) of the 617,025 people who had died from AIDS.

According to the CDC, in *HIV/AIDS Surveillance Report, 2001*, the number of deaths due to AIDS peaked at 51,670 in 1995. Since then the number of deaths each year has been dropping. In 2008 the disease killed 16,769 Americans. (See Figure 3.6.) As a result of more effective treatment, fewer people are dying from AIDS. As fewer people become infected with HIV, the death rate in subsequent years will drop proportionally. However, the statistics for children under the age of 13 years at the time of diagnosis remain grim: half die before their first birthday, whereas the other half do not live to adolescence.

CHAPTER 4
POPULATIONS AT RISK

This chapter examines the prevalence rates of HIV infection—that is, the number of people who have the disease in a specified time period as opposed to (often at the end of a given year) the total number of people in the population being examined. Prevalence rates are based on surveys of selected segments of the general population and the prevalence rates of people in high-risk groups. These are not absolute numbers. The actual number of cases of HIV infection is likely to be higher than those reported in this chapter, because reporting is not universal and, as of August 2011, only 40 U.S. states and five U.S. dependent areas subscribed to confidential reporting practices. However, information on prevalence rates serves as a road map that reveals trends such as the geographic distribution of disease or changes in how the disease is transmitted.

INCREASE IN HIV INFECTION AND AIDS AMONG HETEROSEXUALS

The increase in the number and proportion of HIV/ AIDS cases among heterosexuals signals a major shift in the patterns of the epidemic. In 2009, 41,845 new cases of HIV infection among adults and adolescents were reported to the Centers for Disease Control and Prevention (CDC). (See Table 4.1.) Thirty-one percent were attributed to heterosexual contact. Similarly, 34,233 new cases of AIDS among adults and adolescents were reported to the CDC in 2009. (See Table 2.5 in Chapter 2.) Thirty percent (10,393) of these new AIDS cases were attributed to heterosexual contact. In comparison, the CDC reports in *Weekly Surveillance Report, 1985* (December 30, 1985, http://www.cdc .gov/hiv/topics/surveillance/resources/reports/pdf/surveil lance85.pdf) that 1% of all AIDS cases were attributable to heterosexual transmission in 1985.

The CDC notes that between 1997 and 2001 the number of new AIDS cases dropped significantly and that the proportions of those infected in each exposure category also changed. Cases attributed to male-to-male sexual contact (MSM) represented 35% of all cases in 1997 and 1998; thereafter, they dropped to 34% in 1999, to 32% in 2000, and to 31% in 2001. In 2003 the MSM rate rebounded to 35% and by 2009 it accounted for 67% of new cases among adult and adolescent males. (See Table 2.5 in Chapter 2.) Despite the decline from the late 1990s, MSM continued to represent the largest proportion (46% in both 2000 and 2001, 45% in 2003, and 48% in 2009) of cumulative AIDS cases since 1981.

According to the CDC, in *HIV Surveillance in Women* (May 20, 2011, http://www.cdc.gov/hiv/topics/surveillance/ resources/slides/women/slides/Women.pdf), in 2009 there were 9,973 cases of HIV infection among adult and adolescent women reported by 40 states and five U.S. dependent areas with confidential name-based HIV infection reporting since at least January 2006. The majority of the cases were attributable to high-risk heterosexual contact, which accounted for between 81.5% and 90.4% of cases in female adults and adolescents. (See Table 4.2.) The percentage of cases attributable to injection drug use increased with advancing age, from 9.6% of females aged 13 to 19 years to 17.9% of females aged 45 years and older.

The proportion of women who contracted AIDS through heterosexual contact remained relatively constant at 37% in 2001 and 38% in 2002. However, in 2003 the proportion increased to 45%, and in 2009 it had risen to between 47.9% and 83.9% of cases in female adults and adolescents. (See Table 4.3.)

Risks of Heterosexual Contact

The CDC indicates in *HIV Surveillance in Women* that African-American females continue to be disproportionately affected—in 2009 the largest number of HIV infections in female adults and adolescents was among African-American females—66% (6,627 out of 9,973) of HIV diagnoses were in African-American females (see

Table 4.4), even though African-Americans accounted for just 14% of the female population in the United States. In contrast, white females made up 71% of the female adult and adolescent population in the United States but accounted for just 17% (1,699) of HIV infection diagnoses among females.

High-risk heterosexual contact accounted for an estimated 4,399 cases (14%) of HIV infection among male adults and adolescents in 2009. (See Table 3.2 in Chapter 3.) By contrast, among adult and adolescent males, MSM accounted for three-quarters of HIV diagnoses in 2009.

INJECTION DRUG USERS

In *Preventing HIV Transmission: The Role of Sterile Needles and Bleach* (1995), Jacques Normand, David Vlahov, and Lincoln E. Moses of the National Academy of Sciences concluded that "the HIV epidemic in this country is now clearly driven by infections occurring in the population of injection drug users, their sexual partners, and their offspring." During the 1990s the proportions of both HIV infection and AIDS deaths that were attributable to injection drug use (IDU) among adults and adolescents increased. According to the CDC, in 1995 IDU was the exposure category for 25% of male and 47% of female AIDS deaths. To prevent a rise in IDU-associated HIV infection and AIDS, Normand, Vlahov, and Moses urged policy makers to adequately fund needle exchange programs. Since 1995 the percentage of HIV/AIDS cases attributable to IDU has been steadily decreasing. By 2009 IDU accounted for an estimated 8% of cases of HIV infection in male adults and adolescents and 15% of cases in female adults and adolescents. (See Table 3.2 in Chapter 3.)

How HIV Is Transmitted through Injection Drug Use

HIV can be transmitted through IDU when the blood of an HIV-infected drug user is transferred to a drug user who is not yet infected with HIV. This transfer occurs almost exclusively through the sharing of injecting equipment, primarily needles and syringes.

Blood enters and makes contact with the needle and syringe in two ways. The first occurs when blood is drawn into the syringe to verify that the needle is inside a vein,

TABLE 4.1

HIV infections by transmission category, 2009 and cumulative through 2009

Transmission category	Estimated number of diagnoses of HIV infection, 2009		
	Adult and adolescent males	Adult and adolescent females	Total
Male-to-male sexual contact	23,846	—	23,846
Injection drug use	2,449	1,483	3,932
Male-to-male sexual contact and injection drug use	1,131	—	1,131
Heterosexual contact[a]	4,399	8,461	12,860
Other[b]	47	29	76

HIV = Human immunodeficieny virus.
[a]Heterosexual contact with a person known to have, or to be at high risk for HIV infection.
[b]Includes hemophilia, blood transfusion, prenatal exposure, and risk not reported or not identified.

SOURCE: "Diagnoses of HIV Infection by Transmission Category," in *HIV Surveillance Report: Diagnoses of HIV Infection and AIDS in the United States and Dependent Areas, 2009*, Centers for Disease Control and Prevention, Divisions of HIV/AIDS Prevention, February 28, 2011, http://www.cdc.gov/hiv/topics/surveillance/basic.htm#exposure (accessed June 3, 2011)

TABLE 4.2

HIV Infection among females, by transmission category and age at diagnosis, 2009

[40 states and 5 U.S. dependent areas]

	Age of diagnosis (in years)				
	13–19	20–24	25–34	35–44	≥45
			Population		
Transmission category	476	1,194	2,565	2,741	3,280
	%	%	%	%	%
Injection drug use	9.6	10.0	13.0	15.9	17.9
Heterosexual contact	90.4	89.7	86.9	84.0	81.5
Other[b]	0.0	0.3	0.1	0.1	0.6
Total	**100.0**	**100.0**	**100.0**	**100.0**	**100.0**

HIV = Human immunodeficiency virus.
Note: Data include persons with a diagnosis of HIV infection regardless of stage of disease at diagnosis. All displayed data have been statistically adjusted to account for reporting delays and missing risk-factor information, but not for incomplete reporting.
[a]Heterosexual contact with a person known to have, or to be at high risk for, HIV (human immunodeficiency virus) infection.
[b]Includes blood transfusion, perinatal exposure, and risk factor not reported or not identified.

SOURCE: "Diagnoses of HIV Infection among Adult and Adolescent Females, by Transmission Category and Age at Diagnosis, 2009—40 States and 5 U.S. Dependent Areas," in HIV Surveillance in Women, Centers for Disease Control and Prevention, May 20, 2011, http://www.cdc.gov/hiv/topics/surveillance/resources/slides/women/slides/Women.pdf (accessed June 6, 2011)

TABLE 4.3

AIDS diagnoses among females, by transmission category and age at diagnosis, 2009

[United States and dependent areas]

	Age of diagnosis (in years)				
	13–19	20–24	25–34	35–44	≥45
			Population		
Transmission category	195	391	1,916	2,796	3,580
	%	%	%	%	%
Injection drug use	6.4	12.3	15.7	22.4	27.8
Heterosexual contact[a]	47.9	81.0	83.9	77.4	71.4
Other[b]	45.6	6.7	0.3	0.2	0.8
Total	**100.0**	**100.0**	**100.0**	**100.0**	**100.0**

Note: All displayed data have been statistically adjusted to account for reporting delays and missing risk-factor information, but not for incomplete reporting.
[a]Heterosexual contact with a person known to have, or to be at high risk for, HIV (human immunodeficiency virus) infection.
[b]Includes blood transfusion, perinatal exposure, and risk factor not reported or not identified.

SOURCE: "AIDS Diagnoses among Adult and Adolescent Females, by Transmission Category and Age at Diagnosis, 2009—United States and Dependent Areas," in *HIV Surveillance in Women*, Centers for Disease Control and Prevention, May 20, 2011, http://www.cdc.gov/hiv/topics/surveillance/resources/slides/women/slides/Women.pdf (accessed June 6, 2011)

TABLE 4.4

HIV diagnoses among adult and adolescent females by race/ethnicity, 2009

[40 states]

Race/ethnicity	No.	Rate
American Indian/Alaska Native	51	6.6
Asian	103	3.4
Black/African American	6,627	47.8
Hispanic/Latino*	1,352	11.9
Native Hawaiian/other Pacific Islander	8	13.3
White	1,699	2.4
Multiple races	132	13.4
Total	**9,973**	**9.8**

HIV = Human immunodeficiency virus.
Note: Data include persons with a diagnosis of HIV infection regardless of stage of disease at diagnosis. All displayed data have been statistically adjusted to account for reporting delays, but not for incomplete reporting. Rates are per 100,000 population.
*Hispanics/Latinos can be of any race.

SOURCE: "Diagnoses of HIV Infection among Adult and Adolescent Females, by Race/Ethnicity, 2009—40 States," in *HIV Surveillance in Women*, Centers for Disease Control and Prevention, May 20, 2011, http://www.cdc.gov/hiv/topics/surveillance/resources/slides/women/slides/Women.pdf (accessed June 6, 2011)

before the injection of the drug. The second occurs following the injection, when the syringe is refilled several times with blood from the vein to "wash out" any heroin, cocaine, or other drug left in the syringe after the first injection. Even the smallest amount of HIV-infected blood left in the syringe can cause the virus to be transmitted to the next user of the contaminated syringe and needle.

Among IDUs the risk of HIV infection increases in proportion to the duration of IDU. Put another way, the longer the drug use, the greater the risk of infection. Diseases such as hepatitis show this same pattern. Risk also increases with the frequency of needle sharing and

IDU in a geographic area, such as a large city, where there is a high prevalence of HIV infection.

General Trends

Table 2.5 in Chapter 2 shows that, of the cumulative AIDS cases among adults and adolescents reported from 1981 through 2009 (1,099,161), 273,444 (25% of the cumulative total) were attributable to IDU. Cumulatively, 77,213 cases (7%) were attributable to MSM in conjunction with IDU. Table 4.1 shows that in 2009 IDU was responsible for 3,932 HIV infections (9% of the 41,845 infections) and an additional 1,131 HIV infections (3%) were attributable to MSM in conjunction with IDU. In men with HIV infection, IDU was second only to MSM as a risk factor from 2000 through 2009.

HIV is also spread among non-IDUs who trade sex for drugs, especially crack cocaine, as well as the partners of these users. Those who trade sex for drugs often engage in unprotected sex and have multiple sex partners. People who exchange sex for drugs and have a sexually transmitted disease (STD) that causes ulcers or sores on the genitals, such as syphilis or herpes simplex, are at a higher risk for HIV infection. Drug and/or alcohol users may also be at greater risk for infection because these substances often lessen inhibitions and reduce the reluctance to have unsafe, unprotected sex.

WOMEN AND HIV/AIDS

The proportion of women among AIDS sufferers increased steadily, from a reported 7% in 1985 to 25% in 2009. (See Figure 4.1.) One-third (70,856 cases) of the 213,962 cumulative AIDS cases from 1981 through 2009 among females were associated either directly or indirectly with IDU. (See Table 3.3 in Chapter 3.)

FIGURE 4.1

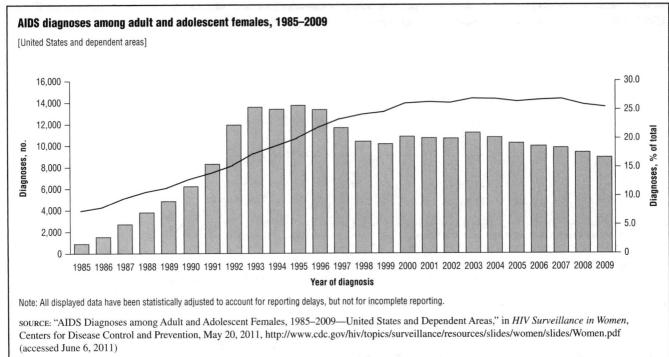

AIDS diagnoses among adult and adolescent females, 1985–2009

[United States and dependent areas]

Note: All displayed data have been statistically adjusted to account for reporting delays, but not for incomplete reporting.

SOURCE: "AIDS Diagnoses among Adult and Adolescent Females, 1985–2009—United States and Dependent Areas," in *HIV Surveillance in Women*, Centers for Disease Control and Prevention, May 20, 2011, http://www.cdc.gov/hiv/topics/surveillance/resources/slides/women/slides/Women.pdf (accessed June 6, 2011)

The racial and ethnic differences among women with HIV/AIDS are striking. Even though African-American and Hispanic women made up 14% and 11%, respectively, of all women in the United States in 2009, they accounted for 66% and 14%, respectively, of the 9,973 adult and adolescent females diagnosed with HIV infection in 2009. (See Table 4.4.) In contrast, white females made up 71% of the U.S. female population but just 17% of women diagnosed with HIV. The difference was comparable in AIDS diagnoses. In 2009, 5,639 (65%) of the AIDS diagnoses in females were among African-Americans, 1,357 (16%) were among Hispanics, and 1,344 (15%) were among whites. (See Table 4.5.)

Women can infect their unborn children with HIV during the course of pregnancy, during delivery, or by breastfeeding after birth. The 48% decrease in the number of women who gave birth to HIV-infected babies during the 1990s was largely attributable to the introduction of the antiretroviral drug zidovudine (ZDV; previously called azidothymidine). Women of childbearing age can be tested for HIV perinatally (before and during pregnancy), and, if they are positive, they have the option of receiving ZDV to prevent transmitting the virus to their unborn children.

According to the CDC, in "One Test, Two Lives" (May 25, 2011, http://www.actagainstaids.org/provider/ottl/index.html), 91% of all AIDS cases among children in the United States result from perinatal transmission. The CDC notes that "antiretroviral therapy during pregnancy can reduce the transmission rate to 2% or less. The transmission rate is 25% without treatment."

TABLE 4.5

AIDS diagnoses among adult and adolescent females by race/ethnicity, 2009

[United States]

Race/ethnicity	No.	Rate
American Indian/Alaska Native	28	2.9
Asian[a]	80	1.3
Black/African American	5,639	35.1
Hispanic/Latino[b]	1,357	7.9
Native Hawaiian/other Pacific Islander	7	4.0
White	1,344	1.5
Multiple races	192	12.7
Total	**8,647**	**6.7**

Note: All displayed data have been statistically adjusted to account for reporting delays, but not for incomplete reporting. Rates are per 100,000 population.
[a]Includes Asian/Pacific Islander legacy cases.
[b]Hispanics/Latinos can be of any race.

SOURCE: "AIDS Diagnoses among Adult and Adolescent Females, by Race/Ethnicity, 2009—United States," in *HIV Surveillance in Women*, Centers for Disease Control and Prevention, May 20, 2011, http://www.cdc.gov/hiv/topics/surveillance/resources/slides/women/slides/Women.pdf (accessed June 6, 2011)

Along with antiretroviral therapy, which lowers the mother's viral load to undetectable levels, deliveries via elective cesarean section (the surgical delivery of a baby) rather than vaginal births may also help reduce mother-to-child transmission. States with HIV case surveillance data are better able to direct resources (e.g., targeted public health education programs, health professionals, and prenatal care) that are aimed at eliminating prenatal (before birth) transmission of HIV.

FIGURE 4.2

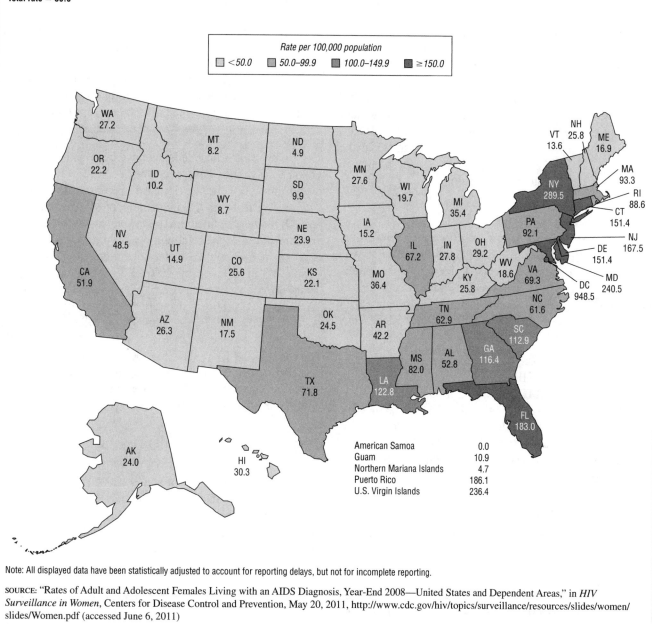

Rates of females living with diagnosed AIDS, 2008

[United States and dependent areas. Population = 115,781.]

Total rate = 89.0

Rate per 100,000 population

☐ <50.0   ☐ 50.0–99.9   ☐ 100.0–149.9   ■ ≥150.0

American Samoa	0.0
Guam	10.9
Northern Mariana Islands	4.7
Puerto Rico	186.1
U.S. Virgin Islands	236.4

Note: All displayed data have been statistically adjusted to account for reporting delays, but not for incomplete reporting.

SOURCE: "Rates of Adult and Adolescent Females Living with an AIDS Diagnosis, Year-End 2008—United States and Dependent Areas," in *HIV Surveillance in Women*, Centers for Disease Control and Prevention, May 20, 2011, http://www.cdc.gov/hiv/topics/surveillance/resources/slides/women/slides/Women.pdf (accessed June 6, 2011)

HIV/AIDS in Women in Small Towns and Rural Areas

Most HIV/AIDS cases occur among women who live in large metropolitan areas with populations of greater than 500,000. However, the number of HIV/AIDS cases is increasing in rural areas, especially through heterosexual transmission. Figure 4.2 reveals that at the end of 2008 the highest rates of women living with AIDS were reported in the District of Columbia (948.5 cases per 100,000 population), New York (289.5), Maryland (240.5), the U.S. Virgin Islands (236.4), Puerto Rico (186.1), and Florida (183). In contrast, the lowest rates were reported by states in the Midwest. Because many women live in states that do not have HIV/AIDS surveillance, it is likely that there are many who have not been tested. As a result, the numbers of women with HIV/AIDS may be underestimated.

Sexually Transmitted Diseases

Preventing, identifying, and promptly treating STDs is vitally important for the health of young women. Most HIV in women is spread through heterosexual sex (see Table 4.3), and the increase in STDs parallels that of HIV/AIDS.

In "The Role of STD Detection and Treatment in HIV Prevention—CDC Fact Sheet" (September 1, 2010, http://www.cdc.gov/std/Hiv/STDFact-STD-HIV.htm), the CDC explains that women with STDs are "at least two to five times more likely than uninfected [women] to acquire HIV infection if they are exposed to the virus through sexual contact" because they have an increased number of HIV target cells (CD4+ T cells) present in their cervical secretions. These cells facilitate the entrance of HIV into the body. Furthermore, women with STDs are more likely to shed HIV in both ulcer-forming and inflammatory genital secretions. They are also more likely to shed HIV in greater amounts than people infected with HIV alone, which contributes to the spread of HIV. By treating an STD, the shedding of HIV on sexual contact is lessened, which in turn reduces the spread of HIV infection.

MSM SEXUAL CONTACT

MSM is still the major risk category for HIV infection, although the increase in the number of cases has slowed steadily over the past few years. Epidemiologists (public health researchers who analyze the extent and types of illnesses in a population and the factors that influence their distribution) believe that HIV/AIDS among MSM may have peaked in 1992.

As in previous years, in 2009 MSM contact accounted for more than half of HIV exposure and transmission for males with or without IDU (16,120, or 59%, of the 27,153 cases). (See Table 3.6 in Chapter 3.) In 2009, 72% of white males, 58% of Hispanic males, and 50% of African-American males were infected with HIV via MSM contact, with or without IDU. MSM was also the leading mode of HIV exposure for all these groups.

PRISONERS AND AIDS

According to Laura M. Maruschak of the Bureau of Justice Statistics, in *HIV in Prisons, 2007–08* (December 2009, http://bjs.ojp.usdoj.gov/content/pub/pdf/hivp08.pdf), the number of HIV-positive state and federal prisoners has declined each year since 1999, when there were 25,807 infected prisoners. Between 2006 and 2008 the number of HIV-positive inmates in state and federal prisons fell from 21,985 to 21,462. However, confirmed AIDS cases as a percent of the total custody population remained constant at 1.5% for males and 1.8% for females at year-end 2008. (See Table 4.6.) Furthermore, the rate of HIV/AIDS cases in state and federal prisoners (0.41%) continued to be over two times higher than the case rate in the total U.S. population (0.17% of the general U.S. population) at year-end 2007. (See Table 4.7.)

Every year since statistics have been gathered, AIDS-related conditions have been the second-leading cause of death for state prison inmates, behind "illness/natural causes." However, the proportion of deaths attributable to AIDS has declined markedly since 1995. Maruschak notes that out of the total number of inmate deaths in state prisons in 1995, 34.2% of the total were from AIDS. (See Table 4.8.) However, by 2007, 3.5% of inmate deaths in state prisons were from AIDS. This remarkable decline in AIDS-related deaths is also reflected by the statistics in the rate of deaths per 100,000 inmates. In 1995 the death rate in state prisons due to AIDS was 100 per 100,000 inmates. (See Table 4.9.) By 2007 the rate had decreased to 9 per 100,000 inmates. This sharp drop is likely attributable to effective treatment with protease inhibitors and combination antiretroviral therapies.

An examination of inmate death figures in federal prisons in 2007 and 2008 reveals relatively low, stable death rates attributable to AIDS. Of the total number of inmate deaths in federal prisons in 2007 (368), 313 (85%) were from natural causes other than AIDS and 10 (3%) were from AIDS. In 2008, 345 (86%) out of a total of 399 deaths were from natural causes other than AIDS, and just 13 (3%) were from AIDS.

TABLE 4.6

HIV/AIDS cases among prison inmates, by gender, 2007 and 2008

	Male HIV/AIDS cases				Female HIV/AIDS cases			
	2007		2008		2007		2008	
	Number	Percent	Number	Percent	Number	Percent	Number	Percent
U.S. total								
Comparable reporting[a]	19,534	:	19,604	:	2,110	:	1,871	:
Reported[b]	19,534	1.5%	20,075	1.5%	2,110	2.1%	1,912	1.9%
Federal[c]	1,576	0.9	1,460	0.8	103	0.9	78	0.7
State	17,958	1.6	18,615	1.5	2,007	2.3	1,834	2.0

:Not calculated.
[a]Excludes data from Illinois and Oregon for both years due to incomplete reporting.
[b]Excludes inmates in jurisdictions that did not report HIV/AIDS infection by gender.
[c]Counts for 2008 may not be comparable to previous year counts due to implementation of a new record-keeping system.

SOURCE: Laura M. Maruschak, "Table 2. Inmates in Custody of State and Federal Prison Authorities Reported to Be HIV Positive or to Have Confirmed AIDS, by Gender, Yearend 2007 and 2008," in *HIV in Prisons, 2007–08*, Bureau of Justice Statistics, January 28, 2010, http://bjs.ojp.usdoj.gov/content/pub/pdf/hivp08.pdf (accessed June 6, 2011)

Geographic Differences

Maruschak indicates that 21,987 U.S. inmates were confirmed as infected with HIV or diagnosed with AIDS in 2008. (See Table 4.10.) This represented 1.5% of the custody population at that time—a slight decrease from the 1.7% of inmates known to be HIV infected in 2006. This modest decrease has not been geographically uniform, however. In 2008 New York held nearly a fifth (3,500, or 5.8%) of all inmates known to be HIV positive or diagnosed with AIDS. The majority of prisoners with

HIV/AIDS were held in four states in 2008: New York, Florida (3,626, or 3.6%), Texas (2,450, or 1.5%), and California (1,402, or 0.8%) of all HIV-positive inmates.

Sex, Racial, and Age Differences

In 2008, 21,987 U.S. inmates were reported as infected with HIV or had confirmed cases of AIDS, which was a slight increase from the previous year's estimate of 21,644 HIV/AIDS cases. (See Table 4.10.) However, the numbers of AIDS-related deaths in state prison decreased slightly—from 176 in 2005, to 155 in 2006, to 120 in 2007. (See Table 4.11.)

Male inmates make up the overwhelming majority of HIV-infected or confirmed cases of AIDS among inmates in state and federal prisons. In 2008 an estimated 20,075 male inmates were known to be HIV positive or diagnosed with AIDS, compared to 1,912 female inmates. (See Table 4.12.) However, as a percent of the U.S. inmate population, a higher percentage of female inmates were reported with HIV/AIDS (1.9% compared to 1.5% of male inmates).

The AIDS-related deaths in state prisons occurred largely among males, who accounted for 93% (112) of such deaths in 2007. (See Table 4.11.) The majority of these deaths (78, or 65%) were among African-American inmates. Female inmates accounted for 8 (7%) of the AIDS-related deaths, and one death was of an inmate who was aged 20 to 24 years.

Even though nearly twice as many AIDS-related deaths occurred in state prisons (9 per 100,000 people), compared to AIDS-related deaths in the U.S. general population (6 per 100,000 people) in 2007, the gap has narrowed considerably since 1995, when more than three times as many inmate deaths (100 per 100,000 people)

TABLE 4.7

Percentage of AIDS cases in the general population and among state and federal prisoners, 1999–2008

Yearend	Percent of population estimated to have confirmed AIDS		Ratio of AIDS cases in prisons to cases in U.S. general population[b]
	State and federal prisoners	U.S. general population[a]	
1999	0.58%	0.12%	4.8
2000	0.51	0.13	3.9
2001	0.50	0.14	3.6
2002	0.45	0.14	3.2
2003	0.47	0.15	3.1
2004	0.46	0.15	3.1
2005	0.43	0.16	2.7
2006	0.46	0.17	2.7
2007	0.41	0.17	2.4
2008	0.39	—	—

— = Not available.

[a]Based on persons age 13 or older in 1999 and persons age 15 or older thereafter. Excludes confirmed AIDS cases reported in state and federal prisons.

[b]Calculation based on percent of AIDS cases in state prisons divided by percent in U.S. general population.

SOURCE: Laura M. Maruschak, "Table 4. Percent with Confirmed AIDS among State and Federal Prisoners and the U.S. General Population, 1999–2008," in *HIV in Prisons, 2007–08*, Bureau of Justice Statistics, January 28, 2010, http://bjs.ojp.usdoj.gov/content/pub/pdf/hivp08.pdf (accessed June 6, 2011)

TABLE 4.8

Percentage of AIDS-related deaths among all deaths in state prisons and the U.S. general population, selected years 1995–2007

Year	Percent of deaths		Ratio of state prison deaths to deaths in U.S. general population[d]
	State prisons[a, b]	U.S. general population ages 15 to 54[c]	
1995	34.2%	12.9%	2.6
2001	10.3	4.3	2.4
2002	9.1	4.1	2.2
2003	8.0	4.2	1.9
2004	5.6	4.3	1.3
2005	5.3	3.8	1.4
2006	4.6	3.4	1.4
2007	3.5	—	:

— = Not available.

: = Not calculated.

[a]Percentages were based on the number of inmate deaths, excluding those in jurisdictions not reporting AIDS-related deaths.

[b]For 2007, the number of AIDS-related deaths used to calculate the percent was based on individual reports submitted to the Deaths in Custody Reporting Program (DCRP). For 2001–2006 AIDS-related deaths were based on a combination of National Prisoner Statistics (NPS-1) data. For 1995, AIDS-related deaths were based on data submitted in the NPS-1.

[c]Excludes deaths reported in state prisons.

[d]Calculation based on percent of state prison deaths divided by percent deaths in the U.S. general population ages 15 to 54.

SOURCE: Laura M. Maruschak, "Table 6. Percent of AIDS-Related Deaths among All Deaths in State Prison and the U.S. General Population," in *HIV in Prisons, 2007–08*, Bureau of Justice Statistics, January 28, 2010, http://bjs.ojp.usdoj.gov/content/pub/pdf/hivp08.pdf (accessed June 6, 2011)

TABLE 4.9

Ratio of AIDS-related deaths in state prisons and the U.S. general population, selected years 1995–2007

Year	Rate per 100,000 persons		Ratio of deaths in state prisons to deaths in U.S. general population[c]
	State prisons[a]	U.S. general population ages 15 to 54[b]	
1995	100	29	3.5
2001	25	9	2.9
2002	22	9	2.6
2003	21	9	2.4
2004	14	9	1.7
2005	13	8	1.7
2006	11	6	1.8
2007	9	6	1.5

[a]For 2007, the number of AIDS-related deaths used to calculate the rate was based on individual reports submitted to the Deaths in Custody Reporting Program (DCRP). For 2001–2006 AIDS-related deaths were based on a combination of National Prisoner Statistics (NPS-1) data. For 1995, AIDS-related deaths were based on data submitted in the NPS-1.
[b]Excludes deaths reported in state prisons.
[c]Calculation based on rate of deaths in state prisons divided by rate in the U.S. general population, ages 15 to 54.

SOURCE: Laura M. Maruschak, "Table 7. Ratio of AIDS-Related Deaths in State Prisons and the U.S. General Population," in *HIV in Prisons, 2007–08*, Bureau of Justice Statistics, January 28, 2010, http://bjs.ojp.usdoj.gov/content/pub/pdf/hivp08.pdf (accessed June 6, 2011)

than deaths in the general population (29 per 100,000) were attributable to AIDS. (See Table 4.9.)

Drug and Needle Use among Prisoners

Public education campaigns about the "safer" use of drugs and syringes appear to be reducing HIV infection in the general public. However, these measures seem to be having no effect in prisons. Many incarcerated IDUs continue to inject while in prison, often sharing needles because injection equipment is in short supply. Indeed, Ralf Jürgens, Andrew Ball, and Annette Verster note in "Interventions to Reduce HIV Transmission Related to Injecting Drug Use in Prison" (*Lancet Infectious Diseases*, vol. 9, no. 1, January 2009) that most incarcerated IDUs report borrowing syringes while in prison, which makes prisons a high-risk environment for the transmission of HIV.

This is a dilemma for prisons, where syringes and needles are prohibited, as are illegal drugs, and chemicals for disinfecting the illicit needles are not readily available to prisoners. Even though state and federal prison officials in the United States want to stop the spread of HIV among inmates, most cannot keep pace with or stem the flow of illegal drugs into prisons. To minimize the spread of HIV in prisons, countries such as Switzerland and the United Kingdom provide prisoners with disinfectant or clean needles. U.S. officials believe these actions endorse illegal drug use. Instead, they focus on providing treatment and rehabilitation programs for drug-addicted prisoners.

Nonetheless, Jürgens, Ball, and Verster observe that prison systems can and should do more to prevent HIV transmission related to IDU. They assert that needle and syringe programs and drug substitution therapy, such as methadone maintenance (the use of methadone as treatment for a person who is addicted to heroin), sharply reduce the sharing of injecting equipment and the spread of HIV and other bloodborne pathogens.

U.S. Prison Systems Take Action to Prevent HIV Infection

In "Sex, Drugs, Prisons, and HIV" (*New England Journal of Medicine*, vol. 356, no. 2, January 11, 2007), Susan Okie states that the Rhode Island prison system's HIV testing practices are highly regarded by U.S. public health experts and are considered to be among the best in the country. Nonetheless, Okie observes that even the Rhode Island program fails to meet international guidelines for reducing the risk of HIV in prisons. The World Health Organization and the Joint United Nations Program on HIV/AIDS recommend that prisoners have access to bleach to clean injecting equipment and that drug treatment, methadone maintenance, and needle exchange programs be offered to inmates. Okie notes that in 2007 condoms were provided on a limited basis in just two state prison systems (Vermont and Mississippi) and five county jail systems (New York, Philadelphia, San Francisco, Los Angeles, and the District of Columbia). Mary Sylla of the Policy and Advocacy for the Center for Health Justice explains in "HIV Treatment in U.S. Jails and Prisons" (*The Body*, Winter 2008) that as of 2008 there were just a few methadone maintenance programs and no U.S. prison had even tested the feasibility of a needle exchange program.

Table 4.13 shows the various circumstances under which inmates received HIV testing in federal and state jurisdictions in 2008. Even though nearly all state jurisdictions reported testing when requested by the inmate or court order or when there was a clinical indication or accident, only a few routinely tested inmates who were considered at high risk for infection, and just six (Missouri, Alabama, Arkansas, Florida, Texas, and Nevada) tested inmates before their release.

In 2009 the Georgia state senate passed a bill requiring that inmates receive HIV testing before their release from state prison. The state already required HIV testing before inmates enter the prison system. According to the

TABLE 4.10

Inmates with HIV/AIDS by jurisdiction, 2006–08

Jurisdiction	Total HIV/AIDS cases[a]			HIV/AIDS cases as a percent of custody population		
	2006	2007	2008	2006	2007	2008
U.S. total						
Comparable reporting[b]	21,985	21,615	21,462	:	:	:
Reported[c]	21,985	21,644	21,987	1.7%	1.5%	1.5%
Federal[d]	1,530	1,679	1,538	0.9	0.9	0.8
State	20,455	19,965	20,449	1.8	1.6	1.6
Northeast	**6,099**	**5,940**	**5,484**	**3.6%**	**3.4%**	**3.2%**
Connecticut	423	415	380	2.2	2.1	2.0
Maine	13	10	9	0.6	0.5	0.4
Massachusetts	268	219	264	2.5	2.0	2.4
New Hampshire	16	18	16	0.6	0.7	0.6
New Jersey	612	550	520	2.7	2.2	2.1
New York	4,000	3,950	3,500	6.3	6.3	5.8
Pennsylvania	697	689	727	1.6	1.5	1.6
Rhode Island	58	67	54	1.6	1.8	1.4
Vermont	12	22	14	0.7	1.0	0.7
Midwest	**1,574**	**1,337**	**1,814**	**0.9%**	**0.7%**	**0.8%**
Illinois	/	/	457	/	/	1.0
Indiana	/	/	/	/	/	/
Iowa	42	56	41	0.5	0.6	0.5
Kansas	61	22	46	0.7	0.3	0.5
Michigan	490	359	341	1.0	0.7	0.7
Minnesota	47	45	44	0.6	0.5	0.5
Missouri	301	292	304	1.0	1.0	1.0
Nebraska	17	14	16	0.4	0.3	0.4
North Dakota	3	4	6	0.2	0.3	0.4
Ohio	447	377	414	1.0	0.8	0.8
South Dakota	14	14	13	0.4	0.4	0.4
Wisconsin	152	154	132	0.7	0.7	0.6
South	**10,953**	**10,784**	**11,003**	**2.1%**	**1.9%**	**1.9%**
Alabama	297	292	275	1.2	1.2	1.1
Arkansas	101	121	118	0.8	0.9	0.9
Delaware	108	119	132	1.5	1.7	1.9
Florida	3,412	3,460	3,626	4.1	3.6	3.6
Georgia	944	970	961	1.8	1.8	1.8
Kentucky	104	103	131	0.8	0.8	0.9
Louisiana	525	512	458	2.5	2.5	2.2
Maryland	612	636	588	2.7	2.7	2.5
Mississippi	279	246	246	2.4	1.4	1.4
North Carolina	688	722	824	1.8	1.9	2.1
Oklahoma	163	148	139	0.9	0.6	0.6
South Carolina	454	438	409	2.0	1.9	1.7
Tennessee	190	187	188	1.3	1.0	1.0
Texas	2,693	2,458	2,450	1.9	1.6	1.5
Virginia	368	358	433	1.3	1.1	1.3
West Virginia	15	14	25	0.3	0.3	0.5
West	**1,829**	**1,904**	**2,148**	**0.7%**	**0.6%**	**0.7%**
Alaska	/	29	13	/	0.6	0.3
Arizona	169	178	179	0.6	0.5	0.5
California	1,155	1,156	1,402	0.7	0.7	0.8
Colorado	165	150	173	1.0	0.7	0.7
Hawaii	15	26	23	0.4	0.5	0.4
Idaho	22	24	28	0.5	0.3	0.4
Montana	6	4	6	0.3	0.1	0.2
Nevada	126	165	116	1.0	1.2	0.9
New Mexico	36	38	33	0.5	0.6	0.5

article "Senate Passes Bill Requiring HIV Testing in Prisons" (Georgia Public Broadcasting News, March 10, 2009), Senator Kasim Reed (1969–), a Democrat, asserted that informing inmates of their HIV status when they are released will help protect the communities to which they are released. Reed opined that "the data suggests that when people know their status, they change their behavior." Senator John F. Douglas (1953–), a Republican, questioned the veracity of this statement, observing that "once these people are released from prison, . . . there is nothing to force them to tell their partner that they have HIV."

In 2011 the Virginia General Assembly passed legislation that requires prison inmates to be offered HIV testing within 60 days of their release from a correctional facility. According to Sabrina Barekzai, in "Prisons to Offer Inmates HIV Testing" (*Virginia Gazette* [Williamsburg,

TABLE 4.10

Inmates with HIV/AIDS by jurisdiction, 2006–08 [CONTINUED]

Jurisdiction	Total HIV/AIDS cases[a]			HIV/AIDS cases as a percent of custody population		
	2006	2007	2008	2006	2007	2008
Oregon[e]	/	/	55	/	/	0.4
Utah	44	33	36	0.9	0.6	0.7
Washington	84	93	79	0.5	0.5	0.4
Wyoming	7	8	5	0.6	0.4	0.3

/ = Not reported.
: = Not calculated.
HIV = Human immunodeficiency virus.
[a]Counts published in previous reports may have been revised.
[b]Excludes data from Illinois, Indiana, Alaska, and Oregon for all 3 years due to incomplete reporting.
[c]Excludes inmates in jurisdictions that did not report data.
[d]Counts for 2008 may not be comparable to previous year counts due to the implementation of a new record-keeping system.
[e]The number of HIV/AIDS cases in Oregon was based on a 3/9/09 count.

SOURCE: Laura M. Maruschak, "Appendix Table 1. Inmates in Custody of State or Federal Prison Authorities and Reported to Be HIV Positive or to Have Confirmed AIDS, by Jurisdiction 2006–2008," in *HIV in Prisons, 2007–08*, Bureau of Justice Statistics, January 28, 2010, http://bjs.ojp.usdoj.gov/content/pub/pdf/hivp08.pdf (accessed June 6, 2011)

TABLE 4.11

Inmate deaths in state prisons by age and race/ethnicity, 2005–07

Characteristic	Number of AIDS-related deaths[a]			Rate of AIDS-related deaths per 100,000 inmates[b]		
	2005	2006	2007	2005	2006	2007
State total	176	155	120	13	11	9
Gender						
Male	166	148	112	14	12	9
Female	10	7	8	12	8	8
Age						
19 or younger	0	1	0	0	5	0
20–24	0	2	1	0	1	0
25–34	25	18	13	6	4	3
35–44	82	62	43	21	16	11
45–54	55	58	45	31	32	24
55 or older	14	14	18	22	22	27
Race/Hispanic origin						
White[c]	33	29	28	8	6	5
Black[c]	120	114	78	24	21	14
Hispanic	21	12	14	9	5	7

[a]For 2005 and 2006, estimates of the number of AIDS-related deaths by gender, age, and race/Hispanic origin were made by applying the percentages based on Deaths in Custody Reporting Program (DCRP) data to the estimated total number of AIDS-related deaths. For 2007, the number of AIDS-related deaths by gender, age, and race/Hispanic origin were based on DCRP data.
[b]To calculate the age rates, the number of state prisoners by age was first estimated by applying the age distribution reported in the 2004 Survey of Inmates in State Correctional Facilities to the 2005–2007 midyear custody counts in NPS-1.
[c]Excludes persons of Hispanic or Latino origin.

SOURCE: Laura M. Maruschak, "Table 5. Profile of Inmates Who Died from AIDS-Related Causes in State Prisons, 2005–2007," in *HIV in Prisons, 2007–08*, Bureau of Justice Statistics, January 28, 2010, http://bjs.ojp.usdoj.gov/content/pub/pdf/hivp08.pdf (accessed June 6, 2011)

Virginia], March 21, 2011), this initiative will test about 8,000 prisoners per year at a cost of approximately $33,000.

HEMOPHILIACS

Hemophilia is a group of genetic disorders in which defects in a number of genes located on the X chromosome disrupt the proper clotting of blood. The most common type of hemophilia—hemophilia A—is a deficiency of a clotting substance designated Factor VIII. Varying severities of hemophilia can occur, depending on the level of Factor VIII present in the patient's plasma. Treatment of hemophilia involves close attention to injury prevention and periodic intravenous administration of Factor VIII concentrates, commonly known as clotting factors.

Because screening for HIV antibodies was not available until 1985, many hemophiliacs were exposed to HIV-contaminated blood and clotting factors before widespread use of screening procedures. The national distribution of clotting factor concentrates before 1985 led to a high prevalence of HIV infections among hemophiliacs.

TABLE 4.12

Inmates with HIV/AIDS by sex and jurisdiction, 2007–08

	Male HIV/AIDS cases				Female HIV/AIDS cases			
	2007		2008		2007		2008	
Jurisdiction	Number	Percent	Number	Percent	Number	Percent	Number	Percent
U.S. total								
Comparable reporting[a]	19,534	:	19,604	:	2,110	:	1,871	:
Reported[b]	19,534	1.5%	20,075	1.5%	2,110	2.1%	1,912	1.9%
Federal[c]	1,576	0.9	1,460	0.8	103	0.9	78	0.7
State	17,958	1.6	18,615	1.5	2,007	2.3	1,834	2.0
Northeast	**5,383**	**3.3%**	**4,988**	**3.1%**	**557**	**6.0%**	**496**	**5.3%**
Connecticut	365	2.0	328	1.9	50	3.9	52	4.1
Maine	10	0.5	8	0.4	0	0	1	0.7
Massachusetts	202	2.0	242	2.3	17	2.1	22	2.9
New Hampshire	18	0.7	16	0.6	0	0	0	0
New Jersey	487	2.0	468	2.0	63	4.7	52	4.2
New York	3,600	6.0	3,200	5.6	350	12.7	300	11.6
Pennsylvania	624	1.4	664	1.6	65	2.7	63	2.3
Rhode Island	59	1.7	48	1.4	8	3.6	6	3.1
Vermont	18	0.9	14	0.7	4	2.5	0	0
Midwest	**1,251**	**0.7%**	**1,688**	**0.8%**	**86**	**0.7%**	**126**	**0.8%**
Illinois	/	/	419	1.0	/	/	38	1.4
Indiana	/	/	/	/	/	/	/	/
Iowa	50	0.6	37	0.5	6	0.8	4	0.5
Kansas	19	0.2	39	0.5	3	0.5	7	1.2
Michigan	344	0.7	326	0.7	15	0.7	15	0.8
Minnesota	42	0.5	41	0.5	3	0.5	3	0.5
Missouri	272	1.0	289	1.0	20	0.8	15	0.6
Nebraska	13	0.3	16	0.4	1	0.3	0	0
North Dakota	3	0.2	6	0.5	1	0.7	0	0
Ohio	351	0.8	385	0.8	26	0.7	29	0.8
South Dakota	11	0.4	12	0.4	3	0.8	1	0.3
Wisconsin	146	0.7	118	0.6	8	0.5	14	1.0
South	**9,589**	**1.8%**	**9,991**	**1.9%**	**1,195**	**2.9%**	**1,012**	**2.4%**
Alabama	275	1.2	260	1.1	17	1.1	15	1.0
Arkansas	110	0.9	106	0.9	11	1.1	12	1.2
Delaware	108	1.6	108	1.7	11	2.0	24	4.5
Florida	3,059	3.5	3,292	3.5	401	6.0	334	4.8
Georgia	882	1.7	871	1.8	88	2.5	90	2.4
Kentucky	94	0.8	118	0.9	9	1.1	13	0.9
Louisiana	475	2.5	406	2.1	37	3.2	52	4.5
Maryland	518	2.4	544	2.5	118	10.1	44	4.2
Mississippi	158	1.0	212	1.3	88	5.0	34	2.0
North Carolina	664	1.9	771	2.1	58	2.1	53	1.9
Oklahoma	134	0.6	129	0.6	14	0.6	10	0.4
South Carolina	400	1.8	380	1.7	38	2.4	29	1.8
Tennessee	178	1.0	172	0.9	9	0.8	16	1.4
Texas	2,199	1.5	2,201	1.5	259	2.1	249	2.0
Virginia	322	1.1	398	1.3	36	1.5	35	1.5
West Virginia	13	0.3	23	0.5	1	0.2	2	0.4

The prevalence of HIV infection differs by the type and severity of the coagulation (clotting) disorder.

According to the National Hemophilia Foundation (NHF), in "NHF—Guardian of the Nation's Blood Supply" (2006, http://www.hemophilia.org/blood_safety/index .htm), during the early 1980s about half of all people with hemophilia became infected with HIV through blood products. Many of these people developed AIDS. Even though precise statistics are unavailable, many health officials— such as those cited in *FDA Workshop on Behavior-Based Donor Deferrals in the NAT Era* (March 8, 2006, http:// www.fda.gov/downloads/BiologicsBloodVaccines/News-Events/WorkshopsMeetingsConferences/TranscriptsMinutes/ UCM054430.pdf)—believe that 70% to 90% of the approximately 17,000 Americans with hemophilia A are HIV positive. The 8,000 or so Americans with the less clinically severe hemophilia B most likely have a lower prevalence rate because they required fewer treatments with the clotting factor and, therefore, were less exposed to HIV-contaminated products. According to the CDC, hemophilia A rates may be overrepresented because the studies were performed at hemophilia treatment centers where the more severe hemophilia A cases are likely to be found.

In "Prognostic Factors for All-Cause Mortality among Hemophiliacs Infected with Human Immunodeficiency Virus" (*American Journal of Epidemiology*, vol. 142, no. 3, August 1, 1995), Laura S. Diamondstone et al. note that before the 1980s most hemophiliacs died from intracranial hemorrhage (bleeding within the brain). However, by 1995 one-third of all deaths were related to HIV infection and

TABLE 4.12

Inmates with HIV/AIDS by sex and jurisdiction, 2007–08 [CONTINUED]

Jurisdiction	Male HIV/AIDS cases				Female HIV/AIDS cases			
	2007		2008		2007		2008	
	Number	Percent	Number	Percent	Number	Percent	Number	Percent
West	**1,735**	**0.6%**	**1,948**	**0.7%**	**169**	**0.7%**	**200**	**0.8%**
Alaska	23	0.5	11	0.2	6	1.1	2	0.4
Arizona	164	0.5	159	0.4	14	0.4	20	0.5
California	1,076	0.7	1,308	0.8	80	0.7	94	0.8
Colorado	129	0.6	149	0.7	21	0.9	24	1.1
Hawaii	24	0.5	18	0.4	2	0.3	5	0.8
Idaho	24	0.4	23	0.4	0	0	5	0.7
Montana	4	0.2	6	0.2	0	0	0	0
Nevada	140	1.2	89	0.7	25	2.1	27	2.7
New Mexico (male-33 female-3)	38	0.6	33	0.6	0	0	0	0
Oregon	/	/	52	0.4	/	/	3	0.3
Utah	30	0.6	28	0.6	3	0.6	8	1.5
Washington	78	0.5	68	0.4	15	1.0	11	0.8
Wyoming	5	0.3	4	0.3	3	1.2	1	0.5

/ = Not reported.
: = Not calculated.
HIV = Human immunodeficiency virus.
[a]Excludes data from Illinois and Oregon for both years due to incomplete reporting.
[b]Excludes inmates in jurisdictions that did not report HIV/AIDS infection by gender.
[c]Counts for 2008 may not be comparable to previous year counts due to the implementation of a new record-keeping system.

SOURCE: Laura M. Maruschak, "Appendix Table 2. Inmates in Custody of State and Federal Prison Authorities and Reported to Be HIV Positive or to Have Confirmed AIDS, by Jurisdiction and Gender, Yearend 2007 and 2008," in *HIV in Prisons, 2007–08*, Bureau of Justice Statistics, January 28, 2010, http://bjs .ojp.usdoj.gov/content/pub/pdf/hivp08.pdf (accessed June 6, 2011)

one-fourth were related to hemorrhage. Hemophiliacs often report that virtually all their fellow hemophiliacs are infected with the virus. Many sexual partners of hemophiliacs have also contracted the virus from sexual intercourse. In the case of females, the virus can be passed to their offspring.

Thomas Tencer et al. explain in "Medical Costs and Resource Utilization for Hemophilia Patients with and without HIV or HCV Infection" (*Journal of Managed Care Pharmacy*, vol. 13, no. 9, November–December 2007) that even though the possibility of contracting HIV or the hepatitis C virus has been virtually eliminated in the United States, at the close of 2007 about one-third of hemophiliacs were believed to be HIV infected or infected with both HIV and hepatitis C. Coinfected people have been found to have higher rates of illness, death, and utilization of clotting factor.

A Slow Reaction

Concentrated clotting factor, which is derived from human blood obtained from as many as 2,000 donors, became available during the mid-1970s. Its success at stopping bleeding was so dramatic that hemophilia changed from a disease that produced intense pain, disability, and the possibility of premature death to one that allowed sufferers to lead nearly normal lives. Hemophiliacs could infuse clotting factors into their own blood if they felt bleeding was about to start. Patients were advised by their physicians to "infuse early and often."

During the late 1970s and early 1980s some clotting factor concentrates were inadvertently infected with HIV.

Even after the first cases of HIV/AIDS appeared in people with hemophilia and the CDC, along with the NHF, identified this new disease as being bloodborne, physicians did not advise their patients to alter their clotting factor treatments. Hemophiliacs were encouraged to continue using their clotting factor because researchers and physicians were not sure there would be a major epidemic.

Anecdotal comments from hemophiliacs indicate that when many of them became infected, primary care doctors were slow to respond and supplied little information. There was no warning to practice safe sex to prevent the spread of HIV. Some hemophiliacs reported receiving more information from gay men's organizations than from their own hematologists (physicians who specialize in diseases and disorders of the blood).

In "The Aging Patient with Hemophilia: Complications, Comorbidities, and Management Issues" (*Hematology*, December 2010), Claire Philipp of the University of Medicine and Dentistry of New Jersey–Robert Wood Johnson Medical School explains that even though clotting factor concentrates free of HIV contamination have been available since 1985, many older hemophiliacs are infected. However, since the advent of highly active antiretroviral therapy, the survival rate of HIV-infected hemophiliacs has improved, with 27% to 39% surviving 20 to 25 years.

ANGER AND COMPENSATION. Many hemophiliacs feel they are entitled to compensation or, at the very least, assistance in paying the overwhelming medical expenses they incur as a result of HIV infection and

TABLE 4.13

Circumstances under which inmates received HIV testing, by jurisdiction, 2008

	All inmates									
	Entering	In custody	Upon release	Random	High-risk	Inmate request	Court order	Clinical indication	Involvement in incident	Other
Federal					X	X	X	X	X	
Northeast										
Connecticut					X	X	X	X	X	
Maine						X	X	X		
Massachusetts						X			X	
New Hampshire	X						X	X		
New Jersey						X	X	X	X	
New York				X	X	X	X	X	X	
Pennsylvania						X	X	X	X	
Rhode Island	X					X	X	X	X	
Vermont						X		X	X	
Midwest										
Illinois					X	X	X	X	X	X
Indiana	X				X	X	X	X	X	
Iowa	X	X				X	X	X	X	
Kansas					X	X	X	X	X	X
Michigan	X					X	X		X	
Minnesota	X					X	X	X	X	
Missouri	X	X	X		X		X	X	X	
Nebraska	X					X	X	X	X	
North Dakota	X	X				X	X	X	X	
Ohio	X					X	X	X	X	
South Dakota						X	X	X	X	X
Wisconsin					X	X	X	X	X	
South										
Alabama	X		X	X		X	X	X	X	X
Arkansas	X		X	X	X	X	X	X	X	X
Delaware						X	X	X	X	
Florida			X			X	X	X	X	
Georgia	X					X	X		X	
Kentucky					X			X	X	
Louisiana						X		X	X	
Maryland					X	X	X	X	X	X
Mississippi	X				X	X	X	X	X	
North Carolina						X	X	X		X
Oklahoma	X					X	X	X	X	X
South Carolina	X					X	X	X	X	X
Tennessee					X	X	X	X	X	
Texas	X		X		X	X	X	X	X	
Virginia						X	X	X	X	X
West Virginia						X				
West										
Alaska					X	X		X	X	
Arizona					X	X	X	X		
California						X	X	X	X	
Colorado	X					X	X	X	X	
Hawaii						X		X	X	
Idaho	X	X			X	X	X	X	X	
Montana						X	X	X	X	
Nevada	X	X	X			X	X	X	X	
New Mexico						X		X		
Oregon						X	X			
Utah	X				X			X	X	
Washington	X				X	X	X	X	X	
Wyoming	X					X		X		

HIV = Human immunodeficiency virus.

SOURCE: Laura M. Maruschak, "Appendix Table 5. Circumstances under Which Inmates Were Tested for the Antibody to HIV, by Jurisdiction, 2008," in *HIV in Prisons, 2007–08*, Bureau of Justice Statistics, January 28, 2010, http://bjs.ojp.usdoj.gov/content/pub/pdf/hivp08.pdf (accessed June 6, 2011)

AIDS treatment. They maintain that the companies that produced the clotting factors were slow to warn the public about HIV and slow to use heat treatment to eliminate the live virus from the clotting factors (although this procedure has not gained widespread acceptance among scientists as an adequate method to inactivate HIV).

Hemophilia foundations in some countries have convinced government pharmaceutical or insurance companies to compensate HIV-infected hemophiliacs. Peter D. Weinberg et al. report in "Legal, Financial, and Public Health Consequences of HIV Contamination of Blood and Blood Products in the 1980s and 1990s" (*Annals of Internal*

Medicine, vol. 136, no. 4, February 19, 2002) that Armour Pharmaceuticals agreed to pay six Canadians $1.5 million each; Germany offered people infected with HIV and those who became ill with AIDS annual compensation; and Switzerland extended annual compensation of $12,216 to people with AIDS. France gave one-time compensation of $87,735 to hemophiliacs at the time they were diagnosed with AIDS due to tainted blood products. During the first decade of the 21st century, more than 20 developed countries had acted to compensate HIV-infected hemophiliacs. In contrast, developing countries continued to grapple with blood-supply safety issues.

In 1995 the U.S. Supreme Court refused to hear a class action suit brought by hemophiliacs against a pharmaceutical company and other blood-product manufacturers (*Barton v. American Red Cross*, 826 F. Supp. 412 and 826 F. Supp. 407, append 43 F. 3rd 678, certiorari denied 116 S. Ct. 84). Regardless, some companies have reached out-of-court settlements with affected people. For example, according to the article "4 Drug Companies Ordered to Pay Hemophiliacs" (*New York Times*, May 8, 1997), in 1997 four manufacturers of blood clotting products were ordered by a federal judge to pay approximately $670 million to settle cases on behalf of more than 6,000 hemophiliacs who were infected in the United States during the early 1980s. The settlement compensated each infected hemophiliac with an estimated $100,000 payment.

The NHF explains in "Ricky Ray Program Office Set to Close" (2005, http://www.hemophilia.org/NHFWeb/MainPgs/MainNHF.aspx?menuid=117&contentid=360) that the international catastrophe of HIV/AIDS in the hemophilia community was recognized by the U.S. federal government in 1998 with passage of the Ricky Ray Hemophilia Relief Fund Act, named for a Florida boy with hemophilia who died from HIV/AIDS. According to the NHF, the act provided "payments of $100,000 to individuals with hemophilia who were treated with HIV-contaminated clotting factor products between July 1, 1982, and December 31, 1987. Spouses and children who contracted HIV from these individuals, as well as specified family survivors were also eligible for compassionate payment." When the program closed in October 2005, it had paid over $559 million to more than 7,171 eligible individuals and survivors.

CHAPTER 5

CHILDREN, ADOLESCENTS, AND HIV/AIDS

HIV/AIDS IN CHILDREN: DIFFERENT FROM HIV/AIDS IN ADULTS

HIV causes AIDS in both adults and children. The virus attacks and damages the immune and central nervous systems of all infected people. However, the development and course of the disease in children differs considerably from its progression in adults.

Before the use of highly active antiretroviral therapy (HAART) and early intervention strategies, there were two patterns of HIV progression among children. The first pattern, which is called severe immunodeficiency, is apparent as recurring serious infections or encephalopathy (any of various diseases of the brain). The National Institute of Allergy and Infectious Diseases (NIAID) reports in the fact sheet "HIV Infection in Infants and Children" (September 10, 2008, http://www.niaid.nih.gov/topics/HIVAIDS/ Understanding/Population%20Specific%20Information/ Pages/children.aspx) that severe immunodeficiency develops in 20% of infected infants during their first year of life. The second pattern of HIV progression, which occurs in the other 80% of infected children, is more gradual and is similar to the development and progression of the disease that is observed in adults.

HIV nucleic acid detection tests can detect the presence of HIV in nearly all infants aged one month and older. Before the development of these tests, detecting HIV infection, especially in babies, was difficult. This is because the earlier tests involved the detection of antibodies formed by the infant in response to HIV. However, infants have often not developed the full capacity to produce antibodies at the time of testing. Furthermore, HIV-infected mothers may transmit antibodies alone, without the virus, to their babies. In the latter instance, infants with positive results from antibody tests at birth may later test negative, indicating that the mother transmitted the HIV antibodies to the baby, but not the virus itself.

In adults, symptoms of fully developed AIDS include the presence of opportunistic infections (OIs) that may or may not be accompanied by rare forms of several types of cancers. The OIs or the cancers can ultimately prove to be the cause of death. The most common diseases associated with AIDS in adults are *Pneumocystis carinii* pneumonia (PCP) and Kaposi's sarcoma. The latter is a normally rare skin carcinoma that can spread to internal organs. Many adult AIDS patients have one or both of these conditions. Other disorders found in adult AIDS patients are lymphomas (lymph gland cancers), prolonged diarrhea causing severe dehydration, weight loss, and central nervous system infections that can lead to dementia.

Among infants and children, the disease is characterized by wasting syndrome, the failure to thrive, and unusually severe bacterial infections. Except for PCP, children with symptomatic HIV infection rarely develop the same OIs that adults contract. Though adults and children with HIV may both suffer from chronic or recurrent diarrhea, its dehydrating effect may be particularly debilitating and life-threatening to children. Instead of other symptoms that are common to adults, children are plagued with recurrent bacterial infections such as severe forms of conjunctivitis (pink eye), ear infections, tonsillitis, and persistent or recurrent oral thrush (an infection of the mouth or throat that is caused by the fungus *Candida albicans*). Children may also suffer from enlarged lymph nodes, chronic pneumonia, developmental delays, and neurological abnormalities. Put simply, the immune system of HIV-infected children is destroyed even as it matures.

Whether HIV positive or not, babies born to HIV-infected mothers appear to be predisposed to a variety of heart problems. In the landmark study "Cardiovascular Status of Infants and Children of Women Infected with HIV-1 (P2C2 HIV): A Cohort Study" (*Lancet*, vol. 360, no. 9330, August 3, 2002), Steven E. Lipshultz et al.

examined more than 500 infants born to HIV-positive women. They discovered that the babies suffered from significantly higher rates of abnormalities, such as defects in the heart wall and valve and reduced pumping action. These defects occurred in less than 1% of healthy children whose mothers were not infected with HIV. Lipshultz et al. recognize that HIV alone did not necessarily cause these anomalies. They observe that a mother's alcohol, drug, or nutrition problems can also interfere with fetal heart development.

Hamisu M. Salihu et al. analyzed over 1.6 million birth records in Florida. In "Maternal HIV/AIDS Status and Neurological Outcomes in Neonates: A Population-Based Study" (*Maternal and Child Health Journal*, April 20, 2011), the researchers report that babies born to HIV-infected mothers are at higher risk of having feeding difficulties and seizures (sudden loss of consciousness).

A CASE DEFINITION FOR CHILDREN

Because data were limited during the first few years of HIV's acknowledged presence in the United States, the Centers for Disease Control and Prevention's (CDC) definition of AIDS did not differentiate between adults and children until 1987, when the classification system was revised. The CDC Division of HIV/AIDS Prevention, National Center for HIV/AIDS, Viral Hepatitis, STD, and TB Prevention updated the pediatric definition in 1994, 1999, and 2008 as more information about HIV and AIDS became available. The 2008 revision, which takes into account new testing technologies, is intended for public health surveillance purposes and not as a guide for clinical diagnosis.

Changes to the case definitions were published by Eileen Schneider et al. of the CDC in "Revised Surveillance Case Definitions for HIV Infection among Adults, Adolescents, and Children Aged <18 Months and for HIV Infection and AIDS among Children Aged 18 Months to <13 Years—United States, 2008" (*Morbidity and Mortality Weekly Report*, vol. 57, no. RR-10, December 5, 2008). No changes were made to the 27 AIDS-defining conditions listed in Table 5.1. However, the 2008 criteria stipulate that:

- Because of the greater uncertainty that is associated with diagnostic testing for HIV in this population (maternal antibodies from the HIV-infected mother might exist in the infant after birth, possibly affecting HIV diagnostic testing of the infant that occurs soon after birth), children whose illness meets clinical criteria for the AIDS case definition but does not meet laboratory criteria for definitive or presumptive HIV infection are still categorized as HIV infected when the mother has laboratory-confirmed HIV infection.

- For children aged 18 months to less than 13 years, laboratory-confirmed evidence of HIV infection is

TABLE 5.1

AIDS-defining conditions

- Bacterial infections, multiple or recurrent[a]
- Candidiasis of bronchi, trachea, or lungs
- Candidiasis of esophagus[b]
- Cervical cancer, invasive[c]
- Coccidioidomycosis, disseminated or extrapulmonary
- Cryptococcosis, extrapulmonary
- Cryptosporidiosis, chronic intestinal (>1 month's duration)
- Cytomegalovirus disease (other than liver, spleen, or nodes), onset at age >1 month
- Cytomegalovirus retinitis (with loss of vision)[b]
- Encephalopathy, HIV related
- Herpes simplex: chronic ulcers (>1 month's duration) or bronchitis, pneumonitis, or esophagitis (onset at age >1 month)
- Histoplasmosis, disseminated or extrapulmonary
- Isosporiasis, chronic intestinal (>1 month's duration)
- Kaposi sarcoma[b]
- Lymphoid interstitial pneumonia or pulmonary lymphoid hyperplasia complexa[a, b]
- Lymphoma, Burkitt (or equivalent term)
- Lymphoma, immunoblastic (or equivalent term)
- Lymphoma, primary, of brain
- *Mycobacterium avium* complex or *mycobacterium kansasii*, disseminated or extrapulmonary[b]
- *Mycobacterium tuberculosis* of any site, pulmonary,[b, c] disseminated,[b] or extrapulmonary[b]
- *Mycobacterium*, other species or unidentified species, disseminated[b] or extrapulmonary[b]
- *Pneumocystis jirovecii* pneumonia[b]
- Pneumonia, recurrent[b, c]
- Progressive multifocal leukoencephalopathy
- *Salmonella* septicemia, recurrent
- Toxoplasmosis of brain, onset at age >1 month[b]
- Wasting syndrome attributed to HIV

[a]Only among children aged <13 years.
[b]Condition that might be diagnosed presumptively.
[c]Only among adults and adolescents aged >13 years.

SOURCE: Eileen Schneider et al., "Appendix A. AIDS-Defining Conditions," in "Revised Surveillance Case Definitions for HIV Infection among Adults, Adolescents, and Children Aged <18 Months and for HIV Infection and AIDS among Children Aged 18 Months to <13 Years—United States, 2008," *Morbidity and Mortality Weekly Report*, vol. 57, no. RR-10, December 5, 2008, http://www.cdc.gov/mmwr/PDF/rr/rr5710.pdf (accessed June 6, 2011)

required to meet the surveillance case definition for HIV infection and AIDS.

- Diagnostic confirmation of an AIDS-defining condition alone, without laboratory-confirmed evidence of HIV infection, is no longer sufficient to classify a child as HIV infected for surveillance purposes.

Table 5.2 presents the criteria for HIV infection in children. These include laboratory criteria such as the results of the screening test for HIV antibodies or detection of HIV using a virologic (nonantibody) test. Diagnosis of HIV infection based on confirmed laboratory test results and documented in a medical record also meets the criteria for HIV infection. Children aged 18 months to less than 13 years are categorized for surveillance purposes as having AIDS if the criteria for HIV infection are met and at least one of the AIDS-defining conditions listed in Table 5.1 has been documented.

There are three categories of HIV-infected children: those younger than 18 months who were perinatally

TABLE 5.2

Surveillance case definitions for HIV infection in children aged 18 months to <13 years, 2008

These 2008 surveillance case definitions of HIV infection and AIDS supersede those published in 1987 and 1999 and apply to all variants of HIV (e.g., HIV-1 or HIV-2). They are intended for public health surveillance only and are not a guide for clinical diagnosis.

The 2008 laboratory criteria for reportable HIV infection among persons aged 18 months to <13 years exclude confirmation of HIV infection through the diagnosis of AIDS-defining conditions alone. Laboratory-confirmed evidence of HIV infection is now required for all reported cases of HIV infection among children aged 18 months to <13 years.

Criteria for HIV infection

Children aged 18 months to <13 years are categorized as HIV infected for surveillance purposes if at least one of laboratory criteria or the other criterion is met.

Laboratory criteria

Positive result from a screening test for HIV antibody (e.g., reactive EIA), confirmed by a positive result from a supplemental test for HIV antibody (e.g., Western blot or indirect immunofluorescence assay).

or

Positive result or a detectable quantity by any of the following HIV virologic (non-antibody) tests:—HIV nucleic acid (DNA or RNA) detection (e.g., PCR)—HIV p24 antigen test, including neutralization assay—HIV isolation (viral culture)

Other criterion (for cases that do not meet laboratory criteria)

HIV infection diagnosed by a physician or qualified medical-care provider based on the laboratory criteria and documented in a medical record. Oral reports of prior laboratory test results are not acceptable.

EIA = enzyme immunoassay. PCR = polymerase chain reaction.

SOURCE: Eileen Schneider et al., "2008 Surveillance Case Definitions for HIV Infection and AIDS among Children Aged 18 Months to <13 Years," in "Revised Surveillance Case Definitions for HIV Infection among Adults, Adolescents, and Children Aged <18 Months and for HIV Infection and AIDS among Children Aged 18 Months to <13 Years—United States, 2008," *Morbidity and Mortality Weekly Report*, vol. 57, no. RR-10, December 5, 2008, http://www.cdc.gov/mmwr/PDF/rr/rr5710.pdf (accessed June 6, 2011)

exposed (acquired the virus from their mother), children older than 18 months with perinatal infection, and infants and children of all ages who acquired the virus through other types of exposure.

Children Younger Than 18 Months

The screening and confirmatory blood tests that accurately diagnose HIV in adults are not reliable for detecting HIV in children younger than 18 months old due to the presence of passively acquired maternal antibodies. Early recognition of HIV infection in infants younger than 18 months is accomplished using polymerase chain reaction (PCR). PCR amplifies the amounts of viral genetic material to detectable levels by the direct isolation of the HIV virus using viral culture techniques or by the detection of the p24 viral antigen. According to the NIAID, in "HIV Infection in Infants and Children," these tests can identify about 33% of infected babies at birth and 95% at three months of age. Those who are HIV-antibody positive and asymptomatic (without symptoms) without immune abnormalities have an HIV-infection status that cannot be determined unless a virus culture or other antigen-detection test is positive. As with any diagnostic test, the accuracy of detection is not

absolute. The test does not detect 100% of people who are HIV positive because low levels of virus may escape detection. This possibility of a "false negative" result means that a negative culture does not necessarily rule out an infection. A small percentage of people who are infected with HIV can produce a negative result during testing.

Infants and children who are known to have been perinatally exposed (in other words, their mother is known to be HIV positive) but who lack one of the diagnostic criteria for HIV infection should be observed further for HIV-related illnesses and tested at regular intervals. The U.S. Public Health Service recommends that all infants of HIV-infected mothers be given the drug zidovudine (ZDV; previously called azidothymidine) for six weeks and that HIV-infected mothers be warned about the risks of transmission through breastfeeding. Infants with negative ZDV tests at birth should be retested periodically during the first 18 months of life. Studies suggest that ZDV therapy does not influence the accuracy of virus detection tests and consequently does not delay the diagnosis of HIV infection.

The 2008 criteria for indeterminate HIV infection stipulate that a child who is aged less than 18 months and who was born to an HIV-infected mother is categorized as having perinatal exposure with an indeterminate HIV infection status if the criteria for infected with HIV and uninfected with HIV are not met. The CDC advises monitoring children with perinatal HIV exposure for potential complications of exposure to antiretroviral medications during the perinatal period and confirming the absence of HIV infection with repeat clinical and laboratory evaluations.

Classification

The 2008 changes in diagnostic criteria did not alter the existing classification system that was developed in 1994 for HIV infection in children less than 18 months or children aged 18 months to less than 13 years old. Table 5.3 shows the three categories of HIV infection that correspond to no evidence of immunological suppression, moderate immunosuppression, and severe suppression as defined by CD4+ T-lymphocyte counts and the percent of total lymphocytes for children less than one year old, one to five years old, and six to 12 years old.

PERINATAL INFECTION

According to the CDC, in *HIV Surveillance Report: Diagnoses of HIV Infection and AIDS in the United States and Dependent Areas, 2009* (February 2011, http://www.cdc .gov/hiv/surveillance/resources/reports/2009report/pdf/2009 SurveillanceReport.pdf), the overwhelming majority (88%) of the cumulative total number of children under the age of 13 years who were reported to have HIV infection through 2008 were infected perinatally. A number of factors are

TABLE 5.3

Pediatric human immunodeficiency virus (HIV) classification

	Age of child					
	<12 mos		1–5 yrs		6–12 yrs	
Immunologic category	μL	(%)	μL	(%)	μL	(%)
1: No evidence of suppression	≥1,500	(≥25)	≥1,000	(≥25)	≥500	(≥25)
2: Evidence of moderate suppression	750–1,499	(15–24)	500–999	(15–24)	200–499	(15–24)
3: Severe suppression	<750	(<15)	<500	(<15)	<200	(<15)

μL = microliter.

SOURCE: M. Blake Caldwell et al., "Table 2. Immunologic Categories Based on Age-Specific CD4+ T-Lymphocyte Counts and Percent of Total Lymphocytes," in "1994 Revised Classification System for Human Immunodeficiency Virus Infection in Children Less Than 13 Years of Age," *Morbidity and Mortality Weekly Report*, vol. 43, no. RR-12, September 30, 1994, http://www.cdc.gov/mmwr/preview/mmwrhtml/00032890.htm (accessed June 6, 2011)

associated with an increased risk of an HIV-positive mother passing the infection to her baby. They include a low CD4+ T cell count, a high viral load (the concentration of the virus in the blood), advanced HIV progression, the presence of a particular HIV protein (p24) in serum, and placental membrane inflammation. Intrapartum (at the time of birth) events that result in increased exposure of the baby to maternal blood—breastfeeding, low vitamin A levels, premature rupture of membranes, prenatal use of illicit drugs, and premature delivery—also increase the risk of mother-to-child transmission. The risk of perinatal transmission also increases when the mother does not know she is infected until late in the course of the illness.

Despite these potential routes of transmission, the number of HIV-infected infants has been declining as a result of the more widespread use of HAART to prevent pregnant women from passing HIV infection to their offspring. Planned cesarean section delivery (C-section; the surgical delivery of a baby), the presence of neutralizing antibodies in the mother, and timely antiretroviral drug therapy (such as with ZDV) further reduce the chances of mother-to-infant HIV transmission. In *HIV Surveillance Report*, the CDC indicates that between 1994 and 2008 there was a downward trend of HIV/AIDS infants born to HIV-infected mothers in the states and U.S. dependent areas with confidential name-based HIV infection reporting. Furthermore, the CDC notes that survival was greatest among children with infection that was attributed to perinatal transmission.

Brenna L. Anderson and Susan Cu-Uvin note in "Pregnancy and Optimal Care of HIV-Infected Patients" (*Clinical Infectious Diseases*, vol. 48, no. 4, February 15, 2009) that there is evidence that planned C-section, with the administration of HAART, prevents some cases of mother-to-child HIV infection. C-section delivery does not expose the baby to potentially HIV-contaminated vaginal tissue.

ZDV

Even without a C-section, drug therapy can be beneficial. Edward M. Connor et al. discuss in "Reduction of

Maternal-Infant Transmission of Human Immunodeficiency Virus Type 1 with Zidovudine Treatment" (*New England Journal of Medicine*, vol. 331, no. 18, November 3, 1994) the results of their study, which was the first examination of perinatal transmission prevention and is considered a landmark study. Connor et al. conducted a randomized, double-blind, placebo-controlled (an inactive substance that does not contain a drug; placebos are used in comparative studies to measure the effectiveness of an experimental drug or regimen) study of antiviral prophylaxis using ZDV. At 18 months there was a 67.5% risk reduction in mother-to-child transmission. HIV transmission occurred in 25.5% of women who had received the placebo, compared to just 8.3% of those who received ZDV.

The NIAID observes in "HIV Infection in Infants and Children" that antiretroviral treatment combined with timely, appropriate prenatal care can reduce the risk of transmission to just 1.5%. In the United States the estimated numbers of perinatally acquired AIDS cases have dropped dramatically as a result of voluntary HIV testing of pregnant women, the use of antiretroviral therapy for pregnant women and newborn infants, and the treatment of HIV infections that slow progression to AIDS. (See Figure 5.1.) In 2009 perinatal exposure accounted for 131 new HIV infections and just 12 new AIDS diagnoses. (See Table 5.4.)

According to the World Health Organization (WHO), in *Children and AIDS: Second Stocktaking Report* (April 2008, http://www.unicef.org/publications/files/ChildrenAIDS_SecondStocktakingReport.pdf), global efforts to reduce the rate of mother-to-child transmission have seen the most significant gains. In 2004 only 11% of HIV-positive pregnant women were getting drugs to prevent transmission, but as of 2006, 31% were receiving treatment.

There have been comparable advances in the care of children with HIV/AIDS. In 2005 only 75,000 children were getting antiretroviral drugs, but in 2006 that number rose to 127,300—a 70% increase. Infection usually occurs during the last stages of pregnancy, most often during labor and delivery.

FIGURE 5.1

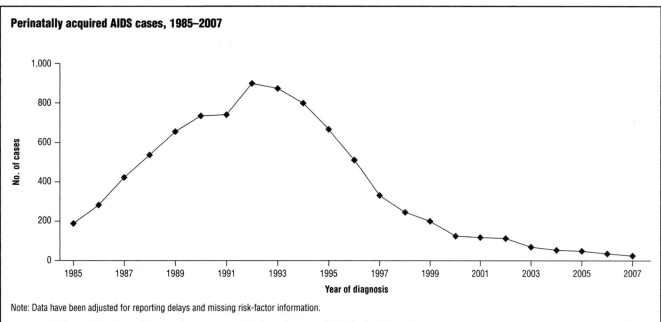

Perinatally acquired AIDS cases, 1985–2007

Year of diagnosis

Note: Data have been adjusted for reporting delays and missing risk-factor information.

SOURCE: "Estimated Numbers of Perinatally Acquired AIDS Cases by Year of Diagnosis, 1985–2007—United States and Dependent Areas," in *Pregnancy and Childbirth*, Centers for Disease Control and Prevention, Divisions of HIV/AIDS Prevention, October 10, 2007, http://www.cdc.gov/hiv/topics/perinatal/index.htm (accessed June 7, 2011)

TABLE 5.4

Perinatally acquired HIV infection and AIDS, 2009

Transmission category	Estimated number of diagnoses of HIV infection, 2009	Estimated number of AIDS diagnoses, 2009	Cumulative estimated number of AIDS diagnoses through 2009[a]
Perinatal	131	12	8,640
Other[b]	35	1	807

HIV = Human immunodeficiency virus.
[a]From the beginning of the epidemic through 2009.
[b]Includes hemophilia, blood transfusion, and risk not reported or not identified.

SOURCE: Adapted from "Diagnoses of HIV Infection by Transmission Category" and "AIDS Diagnoses by Transmission Category," in *HIV Surveillance Report: Diagnoses of HIV infection and AIDS in the United States and Dependent Areas, 2009*, Centers for Disease Control and Prevention, Divisions of HIV/AIDS Prevention, February 28, 2011, http://www.cdc.gov/hiv/topics/surveillance/basic.htm#exposure (accessed June 3, 2011)

Changing Thinking about How to Prevent Mother-to-Child Transmission

In "Effect of Breastfeeding on Mortality among HIV-1 Infected Women: A Randomised Trial" (*Lancet*, vol. 357, no. 9269, May 26, 2001), Ruth Nduati et al. report that the WHO recommended in 2000 that HIV-positive mothers should avoid breastfeeding their infants to prevent transmission of the virus. According to Nduati et al., the WHO stipulated that "when replacement feeding is acceptable, feasible, affordable, sustainable and safe, avoidance of all breastfeeding by HIV-infected women is recommended."

Worldwide, this strategy has had mixed results in terms of its feasibility—specifically, the availability of infant formula and safe, uncontaminated water—and the overall health of infants. Hoosen M. Coovadia et al. find in "Mother-to-Child Transmission of HIV-1 Infection during Exclusive Breastfeeding in the First 6 Months of Life: An Intervention Cohort Study" (*Lancet*, vol. 369, no. 9567, March 31, 2007) that in areas where HIV-infected mothers chose to use formula and breastfeed or to feed their babies formula and soft foods exclusively, there were actually higher rates of mother-to-infant transmission of HIV.

Coovadia et al. indicate that exclusive breastfeeding reduced the risk of HIV transmission by nearly half compared to when formula was given with breast milk, and by more than 10 times compared to when solid foods were also part of the infants' diet. These findings are somewhat surprising. One might expect that the more breast milk the infants consumed, the greater the viral exposure and rate of infection. Coovadia et al. posit several ideas about how exclusive breastfeeding might protect against infection, including:

- Exclusive breastfeeding protects the integrity of the lining of the gastrointestinal tract (the mouth, esophagus, stomach, and intestines), and an intact gastrointestinal tract may prevent the HIV from entering to the blood.

- The consumption of foreign proteins such as cows' milk protein as in formula milk might stimulate the large numbers of immune receptors that ordinarily line the gastrointestinal tract and enable the virus to better adhere to the lining of the gastrointestinal tract and enter into the underlying tissues.

- Exclusive breastfeeding is also associated with a lower amount of HIV virus in the milk, compared to when the mother combines breastfeeding and formula feeding. When mothers supplement their infants' diet with formula, the breast is not entirely emptied and the remaining milk contains higher levels of the virus.

- Breast milk naturally contains several substances that can inhibit virus growth. Even though more breast milk will present more virus, the effects may be countered because the infant also ingests more of the substances that inhibit virus growth.

In "Infant Feeding and HIV: Avoiding Transmission Is Not Enough" (*British Medical Journal*, vol. 334, no. 7592, March 10, 2007), Nigel C. Rollins of the Nelson R. Mandela School of Medicine in South Africa states that, in view of the results of this research, the WHO changed its recommendations in 2007. The new recommendations suggest that decision making be based on individual circumstances and acknowledge that infant survival, as opposed to simply preventing HIV transmission, should be the goal of infant feeding practices.

According to the WHO, in *HIV Transmission through Breastfeeding: A Review of Available Evidence, 2007 Update* (2008, http://whqlibdoc.who.int/publications/2008/9789241596596_eng.pdf), HIV-infected women are recommended to "breastfeed their infants exclusively for the first six months of life, unless replacement feeding is acceptable, feasible, affordable, sustainable and safe for them and their infants before that time. When those conditions are met, WHO recommends avoidance of all breastfeeding by HIV-infected women."

In 2009 the WHO again revised its recommendations about preventing mother-to-infant HIV transmission in response to findings that antiretroviral therapy effectively prevents transmission. According to the press release "New HIV Recommendations to Improve Health, Reduce Infections, and Save Lives" (November 30, 2009, http://www.who.int/mediacentre/news/releases/2009/world_aids_20091130/en/index.html), the WHO explains that the new guidelines advise breastfeeding for a full year, as long as the HIV-positive mother or infant is taking antiretroviral drugs. For HIV-positive women who breastfeed and are not taking antiretroviral drugs, the WHO recommends that nevirapine should be given to the child from birth until breastfeeding is terminated. For those who received drug treatment during pregnancy, treatment should continue until breastfeeding ends.

TREATMENTS FOR CHILDREN

Prescribing drug therapy for children is often more difficult than prescribing for adults because children respond to drugs differently at different ages and because oral medication must have an acceptable taste to ensure that children will take it as prescribed.

In "Approved Antiretroviral Drugs for Pediatric Treatment of HIV Infection" (May 20, 2009, http://www.fda.gov/ForConsumers/ByAudience/ForPatientAdvocates/HIVandAIDSActivities/ucm118951.htm), the U.S. Food and Drug Administration (FDA) lists 28 drugs that are used to treat pediatric HIV patients. Nine of these, called protease inhibitors (PIs; used alone or in combination with other drugs to combat viral infection), were available for children two to 13 years old. PI compounds act by preventing the reproduction of HIV that is already in the host cells. However, safety and effectiveness had not been established for four of the PIs: tipranavir, saquinavir mesylate (SQV), darunavir, and atazanavir sulfate. The PIs approved for use and deemed safe and effective by the FDA are:

- Amprenavir

- Lopinavir/ritonavir

- Fosamprenavir calcium

- Ritonavir

- Nelfinavir mesylate

Another group of drugs approved for pediatric use are known as nucleoside reverse transcriptase inhibitors (NRTIs). NRTIs, which are structurally similar to a nucleoside constituent of deoxyribonucleic acid (DNA), limit HIV replication by incorporating themselves into a strand of DNA, which causes the chain to end. The NRTIs approved for pediatric use are:

- Lamivudine

- Emtricitabine

- Abacavir

- Zalcitabine and dideoxycytidine

- Zidovudine

- Tenofovir disoproxil fumarate

- Enteric-coated didanosine

- Didanosine and dideoxyinosine

- Tenofovir disoproxil/emtricitabine

- Stavudine

Another group of antiretroviral drugs are known as nonnucleoside reverse transcriptase inhibitors (NNRTIs). NNRTIs slow down the functioning of the enzyme that allows the virus to become a part of the infected cell's nucleus. Three NNRTIs are presently approved for pediatric use:

- Delavirdine

- Efavirenz

- Nevirapine

In March 1996 the Antiviral Drugs Advisory Committee of the FDA approved the use of the compound didanosine for pediatric use. The approval was based on the results of two separate U.S. AIDS Clinical Trials Group pediatric studies (one of which was the largest controlled pediatric trial to date) and an Australian study, all of which found that didanosine delayed the progression of AIDS and was superior to ZDV alone. ZDV, which is given to children and adults, had been the only drug widely recognized to help delay the progress of HIV infection and to reduce the risk of perinatal infection.

The study results generated high expectations for the performance of didanosine in both children and adults. Indeed, the didanosine and combination therapies were so much more effective than ZDV alone that the AIDS Clinical Trials Group prematurely discontinued the ZDV-only therapy portion of the study. As promising as these early reports seemed, the effectiveness of didanosine alone or in combination with ZDV was short-lived because HIV susceptibility to the drugs decreased over time. Thus, even though didanosine is still used, it has not proven to be a major breakthrough in HIV infections as was hoped.

In 1999 a study conducted jointly by the United States and Uganda demonstrated that the perinatal transmission of HIV from mother to child could be reduced by the drug nevirapine. The drug is given to the mother in labor and to the child within three days of birth. Initial study results showed the drug to be safe for both mother and child and relatively inexpensive ($4 per mother/child dose). In 2000 the Elizabeth Glaser Pediatric AIDS Foundation, a nonprofit organization that is dedicated to promoting and funding worldwide pediatric AIDS research, secured funds to implement this treatment in developing countries that lack health care resources and infrastructure.

By 2003 the administration of nevirapine to hundreds of thousands of pregnant women in Africa demonstrated the therapeutic potential of the drug in slowing the progression of pediatric AIDS. The WHO, governments throughout sub-Saharan Africa, and the National Institutes of Health have all recommended that nevirapine use be continued to prevent HIV transmission from mothers to infants.

Also in 2003 the drug enfuvirtide was approved for use by children over the age of six. This drug is the first of the fusion inhibitor class of antiretroviral drugs. It acts by inhibiting the fusion of HIV to the host cell membrane.

In late 2007 two additional drugs—maraviroc and raltegravir—joined the FDA-approved list, although neither had, as of August 2011, been established to be safe and effective for children. Maraviroc is an entry inhibitor, meaning that it acts to block a receptor, CCR5, that HIV uses to enter white blood cells. Raltegravir is a HIV integrase strand transfer inhibitor, which means it targets integrase, an HIV enzyme that integrates the viral genetic material into human chromosomes.

CHILDREN ARE AT HIGHER RISK OF DRUG RESISTANCE

In "Risk of Triple-Class Virological Failure in Children with HIV: A Retrospective Cohort Study" (*Lancet*, vol. 377, no. 9777, May 7, 2011), the project team for the Collaboration of Observational HIV Epidemiological Research Europe looked at more than 1,000 children who had been infected with HIV perinatally and became resistant to the three major classes of drugs that are used to treat HIV: NRTIs, NNRTIs, and PIs. The team aimed to estimate the number of children who will need new classes of drugs as they age. It finds that 12% of the children developed resistance to all three drugs within five years of starting antiretroviral therapy. The team also notes that the children who started antiretroviral therapy at older ages were more likely to suffer drug resistance.

HOW MANY CHILDREN ARE INFECTED?

In 2009 an estimated 166 children under the age of 13 years were diagnosed with HIV infection in the United States. (See Table 3.2 in Chapter 3.) Of the estimated 34,247 AIDS diagnoses reported in 2009, just 13 were diagnosed in children under the age of 13 years. (See Table 3.3 in Chapter 3.)

Suzanne K. Whitmore, Xinjian Zhang, and Allan W. Taylor of the CDC estimate in "Estimated Number of Births to HIV-Positive Women, United States, 2006" (February 4, 2009, http://www.retroconference.org/2009/PDFs/924.pdf) that between 8,650 and 8,900 infants were born to HIV-infected women in the United States in 2006. The CDC indicates in *Pediatric HIV Surveillance* (July 2011, http://www.cdc.gov/hiv/topics/surveillance/resources/slides/pediatric/index.htm) that of the 166 pediatric HIV cases reported in 2009 in the United States and dependent areas, 128 cases (representing 77% of the total) were in African-American children.

Geographic Distribution

The CDC reports in *Pediatric HIV/AIDS Surveillance* (May 19, 2009, http://www.cdc.gov/hiv/topics/basic/index.htm) that among children under the age of 13 years in 2007, a total of 87 AIDS cases were reported; this was a decrease from 93 in 2005. As in previous years, most (86%) of these cases were acquired perinatally. In 2007 Florida (13), New York (12), California (11), Georgia (9), and New Jersey (8) reported the highest numbers of cases. (See Figure 5.2.) Twenty-nine states and four dependent areas reported no pediatric AIDS cases in 2007.

FIGURE 5.2

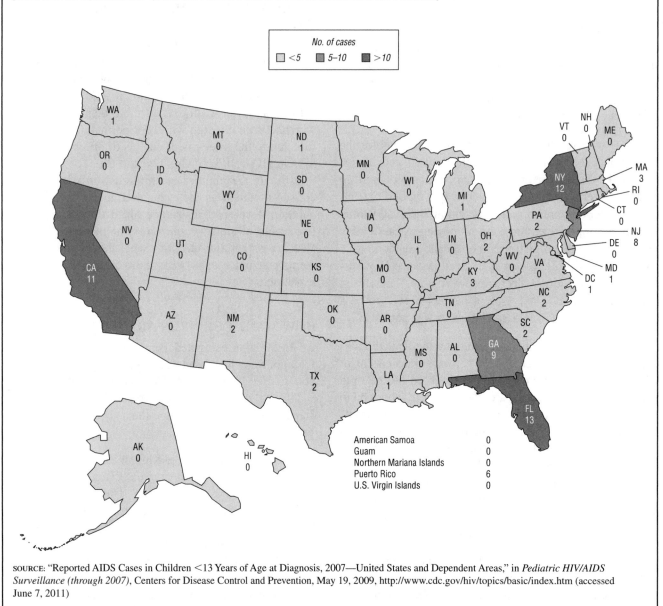

AIDS cases in children under 13 years old, by state, 2007

[United States and dependent areas. Population is 87. Includes 3 cases in children whose area of residence is unknown.]

SOURCE: "Reported AIDS Cases in Children <13 Years of Age at Diagnosis, 2007—United States and Dependent Areas," in *Pediatric HIV/AIDS Surveillance (through 2007)*, Centers for Disease Control and Prevention, May 19, 2009, http://www.cdc.gov/hiv/topics/basic/index.htm (accessed June 7, 2011)

Global Outlook

The United Nations (UN) Children's Fund (UNICEF) observes in *Children and AIDS: Fifth Stocktaking Report, 2010* (November 2010, http://www.unicef.org/publications/files/Children_and_AIDS-Fifth_Stocktaking_Report_2010_EN.pdf) that great strides have been made toward the goal of eliminating mother-to-child transmission of HIV by 2015. Many countries in eastern and southern Africa, Latin America, East Asia, and central and eastern Europe are close to meeting the goal of providing universal treatment to prevent transmission. For example, in 2005 just 15% of HIV-positive pregnant women in low- and middle-income countries received antiretroviral drugs to prevent mother-to-child transmission. By 2009 more than half (53%) of HIV-positive pregnant women received antiretroviral drugs. Similarly, in 2005 only 75,000 children under the age of 15 years received antiretroviral treatment. By 2009 the number had risen to an estimated 356,400, about 28% of children in need of treatment.

The testing, diagnosis, and treatment of HIV infection are also improving. Worldwide, the percentages of expectant mothers tested for HIV have increased. For example, in Latin America and the Caribbean testing of expectant mothers rose from 29% in 2005 to 57% in 2009. Impressive strides have also been made in countries with high HIV prevalence, such as Botswana, Namibia, South Africa, and Zambia, where testing is above 80%.

However, less progress has been made in ensuring that infants receive antiretroviral drugs to prevent transmission. In low- and middle-income countries the provision of antiretroviral drugs to infants inched up from 12% in 2005 to 35% in 2009. UNICEF cites social, cultural, and economic factors that impede the use of antiretroviral therapy and health services, including the high cost of pre- and postnatal care, long waiting times, the inability to pay for transportation to clinics, the lack of partner support, and HIV-related stigma and discrimination.

According to UNICEF, 2.5 million children under the age of 15 years were living with HIV infection in 2009, and just 28% were receiving antiretroviral therapy, compared to 37% of HIV-infected adults. In 2010 the WHO issued new guidelines for children. The updated guidelines stipulate that HIV-infected children less than 24 months of age begin antiretroviral drugs as soon as they are diagnosed. The guidelines also call for the use of PIs in children who were exposed to NNRTIs, such as nevirapine or efavirenz, to prevent mother-to-child transmission. PIs are prohibitively expensive in many low-income countries and because some require refrigeration they are often unavailable for children in rural areas of developing countries. UNICEF explains that even though newer drugs such as raltegravir and etravirine may prove to be as or more effective than PIs for children, these drugs have not been sufficiently tested in infants to conclusively demonstrate their safety and efficacy (the ability of an intervention to produce the intended diagnostic or therapeutic effect in optimal circumstances).

Gene Mutation in Some Babies May Help

A gene mutation that slows the progress of HIV in adults was shown during the late 1990s to help HIV-infected newborns avoid serious AIDS-associated illnesses longer than those who do not have the mutation. Michael Fischereder et al. report in "CC Chemokine Receptor 5 and Renal-Transplant Survival" (*Lancet*, vol. 357, no. 9270, June 2, 2001) that the gene CC chemokine receptor 5 (CCR5) is present in 10% to 15% of whites but is not found in Asian-Americans or African-Americans.

The gene codes for a protein called CCR5. This protein and another one called CXCR4 are located on the surface of a number of human cells. In "Analysis of the Mechanism by Which the Small-Molecule CCR5 Antagonists SCH-351125 and SCH-350581 Inhibit Human Immunodeficiency Virus Type 1 Entry" (*Journal of Virology*, vol. 77, no. 9, May 2003), Fotini Tsamis et al. demonstrate that CCR5 and CXCR4 can be used as receptors by HIV-1 to enter and infect CD4+ T cells, dendritic cells, and macrophages. Furthermore, CCR5 has been shown to be essential for viral transmission and replication during the early phase of the disease, even before symptoms of infection appear. Researchers expect that further investigation of the CCR5

gene will eventually help them develop drugs to prevent or destroy HIV in newborns.

Some researchers, such as Michael Marmor et al., in "Resistance to HIV Infection" (*Journal of Urban Health*, vol. 83, no. 1, January 2006), speculate that because several of the same genetic mutations have been found in both exposed uninfected populations and in long-term nonprogressor populations (people who become infected but do not develop AIDS), a single theory may explain both phenomena—that the genetic traits prevent or hinder HIV-1 entry into cells, which reduces the likelihood of infection and, should infection occur, slows or entirely eliminates the development of serious disease.

According to María Salgado of Hospital Carlos III, in Madrid, Spain, in "The Role of the Host in Controlling HIV Progression" (*AIDS Reviews*, vol. 11, no. 2, April–June 2009), new genetic technology and tools enable researchers to explore the impact of the complex interactions between viral and host factors that result in the control of HIV-induced immunodeficiency in some individuals who are long-term nonprogressors. Different genetic markers that are associated with the host immune system appear to play important roles in the control of HIV progression. These new technologies enable the collection and analysis of vast amounts of information and may help shed light on the precise role of host genetics in HIV disease progression.

ALL PREGNANT WOMEN SHOULD BE TESTED FOR HIV

When HIV-infected pregnant women know their HIV infection status, they are better able to make informed decisions about antiretroviral therapy to reduce perinatal transmission of HIV to their infants. The U.S. Preventive Services Task Force recommends that all pregnant women be offered HIV counseling and voluntary HIV tests.

In September 2008 the American College of Obstetrics and Gynecology's (ACOG) Committee on Obstetric Practice expanded its recommendations about prenatal and perinatal HIV testing in "ACOG Committee Opinion No. 418: Prenatal and Perinatal Human Immunodeficiency Virus Testing: Expanded Recommendations" (*Obstetrics and Gynecology*, vol. 112, no. 3). The committee recommended that all pregnant women be screened for HIV infection as early as possible during each pregnancy and informed that they will receive an HIV test as part of routine prenatal testing unless they decline or opt-out of HIV screening. Repeat conventional or rapid HIV testing during the third trimester of pregnancy is recommended for:

- Women living in areas with high HIV prevalence rates.

- Women known to be at high risk for acquiring HIV.

- Women who declined testing earlier in the pregnancy.

TABLE 5.5

Maternal HIV testing among children with perinatally acquired AIDS, HIV exposure, or HIV infection, 2007

Time of maternal HIV test	Perinatally acquired AIDS Population = 73		HIV exposure[a] Population = 2,361		HIV infection[b] Population = 529	
	No.	%	No.	%	No.	%
Before or at birth	28	38	2,240	95	213	40
After birth	29	40	47	2	138	26
Unknown	16	22	74	3	178	34

[a]From 33 areas that report perinatal exposure.
[b]From 53 areas with confidential name-based HIV infection reporting.

SOURCE: "Slide 11. Time of Maternal HIV Testing among Children with Perinatally Acquired AIDS, HIV Exposure or HIV Infection Reported in 2007—United States and Dependent Areas," in *Pediatric HIV/AIDS Surveillance (through 2007)*, Centers for Disease Control and Prevention, May 19, 2009, http://www.cdc .gov/hiv/topics/basic/index.htm (accessed June 8, 2011)

Of the children who were reported to the CDC in 2007 as being perinatally exposed to HIV (but had not acquired HIV/AIDS), 95% were born to women who were tested before or at the time of birth. (See Table 5.5.) Of the children who were perinatally HIV infected, only 40% of their mothers were tested before or at the time of birth; of the children who were diagnosed with AIDS, only 38% were born to mothers who were tested before or at the time of birth. An additional 26% of mothers who had children reported with HIV infection and 40% of mothers who had children with AIDS were not tested until after the child's birth. These data demonstrate that early testing, which allows the timely ZDV therapy to prevent transmission, can help reduce HIV transmission from mothers to their children.

SURVIVING INTO THEIR TEENS

The CDC indicates in *HIV Surveillance Report* that at the end of 2008, 3,022 children under the age of 13 years were reported to be living with HIV infection in the 40 states and five U.S. dependent areas that conducted confidential name-based HIV infection case surveillance. Even though many HIV-infected children die as infants and toddlers, most infected from birth now survive beyond age five, and it is not uncommon for others to reach their teens.

In "HIV Infection in Infants and Children," the NIAID distinguishes three distinct patterns of disease progression among HIV-infected children. The first group consists of those who display symptoms within their first 18 months following infection. Even with treatment, progression to AIDS in this group is rapid and most children die by age four. Children in the second group experience a less aggressive progression and often have milder or less prolonged symptomatic periods. These children tend to live longer. The third group is a recently emerging group of survivors. These children have grown up with few, if any, symptoms. Researchers are eager to determine precisely why and how these children remain asymptomatic in spite of their infection.

Research indicates that some of the difference in response to HIV is attributable to polymorphisms (common genetic variations). Kumud K. Singh and Stephen Spector find in "Host Genetic Determinants of HIV Infection and Disease Progression in Children" (*Pediatric Research*, vol. 65, May 2009) that HIV-infected children with a specific polymorphism called CCR5-delta32 had half the rate of disease progression compared to children with normal CCR5. They also observe that the most rapid progression of HIV symptoms occurred in children with normal CCR5 plus a polymorphism called 59029-A/A. This particular polymorphism was identified in about 25% of the HIV-infected children studied, representing the genotype that most often accelerated the rate of disease progression in children with normal CCR5. Furthermore, Singh and Spector find that there were some polymorphisms that had an impact in adults but not in children, and some that seemed to have an important impact in children but only a modest impact in adults.

In "Host and Viral Genetic Correlates of Clinical Definitions of HIV-1 Disease Progression" (*PLoS One*, vol. 5, no. 6, June 11, 2010), Concepción Casado et al. describe patterns of HIV disease progression that are based on host genetic markers and viral factors. The researchers attempt to better define long-term nonprogressor elite controllers (HIV-infected people who show no signs of disease progression for over 12 years and remain asymptomatic), viremic controllers (HIV-infected people who progress to AIDS very slowly, after a long period, or in some instances do not progress to AIDS), viremic noncontrollers (HIV-infected people who have high levels of viral load), chronic progressors (HIV-infected people who progress to AIDS within 10 years of diagnosis), and rapid progressors (HIV-infected people who progress to AIDS within four years of diagnosis).

Dealing with Physical and Emotional Problems

When HIV-infected children died during the early years of the HIV/AIDS epidemic, they were generally unaware of what was happening to them. In the 21st century, at the Children's Evaluation and Rehabilitation Center of the Albert Einstein College of Medicine of Yeshiva University in New York City, school-aged children meet with social workers in a support group to handle the physical and emotional ordeals of growing up with HIV and AIDS. These children are part of the increasing number born with HIV who have survived long enough to realize what it means. They must learn to cope with the physical, psychological, and emotional consequences of HIV/AIDS.

In "Living with 'The Monster'" (*Achieve*, Winter 2009), Raven Lopez explains that HIV-positive children deal with problems unique to their situation. For example, she recounts being excluded from class trips at school, being shunned and taunted by classmates, and being fearful of disclosing her HIV status to peers.

Lisa Henry-Reid, Lori Wiener, and Ana Garcia observe in "Caring for Youth with HIV" (*Achieve*, Winter 2009) that adolescents with HIV require significant psychological and emotional support because they face unique challenges including:

- Stigma and fear of rejection

- Side effects of HIV drugs

- Coping with a potentially life-threatening illness and an uncertain life span

- Disclosure and transmission

- The impact of loss

- Effectively navigating the health care system

Henry-Reid, Wiener, and Garcia report that adolescents who share their HIV diagnosis with others fare better psychologically and socially than those who do not disclose their HIV status. They assert that HIV-infected adolescents must deal with the normal challenges of adolescence and illness as well as with additional stressors such as poverty, barriers to care and social services, violence, racism, homophobia, broken families, homelessness, and child abuse.

Global HIV Infection in Young People

In *Opportunity in Crisis: Preventing HIV from Early Adolescence to Early Adulthood* (June 2011, http://www.unicef.org/publications/files/Opportunity_in_Crisis-Report_EN_052711.pdf), UNICEF states that worldwide an estimated 5 million young people aged 15 to 24 years were living with HIV infection in 2009 and that this age group accounted for 41% of new HIV infections in people aged 15 years and older. An estimated 890,000 young people were diagnosed with HIV infection in 2009. Globally, young women accounted for 60% of all young people living with HIV. In sub-Saharan Africa nearly three-quarters of HIV-infected young people were female.

Sub-Saharan Africa accounted for nearly seven out of 10 (69%) new HIV infections globally in young people in 2009. An increase in HIV infection among young people in central and eastern Europe is attributed to escalating injection drug use. UNICEF observes that young people often engage in more than one high-risk behavior, which increases the speed with which infection spreads in the population.

In Asia and the Pacific a higher proportion of cases are attributable to heterosexual contact, and in India the epidemic is fueled by sex workers—nearly 5% are HIV infected. In contrast, young people at risk in Latin America are men who have sex with men (MSM), transgender people, sex workers, and injection drug users.

According to UNICEF, children and young teens aged 10 to 14 years who are sexually active or inject drugs are at especially high risk for HIV infection because they are not knowledgeable and mistakenly believe they are not at risk. UNICEF indicates that abstinence-only education programs have not proven to be effective at preventing or reducing HIV transmission, other sexually transmitted diseases (STDs), or pregnancy. However, there has been greater success in preventing high-risk behaviors with programs that present abstinence as an option and also teach safe-sex strategies such as condom use.

WHO WILL CARE FOR THEM?

The HIV/AIDS epidemic has created many tragedies, including millions of orphans. The UN Joint Program on HIV/AIDS (UNAIDS) estimates in "Global and Regional Trends" (June 2011, http://www.childinfo.org/hiv_aids.html) that by 2010 there were an estimated 16.6 million orphans due to AIDS worldwide. According to UNAIDS, in *Global Report: UNAIDS Report on the Global Aids Epidemic, 2010* (2010, http://www.childinfo.org/files/20101123_Global_Report_em.pdf), nearly 90% of these orphaned children live in sub-Saharan Africa.

It is not always possible to find someone to care for an orphan of parents who died of AIDS, particularly if the child also has HIV or AIDS. Some family members may be hesitant to take in the child for fear he or she may spread the infection. In a growing number of cases, however, grandparents (in most cases, grandmothers) are taking these orphans into their homes. This may be a burden on older people who have lost their own children and may feel too old, tired, or impoverished to rear another family. They may also fear that they will die before their grandchildren do, leaving no one to care for them. It is no less difficult for the children who have lost their parents and fear they will probably miss the advantages they would have had with younger parents, such as being able to play more active childhood games.

Older orphans struggle with the rage, shame, and isolation of losing a parent to AIDS. Observers are finding that the HIV/AIDS epidemic is creating a class of particularly troubled youth. All children who lose a parent suffer to some degree, but for those whose parents die from AIDS, embarrassment and secrecy often compound the trauma. Teens whose parents became infected as a result of injecting drugs or practicing unsafe sex are often torn between feeling sorry for their parents and blaming them for their illness.

ADOLESCENTS, YOUNG ADULTS, AND HIV/AIDS
Patterns of Infection

The transmission and course of AIDS among adolescents aged 13 to 19 years and young adults aged 20 to 24 years follow similar patterns to those over the age of 25 years. The CDC reports in *HIV Surveillance in Men Who Have Sex with Men (MSM)* (June 6, 2011, http://www.cdc.gov/hiv/topics/surveillance/resources/slides/msm/slides/msm.pdf) that from 2006 through 2009, 87% of diagnosed HIV infections in males aged 13 to 24 years were attributed to MSM. Likewise, the sharpest increase in HIV infection attributable to MSM was in those aged 13 to 24 years. (See Figure 5.3.) By contrast, female adolescents and young adults aged 13 to 19 years became infected through

FIGURE 5.3

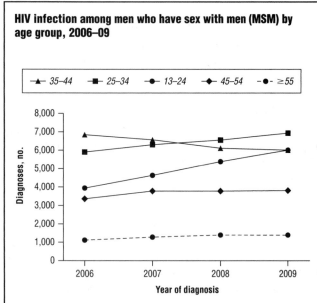

HIV infection among men who have sex with men (MSM) by age group, 2006–09

HIV = Human immunodeficiency virus.
Notes: Data include persons with a diagnosis of HIV infection regardless of stage of disease at diagnosis. All displayed data have been statistically adjusted to account for reporting delays and missing risk-factor information, but not for incomplete reporting. Data exclude men who reported sexual contact with other men and injection drug use.

SOURCE: "Diagnoses of HIV Infection among Men Who Have Sex with Men, by Age Group, 2006–2009—40 States and 5 U.S. Dependent Areas," in *HIV Surveillance in Men Who Have Sex with Men (MSM)*, Centers for Disease Control and Prevention, June 6, 2011, http://www.cdc.gov/hiv/topics/surveillance/resources/slides/msm/slides/msm.pdf (accessed June 8, 2011)

heterosexual contact (90.4%) or injection drug use (9.6%). (See Table 4.2 in Chapter 4.)

The characteristics of adolescence—a time of development, uncertainty, and a misleading sense of bravado and immortality, often combined with pushing the boundaries of good sense—create the potential for some young people to become particularly vulnerable to HIV infection. For many, this is a time of experimentation and risk-taking, often in terms of sexual behavior or use of alcohol and illicit drugs.

Many Adolescents Are Sexually Active

More than one-third of adolescents are sexually active. In *The Youth Risk Behavior Surveillance System (YRBSS): 2009* (June 1, 2011, http://www.cdc.gov/HealthyYouth/yrbs/pdf/us_sexual_trend_yrbss.pdf), the National Youth Risk Behavior Survey, which monitors health risk behaviors of adolescents in grades nine to 12, indicates that in 2009 nearly half (46%) said they had had sexual intercourse and more than half (61.1%) said they had used a condom during their last sexual intercourse. (See Table 5.6.)

In 2009 the overwhelming majority (87%) of teens said they had been taught in school about AIDS or HIV infection, an increase of about five percentage points since 1991. (See Figure 5.4.) Just 12.7% of high school students received HIV testing in 2009, and more females and African-Americans were tested. (See Figure 5.5.)

SEXUALLY TRANSMITTED DISEASES. Teenagers engaging in sexual activity before becoming sufficiently mature, with ineffective contraceptive methods, have led to record high rates of STDs among heterosexuals. According to the CDC, in *Trends in Sexually Transmitted Diseases in the United States: 2009 National Data for Gonorrhea, Chlamydia, and Syphilis* (November 22, 2010, http://www.cdc.gov/std/stats09/trends.htm), 19 million new infections occur each year, almost half of them among young people aged 15 to 24 years, and many in this group are unaware that they are infected.

Even though overall rates of infection for some STDs, such as gonorrhea, declined during the 1990s and leveled off during the first decade of the 21st century, gonorrhea, syphilis, and chlamydia infections among adolescents appeared to be increasing. The CDC notes in "STDs in Adolescents and Young Adults" (November 22, 2010, http://www.cdc.gov/std/stats09/adol.htm) that even though young people aged 15 to 24 years represent only 25% of the sexually experienced population, they acquire nearly half of all new STDs. In 2009 gonorrhea rates for people aged 15 to 19 years and 20 to 24 years decreased by 10.3% and 7.4%, respectively. In contrast, chlamydia rates for young people aged 15 to 19 years and 20 to 24 years rose 2.4% and 4%, respectively.

TABLE 5.6

Trends in the prevalence of sexual behaviors of high school students, selected years 1991–2009

	1991	1993	1995	1997	1999	2001	2003	2005	2007	2009	Changes from 1991–2009[a]	Change from 2007–2009[b]
Ever had sexual intercourse	54.1	53.0	53.1	48.4	49.9	45.6	46.7	46.8	47.8	46.0	Decreased, 1991–2009	No change
Had sexual intercourse with four or more persons (during their life)	18.7	18.7	17.8	16.0	16.2	14.2	14.4	14.3	14.9	13.8	Decreased, 1991–2009	No change
Had sexual intercourse with at least one person (during the 3 months before the survey)	37.5	37.5	37.9	34.8	36.3	33.4	34.3	33.9	35.0	34.2	Decreased, 1991–2009	No change
Used a condom during last sexual intercourse (among students who were currently sexually active)	46.2	52.8	54.4	56.8	58.0	57.9	63.0	62.8	61.5	61.1	Increased, 1991–2003 No change, 2003–2009	No change
Used birth control pills or Depo-Provera before last sexual intercourse to prevent pregnancy (among students who were currently sexually active)	NA[c]	NA	NA	NA	19.5	22.6	20.7	20.5	18.8	22.9	No change, 1999–2009	Increased
Drank alcohol or used drugs before last sexual intercourse (among students who were currently sexually active)	21.6	21.3	24.8	24.7	24.8	25.6	25.4	23.3	22.5	21.6	Increased, 1991–2001 Decreased, 2001–2009	No change
Were ever taught in school about AIDS or HIV infection	83.3	86.1	86.3	91.5	90.6	89.0	87.9	87.9	89.5	87.0	Increased, 1991–1997 Decreased, 1997–2009	Decreased

[a]Based on trend analyses using a logistic regression model controlling for sex, race/ethnicity, and grade.
[b]Based on t-test analyses.
[c]Not available.
Note: The national Youth Risk Behavior Survey (YRBS) monitors priority health risk behaviors that contribute to the leading causes of death, disability, and social problems among youth and adults in the United States. The national YRBS is conducted every two years during the spring semester and provides data representative of 9th through 12th grade students in public and private schools throughout the United States.

SOURCE: "Trends in the Prevalence of Sexual Behaviors National YRBS: 1991–2009," in *The Youth Risk Behavior Surveillance System (YRBSS): 2009*, Centers for Disease Control and Prevention, National Center for Chronic Disease Prevention and Health Promotion, Division of Adolescent and School Health, June 1, 2011, http://www.cdc.gov/HealthyYouth/yrbs/pdf/us_sexual_trend_yrbs.pdf (accessed June 8, 2011)

FIGURE 5.4

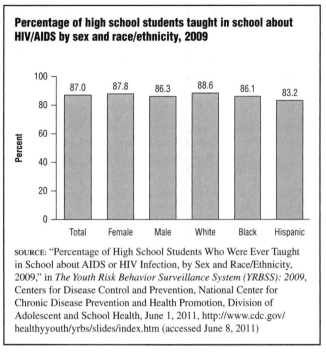

Percentage of high school students taught in school about HIV/AIDS by sex and race/ethnicity, 2009

SOURCE: "Percentage of High School Students Who Were Ever Taught in School about AIDS or HIV Infection, by Sex and Race/Ethnicity, 2009," in *The Youth Risk Behavior Surveillance System (YRBSS): 2009*, Centers for Disease Control and Prevention, National Center for Chronic Disease Prevention and Health Promotion, Division of Adolescent and School Health, June 1, 2011, http://www.cdc.gov/healthyyouth/yrbs/slides/index.htm (accessed June 8, 2011)

FIGURE 5.5

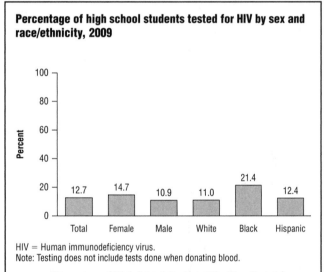

Percentage of high school students tested for HIV by sex and race/ethnicity, 2009

HIV = Human immunodeficiency virus.
Note: Testing does not include tests done when donating blood.

SOURCE: "Percentage of High School Students Who Were Tested for HIV, by Sex and Race/Ethnicity, 2009," in *The Youth Risk Behavior Surveillance System (YRBSS): 2009*, Centers for Disease Control and Prevention, National Center for Chronic Disease Prevention and Health Promotion, Division of Adolescent and School Health, June 1, 2011, http://www.cdc.gov/healthyyouth/yrbs/slides/index.htm (accessed June 8, 2011)

The rates of syphilis infection are similar. Rates among 15- to 19-year-old females increased from 1.9 cases per 100,000 population in 2005 to 3.3 cases per 100,000 population in 2009. Among women aged 20 to 24 years there were 5.6 cases per 100,000 population in 2009. (See Figure 5.6.) Among 15- to 19-year-old males the rate rose from 2.3 cases per 100,000 population in 2005 to 6 cases per 100,000 population in 2009. Men aged 20 to 24 years had the high-est rates of any age group—20.7 cases per 100,000 population in 2009. Figure 5.7 shows increasing rates of syphilis among men aged 15 to 44 years.

LEADING THE WAY: YOUNG PEOPLE AS AIDS ACTIVISTS AND ORGANIZATIONS THAT HELP YOUNG PATIENTS

Almost since the beginning of the HIV/AIDS epidemic, children and teenagers have been among the activists campaigning for HIV/AIDS reforms and awareness of the disease. Their role has been a profoundly personal one. For example, until his death from AIDS on April 8, 1990, Ryan White—an Indiana teenager—generated worldwide attention to the disease and, in particular, to the stigmas and misconceptions surrounding it. White, who contracted the virus during treatment for his hemophilia, was a white, middle-class, heterosexual boy, which ran counter to public perception of AIDS at the time as a disease of gay men.

Being expelled from school because of the supposed health risk to other students galvanized White to educate others on the nature of HIV and AIDS. His legacy includes the Ryan White Comprehensive AIDS Resources Emergency Act, the multibillion-dollar program that funds programs to help provide primary health care and support to those living with HIV/AIDS.

The National Association of People with AIDS, founded in 1983, advocates for people, including children, who live with HIV/AIDS. The nonprofit organization—the oldest national AIDS organization in the United States—is a strong advocate for HIV/AIDS social programs and research funding.

The AIDS Alliance for Children, Youth, and Families was established in 1994 to publicize the concerns of women, children, young people, and families who are affected by HIV/AIDS. The nonprofit organization is also a clearinghouse for relevant information and advocates for public policy changes in the areas of HIV/AIDS social welfare and disease prevention.

Metro TeenAIDS focuses on prevention, education, and treatment needs of teenagers. Through its website (http://www.metroteenaids.org/) and in-person contact at schools, nightclubs, youth centers, shelters, and on the street, Metro TeenAIDS connects with teenagers in a language that is relevant to them. The intent is to help teenagers protect themselves from the risks of HIV exposure and contamination and in securing medical care for HIV infection and AIDS.

Metro TeenAIDS has been working in conjunction with other youth and AIDS activist groups since 1994 to host annual conferences around the country that focus on educating young people about HIV and AIDS. In 1995 the conference became known as the Ryan White National Youth Conference on HIV and AIDS (RWNYC). In 2001 the first

FIGURE 5.6

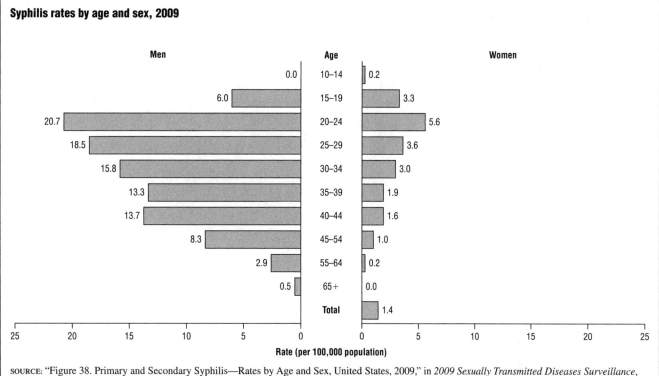

Syphilis rates by age and sex, 2009

SOURCE: "Figure 38. Primary and Secondary Syphilis—Rates by Age and Sex, United States, 2009," in *2009 Sexually Transmitted Diseases Surveillance*, Centers for Disease Control and Prevention, National Center for HIV/AIDS, Viral Hepatitis, STD, and TB Prevention, Division of STD Prevention, November 22, 2010, http://www.cdc.gov/std/stats09/figures/38.htm (accessed June 8, 2011)

FIGURE 5.7

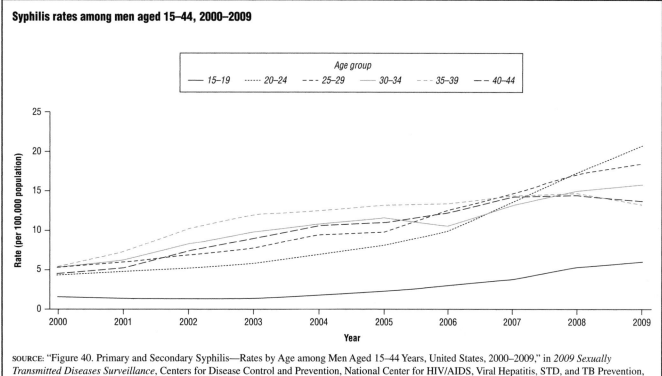

Syphilis rates among men aged 15–44, 2000–2009

SOURCE: "Figure 40. Primary and Secondary Syphilis—Rates by Age among Men Aged 15–44 Years, United States, 2000–2009," in *2009 Sexually Transmitted Diseases Surveillance*, Centers for Disease Control and Prevention, National Center for HIV/AIDS, Viral Hepatitis, STD, and TB Prevention, Division of STD Prevention, November 22, 2010, http://www.cdc.gov/std/stats09/figures/40.htm (accessed June 8, 2011)

Positive Youth Institute—a one-day gathering specifically focusing on the needs of HIV-positive young people—was held before and in conjunction with the RWNYC. Each year several hundred young people, health care workers, and AIDS activists attend the conference. In February 2009 Metro TeenAIDS (2009, http://metroteenaids.org/?p=185) celebrated 20 years of service to more than 200,000 at-risk and HIV-infected adolescents, families, youth workers, and the community-at-large. Deb LeBel notes in "AIDS.gov Microgrant Awardees: Using New Media to Reach Youth" (October 5, 2010, http://blog.aids.gov/2010/10/aidsgov-microgrant-awardees-using-new-media-to-reach-youth .html) that in 2010 Metro TeenAIDS was awarded a grant to extend its use of social media and social networking sites to educate and inform young people. The grant funded creation of videos using poetry, song, and dance to communicate safer sex messages. When the videos aired, Metro TeenAIDS reported an increase in HIV testing and the numbers of young people seeking information.

CHAPTER 6
HIV/AIDS COSTS AND TREATMENT

FINANCING HEALTH CARE DELIVERY

Care for HIV/AIDS patients is expensive. Drug treatments, most prominently highly active antiretroviral therapy (HAART), have high per-unit costs. Nonetheless, their introduction in 1996 reduced total health care spending on AIDS by reducing the rate of hospitalization and outpatient care. According to Samuel A. Bozzette et al., in "Expenditures for the Care of HIV-Infected Patients in the Era of Highly Active Antiretroviral Therapy" (*New England Journal of Medicine*, vol. 344, no. 11, March 15, 2001), the average HIV patient incurred costs of approximately $1,410 per month in 1998. Extended over the full year, a patient's drug treatment for HIV could cost as much as $18,300. People with AIDS could spend up to $77,000 per year on treatment.

Longer survival periods following infection with HIV lead to even greater costs for care and treatment. For example, Bruce R. Schackman et al. note in "The Lifetime Cost of Current Human Immunodeficiency Virus Care in the United States" (*Medical Care*, vol. 44, no. 11, November 2006) that people with HIV can gain as many as 24.2 extra years of life at a total cost of $618,900 (in 2004 dollars).

Schackman et al.'s study illustrates the effects of the increasing treatment costs and enhanced survival. The researchers estimate the monthly cost of care at $2,100, with about 70% of costs attributable to medications. This equates to $25,200 per year. In 1998 the average annual cost was $18,300, according to Bozzette et al. The cost increase is not simply a consequence of inflation, because the increased cost of HIV drugs account for much of the difference. Schackman et al. estimate that these costs are $12.1 billion per year.

Some HIV/AIDS patients rely on health insurance to help pay these costs. However, many patients are not insured. Also, many policies exclude or deny coverage to people with preexisting conditions, and, as a result, many HIV-positive people are denied private health insurance.

In "Can You Afford Your HIV Treatment?" (May 13, 2009, http://www.everydayhealth.com/hiv-aids/can-you-afford-hiv-treatment.aspx), Madeline Vann explains that about half of people living with HIV/AIDS in the United States have the costs of their treatment paid for by Medicaid and Medicare. Medicaid is an entitlement program that is run by the federal and state governments to provide health care insurance to patients under the age of 65 years who cannot afford to pay for private health insurance. Medicare is the federal health insurance program for adults aged 65 years and older and younger adults with permanent disabilities. Medicaid eligibility requirements vary from state to state. Generally, however, Medicaid covers people with very little income who cannot support themselves financially due to a physical or mental impairment—an impairment that is expected to last at least one year or result in death. The operation of Medicaid programs also varies widely by jurisdiction. Many states supplement federal funding with their own funds, and each state determines its eligibility criteria and benefits—the number and type of treatments that are provided through the program.

The toll of HIV/AIDS on Medicaid is huge. The Kaiser Family Foundation estimates in the fact sheet "U.S. Federal Funding for HIV/AIDS: The President's FY 2012 Budget Request" (March 2011, http://www.kff.org/hivaids/upload/7029-07.pdf) that the federal contribution to Medicaid for HIV/AIDS care rose from $4.7 billion in fiscal year (FY) 2010 to $5.4 billion in FY 2012.

Medicare accounts for approximately a quarter of federal spending on HIV/AIDS care in the United States. The Kaiser Family Foundation projects that Medicare spending for HIV/AIDS will grow from $5.1 billion in FY 2010 to $5.8 billion in FY 2012.

A Reverse in Federal Policy

In early 1997 the administration of Bill Clinton (1946–) announced that it hoped to expand Medicaid to cover all low-income HIV-infected people. The administration wanted to give low-income HIV-positive people access to HAART drugs that slow the onset of AIDS. By the end of the year, however, the administration announced that it could not follow through because such a nationwide plan would increase government spending. Both the Clinton administration and the administration of George W. Bush (1946–) forbade the federal government and states to change the Medicaid rules if that change would increase spending over a five-year period. As of August 2011, only patients who had been diagnosed with full-blown AIDS, not those who were HIV positive, were covered by Medicaid.

Even though efforts were made to extend Medicaid benefits to cover people with HIV before they develop AIDS, these efforts were unsuccessful. In March 2009 Representatives Eliot L. Engel (1947–; D-NY), Ileana Ros-Lehtinen (1952–; R-FL), and Speaker of the House Nancy Pelosi (1940–; D-CA) reintroduced H.R. 1616, Early Treatment for HIV Act, to allow states to expand Medicaid coverage to low-income HIV-positive people. This bill had been introduced in previous congressional sessions, but despite broad bipartisan support it never became law. Nevertheless, the health care reform legislation that was passed in 2010 expands Medicaid eligibility to cover people with HIV who do not have an AIDS diagnosis.

State Programs to Provide Drugs

During the late 1980s state-administered programs were established to help AIDS patients pay for azidothymidine (now called zidovudine [ZDV]), the most effective drug at the time. The programs provide free drugs to AIDS patients who are not poor enough to qualify for Medicaid coverage but who do not have private health insurance coverage or who have used up their prescription drug coverage. The federal government provides two-thirds of the funding for the state programs, and the balance comes mostly from the states. In "Utilization and Spending Trends for Antiretroviral Medications in the U.S. Medicaid Program from 1991 to 2005" (*AIDS Research and Therapy*, vol. 4, no. 1, October 16, 2007), Yonghua Jing et al. of the University of Cincinnati report that in 2005 Medicaid spent $1.6 billion for antiretroviral drugs. (Since 2006, when a new Medicare prescription drug benefit, Part D, went into effect, people eligible for both Medicaid and Medicare have had the cost of their drugs covered by the new benefit.)

Until recently, these drug programs did not attract many participants, primarily because ZDV alone was not effective against the disease. During the late 1990s, however, with the development of a new class of antiretroviral drugs—called protease inhibitors—that reduce the amount of virus in the blood, more patients wanted to take advantage of the programs. (According to the Institute of Medicine, in *Public Financing and Delivery of HIV/AIDS Care: Securing the Legacy of Ryan White* [May 2004], a typical three-drug cocktail—one protease inhibitor combined with two other HIV/AIDS medications—cost more than $12,000 per patient in 2004. By 2011 the costs were higher still. For example, according to Margaret Rode, in "Stop Price Increases for H.I.V. and AIDS Prescriptions" [May 12, 2011, http://pharmacycheckerblog.com/stop-price-increases-for-h-i-v-and-aids-prescriptions], the AIDS Healthcare Foundation states that at a retail pharmacy a three-month supply of the drug Atripla [efavirenz, emtricitabine, and tenofovir] cost $6,540.29 in 2011. Similarly, a three-month supply of Truvada [emtricitabine and tenofovir] cost $3,966.97 and of Emtriva [emtricitabine] cost $1,490.99.)

This growing demand has put a financial strain on the programs, and many states have to ration HIV/AIDS drugs or turn patients away to remain solvent. Some states are making it harder for people to qualify for the programs, and a few are beginning to charge small co-payments (a percentage of the total cost that the patient is responsible for paying) to offset the cost of the drugs. Others are attempting to obtain larger price discounts or rebates on HIV/AIDS drugs in an effort to reduce their costs so they can continue to provide the drugs to an expanding population of patients.

The National Alliance of State and Territorial AIDS Directors (NASTAD) reports in *National ADAP Monitoring Project Annual Report Module Two* (May 2011, http://www.nastad.org/) that AIDS Drug Assistance Programs (ADAP) enrollment and utilization peaked during FY 2010. However, in response to the economic recession (which lasted from late 2007 to mid-2009) and reduced state funding, ADAP enrollment decreased by 2% and the use of waiting lists grew between June and December 2010.

In "ADAP Watch" (August 12, 2011, http://www.nastad.org/Docs/041808_NASTAD%20ADAP%20Watch%20-%20August%202011.pdf), NASTAD indicates that 9,217 people in 12 states were on waiting lists for ADAPs in August 2011. According to NASTAD, in *National ADAP Monitoring Project Annual Report: Module Two and Module Two Supplement* (April 2011, http://www.nastad.org/Docs/Public/Resource/201152_Module%20Two%20and%20Module%20Two%20Supplement%20slide%20set%20-%20May%202011.pdf), ADAP spending on prescription drugs totaled over $146 million in June 2010 and 10 states accounted for three-quarters of all drug spending. In 2010 average per client expenditures were $11,388. The ADAP budget grew by 13% from 2009 to 2010, rising to $1.8 billion. Despite this increase, ADAPs faced significant challenges including:

- Increased demand in response to unemployment
- Fluctuations, and often decreases, in state funding

- Increasing HIV testing and new treatment guidelines advising earlier drug treatment

- High drug costs

Changes to the Health Care System

Since the 1960s U.S. government spending on health services has consistently increased. The Centers for Medicare and Medicaid Services' Office of the Actuary reports in *National Health Expenditure Projections 2009–2019* (January 2010, https://www.cms.gov/NationalHealthExpend Data/downloads/proj2009.pdf) that federal health expenditures rose, from $599.8 billion in 2004 to an estimated $984.8 billion in 2011. At the same time health care providers—doctors, hospitals, and other health-related institutions and professions—watched as payments for Medicare, Medicaid, and private insurance coverage, once easily obtained during the 1960s and 1970s, were increasingly restricted and limited. During the 1990s providers also encountered a greater resistance among private insurers to pay. Bureaucratic management, increasing amounts of paperwork to document medical care and claims, and slow reimbursement rates prompted some physicians to stop caring for Medicare and Medicaid patients.

Managed-care plans (also known as managed-care organizations [MCOs]), which control the use of and reimbursement for services in an effort to contain costs, rely heavily on primary care practitioners (general and family physicians). These plans have become the health care providers for increasing numbers of HIV/AIDS patients. Since 2000 many HIV-infected people have enrolled in managed-care plans. This is partly because more companies are only offering employees managed-care plans and partly because government insurance programs are directing Medicaid recipients to such programs.

A MANAGED-CARE PLAN FOR HIV/AIDS PATIENTS: THE TENNESSEE "CENTERS OF EXCELLENCE" PROGRAM. On January 1, 1994, Tennessee withdrew from the federal Medicaid program and began implementing a state health care reform plan called Tennessee Medicaid (TennCare). In May 1998 TennCare introduced a voluntary managed-care plan for its members with HIV or AIDS. The model plan features "Centers of Excellence" providers—practitioners with expertise in the care of HIV/AIDS patients. The providers must agree to adopt and adhere to a clinical protocol (practice and care guidelines) developed by a committee composed of providers, consumers, MCOs, and public health officials. The committee meets up to twice a month to evaluate and recommend new drug therapies as they become available and to inform participating providers about new treatments.

Providers may be individual practitioners with access to needed services or full-service clinics composed of a group of practitioners. There are no financial incentives to participate in the program. However, providers who meet the Centers of Excellence criteria do not have to obtain prior authorization when they prescribe drugs or treatments that fall under the clinical protocols.

The Centers of Excellence program frees MCOs from the clinical and administrative responsibility of keeping close tabs on HIV/AIDS care. It also allows MCOs to remain confident that providers are capable and have access to a wide range of services needed by members. MCO members know that participating providers meet high standards of HIV/AIDS clinical care. Other managed-care plans are developing comparable programs to meet the unique health and social service needs of people living with HIV/AIDS.

TennCare (2011, http://www.tennessee.gov/tenncare/), which provides health care for 1.2 million people with an annual budget of more than $8 billion per year, has endured criticism since its beginning. Doctors and hospitals have complained that it has been underfunded, forcing them to carry an unfair proportion of the costs. However, in *Tenn-Care Presentation on the Governor's FY 2012 Recommended Budget* (April 2011, http://www.tn.gov/tenncare/forms/tenncarebudgetFY12.pdf), TennCare notes that it has been able to reduce spending while simultaneously improving quality. TennCare describes its operations as "part of the budget solution to help the state through the recent economic downturn."

CHALLENGES FOR THE DELIVERY SYSTEM

HIV/AIDS poses a major challenge to health care institutions, health care professionals, and others who provide direct health care services. Since its emergence and identification, HIV infection has undergone a dramatic transformation—it has gone from being an infectious disease that was an almost certain death sentence to a chronic disease that for many can be managed for decades. Furthermore, unlike most chronic diseases that afflict older Americans, HIV/AIDS affects people of all ages, and young adults are disproportionately affected. The health care system cares for more than a million people in the United States suffering from a disease that is still only partly understood. The system must also plan to deliver services to the tens of thousands of people in the United States who are HIV positive and will require specialized health care services during the coming years, even though only a small proportion will need intensive medical care at any one time.

The number of indigent people in need of HIV/AIDS care, particularly those who bring the added complications of drug addiction, homelessness, and other socioeconomic problems, has strained public hospitals in particular. Patients in public hospitals are often different from those in private hospitals. They generally seek care later in the course of the disease's progression and are, therefore, sicker. The scarcity of resources—trained personnel, hospital beds, and support services—in the community, combined with inadequate funding and reimbursement for HIV/AIDS care, are significant obstacles to effective health care delivery for poor HIV/AIDS patients.

Health Care Reform Legislation Promises to Improve Access to Care

In March 2010 President Barack Obama (1961–) signed the Patient Protection and Affordable Care Act (PPACA) into law. The PPACA is considered the most comprehensive and important health care reform legislation since the 1965 passage of Medicare and Medicaid. The provisions of the legislation that aim to improve access to care for people with HIV/AIDS include:

- Eliminating the Medicaid disability requirement (people with HIV no longer must wait for an AIDS diagnosis to be eligible for Medicaid coverage) and extending access to Medicaid to people with an income 133% of the federal poverty line in 2014

- Closing the Medicare Part D donut hole (a gap in Medicare that stops paying for prescriptions and the beneficiary must pay the entire cost) by 2020, and allowing the ADAP to be used to meet the Medicare Part D True Out of Pocket Spending Limit

- Requiring pharmaceutical companies to offer a 50% discount on brand-name drugs in the donut hole

- Increasing access to private health insurance in 2014 by prohibiting discrimination or higher premiums based on health status or gender and banning preexisting condition exclusions and lifetime limits on coverage

- Expanding the scope of coverage in 2014 by mandating benefits that include prescription drugs, mental health and substance abuse treatment, preventive care, and chronic disease management

- Increasing affordability of insurance coverage by providing subsidies for people with incomes up to 400% of the federal poverty line

Hospital Care

The American Hospital Association reports in "Fast Facts on US Hospitals" (December 6, 2010, http://www.aha .org/aha/resource-center/Statistics-and-Studies/fast-facts .html) that in 2009 there were 5,795 hospitals. These hospitals are also feeling the pinch of Medicare rate limits, reduced payments from MCOs, and intense competition from other providers, such as ambulatory surgical centers and hospices. Many are struggling to remain profitable institutions. During the 1970s and 1980s the steady growth of for-profit hospitals lured many privately insured, middle-class patients away from community hospitals, leaving most of the uninsured, sicker patients to seek care from inner-city public hospitals.

Most HIV/AIDS patients are cared for in inner-city public hospitals that are already overburdened with inadequate revenues, staff shortages, lack of referral facilities, and emergency departments that are used by many poor neighborhood residents as sources of primary medical care. Many health care professionals praise a model of hospital care that was pioneered in San Francisco, California. The city was hit hard during the early days of the HIV/AIDS epidemic and developed a range of innovative, effective programs in response to acute need. This model of care relies on extensive outpatient services and volunteer social support services that are provided by the well-established and well-organized gay and lesbian community.

Changes in Health Care Delivery

Even though fewer people are acquiring HIV/AIDS, the evolution of HIV care is altering the ways in which health care is delivered. In the late stages of AIDS, most patients require intermittent hospitalization and home health care. Those who are not as severely affected and have symptoms or conditions that once required intravenous therapy (which had to be administered in a hospital or by home health professionals) are now able to self-medicate at home. Many drugs are now available for oral administration in pill or liquid form. These home care and community-based measures lessen the burden on the health care delivery system and make it easier for HIV/AIDS patients to care for themselves.

People with AIDS (PWAs) who receive informal home health care (such as care from friends and family) often use fewer hospital services, perhaps reflecting a greater desire to remain at home. PWAs who have strong social support systems and who prefer to remain at home may also be less likely to demand an aggressive approach to treating their illness. Those who receive formal home health care (visits from physicians, nurses, therapists, social workers, case managers, and other paid caregivers) often use more hospital services. This may reflect a greater use of all types of health services by PWAs with weaker social support systems and/or an aggressive approach to treatment by medical professionals.

An AIDS Care Alternative

In an effort to offer uninsured AIDS patients in Atlanta, Georgia, treatment equal to that available to patients with private insurance, in 1986 Grady Memorial Hospital (2011, http://www.gradyhealthsystem.org/clinic/ 63/) opened the Ponce De Leon Center, one of the largest centers that is dedicated to the treatment of advanced HIV/AIDS. The Ponce Center provides internal medicine and infectious disease care, mental health counseling, social and support services, HIV research and education, and case management. The program also works closely with many local AIDS service organizations, some housed on-site, to meet the complex needs of people living with HIV/AIDS. The Ponce Center is the largest publicly funded program of its kind in the eastern United States and is consistently named one of the top-three HIV/AIDS outpatient clinics in the country.

Hospice Care

The AIDS epidemic has had a significant impact on hospices. According to the National Center for Health Statistics, in *Health, United States, 2010* (February 2011, http://www.cdc.gov/nchs/data/hus/hus10.pdf), the number of certified hospice care agencies grew 20-fold between 1985 and 2007. Hospice care, both in the home and in specialized centers, offers care that is aimed at comfort rather than cure. This includes expert pain relief, along with emotional, psychological, and spiritual support for patients, their families, and friends. Most hospice patients are older adults who suffer from terminal diseases such as cancer and face imminent death.

At the beginning of the AIDS epidemic, patients did not fit well into the hospices of the day. AIDS patients were younger than traditional hospice patients, and the progression of their disease was less predictable than many cancers. Furthermore, as one hospice administrator noted, because many people with AIDS were accustomed to prejudice, they initially mistrusted the motivation and altruism of hospice workers. However, during the first decade of the 21st century home-based hospice programs were designed to meet the needs of AIDS patients, their partners, and families and gained acceptance in the medical community as well as among HIV-infected people and the voluntary social service agencies that are organized to support them.

HEALTH CARE PROVIDERS
Physicians

There are physicians from many medical specialties—primary care physicians such as family practitioners, internists, and specialists in infectious diseases, pulmonary medicine, and cancer medicine—who care for people infected with HIV or those suffering from AIDS. Physicians who treat AIDS patients often perform a wide variety of services besides providing care to AIDS patients. Many are also AIDS activists and may be involved in developing policies, planning for care needs, and dealing with the media.

One challenge in the training of physicians to treat AIDS patients is that AIDS care requires skills and training in the multitude of conditions that are known to be part of HIV/AIDS. However, the amount of experience—rather than the kind of training—may be a better predictor of the quality of care the physician is able to deliver.

Mari M. Kitahata et al. claim in the landmark study "Physicians' Experience with the Acquired Immunodeficiency Syndrome as a Factor in Patients' Survival" (*New England Journal of Medicine*, vol. 334, no. 11, March 14, 1996) that AIDS patients who were treated by primary care physicians with no previous experience dealing with the disease died more than a year earlier than those whose doctors had treated at least five AIDS patients. The researchers also show that patients had a 43% decrease in relative risk of death at any given time when treated by a physician who had treated other AIDS patients. The difference, according to Kitahata et al., was that the more experienced physicians consulted more frequently with specialists and reported more visits with their AIDS patients.

Since 1996 Kitahata et al.'s findings have been verified by further research, such as William E. Cunningham et al.'s "The Effect of Hospital Experience on Mortality among Patients Hospitalized with Acquired Immunodeficiency Syndrome in California" (*American Journal of Medicine*, vol. 107, no. 2, August 1999) and Kitahata et al.'s "Primary Care Delivery Is Associated with Greater Physician Experience and Improved Survival among Persons with AIDS" (*Journal of General Internal Medicine*, vol. 18, no. 2, February 2003).

There is also a continuing debate about the types of physicians who should treat patients with complex chronic medical conditions such as HIV infection. In "Physician Specialization and the Quality of Care for Human Immunodeficiency Virus Infection" (*Archives of Internal Medicine*, vol. 165, no. 10, May 23, 2005), Bruce E. Landon et al. describe the results of their research to assess the relationship between specialty training and expertise and the quality of care delivered to patients with HIV infection. The researchers looked at 5,247 patients of 177 physicians who responded to a survey. Over four out of 10 (42%) of the physicians were infectious diseases specialists and 58% were general medicine physicians (primary care physicians who are often called generalists). Nearly two-thirds of the generalists (63% of the generalists and 37% overall) considered themselves expert in HIV care. An analysis of the data Landon et al. collected reveals that infectious diseases physicians and generalists who considered themselves expert in HIV care had performed similarly. In contrast, nonexpert generalists delivered lower-quality care. Landon et al. posit that their findings reconfirm the premise that "generalists with appropriate experience and expertise in HIV care can provide high-quality care to patients with this complex chronic illness."

Maria Zolfo et al. describe in "A Telemedicine Service for HIV/AIDS Physicians Working in Developing Countries" (*Journal of Telemedicine and Telecare*, vol. 17, no. 2, March 2011) an Internet-based service to assist physicians and other health care workers in countries where medical resources are limited. Between April 2003 (when it was founded) and December 2009 the service had fielded 1,058 queries from more than 40 countries. Most of the questions were posed in a web-based telemedicine discussion forum and some were submitted via e-mail. About half of the questions were about the use of antiretroviral drugs. A survey of users of the service revealed that it helped them manage specific cases and influenced their future patient management.

Nurses

The effect of HIV/AIDS on nurses can be more difficult to assess than its effect on doctors. Nurses often have different viewpoints than some physicians about their professional obligations to patients with HIV/AIDS. As hospital employees, nurses seldom have the option of choosing whether to treat a particular patient (nor do patients have much choice of nurses). Nurses, however, report that caring for HIV/AIDS patients can take an enormous emotional toll because they are often the primary source of continuous physical and emotional care for these patients, who generally require more intensive care and services than other patients.

Nurses, physicians, and other health care professionals must cope with more than simply their fears of contracting the disease from HIV/AIDS patients and keeping abreast of advances in the treatment of the disease. They also face a wide range of emotional issues when caring for these patients, from feelings of failure when treatment is unsuccessful to grief when witnessing the untimely deaths of patients. In "How Caring for Persons with HIV/AIDS Affects Rural Nurses" (*Issues in Mental Health Nursing*, vol. 30, no. 5, May 2009), Iris L. Mullins of New Mexico State University explains that caring for patients with HIV/AIDS affects nurses in three distinct areas of their personal and professional lives: their personal sense of self as a nurse in practice; their interactions with their family members, friends, and colleagues; and their interactions with patients with HIV/AIDS. Nurses caring for HIV/AIDS patients in rural areas expressed additional concerns including the need for ongoing continued education about the care of people with HIV/AIDS.

Support groups and counselors help many health professionals, especially hospice workers, to share and understand these feelings so that they are better able to care for HIV/AIDS patients and their families.

CDC Guidelines

In response to an incident in which five patients acquired HIV from David J. Acer (1949–1990), a Florida dentist, the CDC addressed occupational exposure to bloodborne pathogens in "Recommendations for Preventing Transmission of Human Immunodeficiency Virus and Hepatitis B Virus to Patients during Exposure-Prone Invasive Procedures" (*Morbidity and Mortality Weekly Report*, vol. 40, RR-8, July 12, 1991). The updated guidelines were intended to prevent the accidental spread of the infection from health care providers to patients and from patients to health care workers. The recommendations stressed the careful and consistent use, with all patients, of standard infection control procedures for bloodborne agents—the so-called universal precautions—that were published by the CDC in 1987.

The CDC guidelines also recommended that HIV-infected health care workers stop performing exposure-prone invasive procedures and that professional medical and dental groups draw up lists of exposure-prone procedures for their disciplines. The CDC recommended that HIV-infected health care workers consult with a panel of experts to determine which, if any, limits should be placed on their medical practices and further advised practitioners to inform patients of their HIV-infection status before performing medical procedures.

The CDC guidelines resulted in some unforeseen consequences. Professional groups, hospital attorneys, state courts, legislatures, and Congress reacted with alarm to a perception of dangers to patients posed by HIV-infected health care professionals totally out of proportion to the largely theoretical risk. Adelisa L. Panlilio et al. of the CDC note in "Updated U.S. Public Health Service Guidelines for the Management of Occupational Exposures to HIV and Recommendations for Postexposure Prophylaxis" (*Morbidity and Mortality Weekly Report*, vol. 54, RR-9, September 30, 2005) that the average risk of HIV infection after skin contact with HIV-infected blood is estimated to be about 0.3%, and the risk for transmission is even lower from contact with body fluids or tissues other than blood. In "Surveillance of Occupationally Acquired HIV/AIDS in Healthcare Personnel, as of December 2010" (May 2011, http://www.cdc.gov/HAI/organisms/hiv/Surveillance-Occupationally-Acquired-HIV-AIDS.html), the CDC states that 57 documented cases had been reported between 1981 and 2010 (though no documented cases were reported between 2000 and 2010), and it was possible that 143 additional cases of HIV infection were linked to occupational exposures.

According to Panlilio et al., the CDC recommends that the following procedures and philosophies would best serve patients and health care workers:

- The universal and meticulous use of well-understood infection-control procedures, particularly those developed from the study of hepatitis B (another bloodborne infection that is 100 times more infectious and 10 times more common in health professionals), should be applied in all health care settings, whether hospital, office, or home based.

- Operative or other invasive procedures, in which injury to health care professionals occurs with any frequency, should be discontinued or modified to the greatest extent possible. This involves developing new instruments and investigating new operative techniques.

- All health care professionals should consider being tested for HIV. However, an HIV-positive result should not justify restricting the practice of health care professionals.

Should Doctors Tell Patients?

Since 1991 the American College of Surgeons (ACS), the nation's largest professional organization of surgeons, has refused to draw up a list of procedures that might pose a high risk of transmitting HIV from doctor to patient. The group maintains that because not a single documented case of surgeon-to-patient transmission has been established, there is no scientific basis for suggesting that a particular surgical procedure increases the risk of viral transmission. The ACS also notes that surgical patients are at greater risk for other surgery-related infections than for HIV, even from an HIV-infected physician.

Panlilio et al. note that the CDC guidelines instruct HIV-infected health care workers to avoid contact with patients that could potentially bring the worker's blood into contact with a patient's body cavities or mucous membranes.

HEALTH CARE WORKERS AND INFECTION
Health Care Workers with HIV and AIDS

In "Surveillance of Occupationally Acquired HIV/AIDS in Healthcare Personnel, as of December 2010," the CDC indicates that as of 2010 it was aware of only 57 documented cases of health care workers other than surgeons in the United States who had become infected with HIV as a result of occupational exposures. The breakdown of those who were infected was as follows:

- Nurses (24)
- Clinical laboratory workers (16)
- Nonsurgical physicians (6)
- Nonclinical laboratory technicians (3)
- Housekeeper/maintenance workers (2)
- Surgical technicians (2)
- Dialysis technician (1)
- Embalmer/morgue technician (1)
- Health aide/attendant (1)
- Respiratory therapist (1)

As of 2010, the CDC was also aware of 143 cases of HIV infection or AIDS that were possibly linked to occupational exposure among health care workers. These workers had not reported other risk factors for HIV infection. They reported a history of occupational exposure to blood, body fluids, or HIV-infected laboratory material, but they did not document infection after a specific exposure.

The known and possible cases of occupational acquisition of HIV undoubtedly represent an underestimate. There are likely unknown numbers of people who acquired their infection through occupational exposures, although, even in 2011, this is purely conjecture.

According to the National Institute for Occupational Safety and Health, in "Overview of State Needle Safety Legislation" (October 27, 2010, http://www.cdc.gov/niosh/topics/bbp/ndl-law.html), as of June 2002, 21 states had enacted needle-safety legislation to safeguard health care workers from bloodborne pathogen (agents that cause disease) exposures. State laws aim to supplement and strengthen the federal standards mandated by the Occupational Safety and Health Administration. Many of the state laws require the creation of a written exposure plan that is periodically reviewed and updated; protocols for safety device identification and selection; logs to document and report injuries with sharp instruments; and strict requirements and training for workers on how to use safety devices.

In "Updated U.S. Public Health Service Guidelines for the Management of Occupational Exposures to HBV, HCV, and HIV and Recommendations for Postexposure Prophylaxis" (*Morbidity and Mortality Weekly Report*, vol. 50, RR-11, June 29, 2001), the U.S. Public Health Service updated the guidelines for treatment to prevent health care workers with occupational exposure to HIV from becoming infected with the virus. Known as postexposure prophylaxis (PEP), the recommendation was that affected workers be given a four-week regimen of two antiretroviral drugs such as ZDV and lamivudine, with the addition of a third drug for HIV exposures that pose an increased risk of transmission. Another update was issued by Panlilio et al. in September 2005 because since publication of the 2001 update, the U.S. Food and Drug Administration (FDA) had approved new antiretroviral agents, and additional information had become available about the use and safety of PEP. Even though the best strategy to protect health care workers is to avoid exposure to HIV and other bloodborne pathogens, PEP has, as of 2011, proven generally effective in preventing HIV infection in workers who have been exposed.

Risks to Patients

Health care officials are not the only ones worried about HIV transmission in the health care setting. Patients also fear that infected health care workers can transmit the virus to them. In the landmark study "HIV Transmission from Health Care Worker to Patient: What Is the Risk?" (*Annals of Internal Medicine*, vol. 116, no. 10, May 15, 1992), Mary E. Chamberland and David M. Bell of the CDC develop a model of the risk of HIV transmission to patients and estimate that the risk of a patient becoming infected by an HIV-positive surgeon during a single operation is anywhere from 1 out of 42,000 to 1 out of 420,000. This risk is considerably less than the risks that are associated with many other medical procedures.

The CDC indicates in "HIV and Its Transmission" (July 1999, http://www.hivlawandpolicy.org/resources/download/360) that of more than 22,000 patients of 63 HIV-infected health care workers, no documented evidence has been found that links HIV infection to medical or dental care, except for the five patients of Acer in 1990. Medical researchers have tried without success to determine how Acer infected his patients and whether the exposure was accidental or deliberate. One theory is that he did not properly sterilize his dental tools; another is that he accidentally cut his finger or jabbed himself with a hypodermic needle, did not notice it, and bled into the patients' mouths. Before his death in 1990, Acer denied intentionally exposing his patients.

Even though HIV transmission through transplanted organs occurs very rarely, in November 2007 the first known cases in 20 years of HIV transmission from a high-risk donor were reported by the national media. The most likely explanation for this transmission is that the donor had tested HIV negative because the infection was recent and antibodies had not yet formed to the virus. In "Provider Response to a Rare but Highly Publicized Transmission of HIV Through Solid Organ Transplantation" (*Archives of Surgery*, vol. 146, no. 1, January 2011), Lauren M. Kucirka et al. examine how transplant surgeons' practices changed following the cases of HIV transmission. The researchers determine that nearly one-third (31.6%) of transplant surgeons said their practices changed following this exceedingly rare event. Over four out of 10 (41.7%) decreased use of high-risk donors, 34.5% intensified efforts to obtain patients' informed consent, and 16.7% increased their use of nucleic acid amplification testing, which is a more difficult and time-consuming test, but it does detect viral infection earlier than traditional antibody tests.

In March 2011 another instance of HIV transmission from a kidney transplant—the first documented case of this kind—was reported. The donor did not develop AIDS, but the recipient did, possibly because the recipient was taking drugs to prevent organ rejection and these drugs suppress the immune system.

WHAT DOES IT COST TO TREAT HIV/AIDS PATIENTS?

The Kaiser Family Foundation states in "U.S. Federal Funding for HIV/AIDS: The President's FY 2012 Budget Request" that in FY 2011 federal government spending for domestic and global HIV-related activities totaled $27 billion. President Obama's federal budget request for FY 2010 included an estimated $28.3 billion—$21.4 billion for domestic programs and $6.9 billion for global initiatives and activities. Federal funding has increased significantly throughout the course of the epidemic, and the FY 2012 federal budget for domestic programs and research represented a 4.8% increase over FY 2011. Much of the federal funding for HIV/AIDS care, as opposed to other assistance such as housing, was for Medicaid and Medicare, which were budgeted for 5.9% and 7.4% increases, respectively, in funding.

HIV/AIDS-related costs are expected to increase in response to the rising costs of hospitalization, home care, insurance premiums and co-payments, physician services, and pharmaceutical drugs. In 2000 certain drugs (including didanosine and ritonavir) rose substantially in price. Growing concern about rising drug prices led to a self-imposed price freeze by some manufacturers in 2002. However, price increases were eventually instituted. For example, Ron Leuty reports in "Gilead Boosts HIV Drug Prices" (*San Francisco Business Times*, April 7, 2011) that in April 2011 Gilead Sciences Inc. announced that the price for Atripla, its best-selling antiretroviral drug, would increase by 5.1% and that Truvada and Emtriva would increase in price by 7.9%.

Regardless, some HIV/AIDS care-related expenses have actually been reduced by relocating services from the hospital to a variety of outpatient settings. Examples of cost-saving services include outpatient transfusions and outpatient treatment for opportunistic infections such as *Pneumocystis carinii* pneumonia and cryptococcal meningitis. Increased volunteer-based social service programs that enable patients to be cared for at home can also prevent expensive hospital stays.

The Ryan White Comprehensive AIDS Resources Emergency Act

As of 2011, the Ryan White Comprehensive AIDS Resources Emergency (CARE) Act was the only federal program that exclusively funded medical and supportive services for people with HIV/AIDS. The act was named after Ryan White, who died of AIDS in 1990. White was an Indiana teenager with hemophilia who became infected through a blood transfusion. Shunned by his community because many people feared becoming infected through any kind of contact with him, White fought to attend school and attain rights for those infected with HIV/AIDS. White's efforts helped change the way the world treated those with the disease. The CARE Act was signed in 1990 and reauthorized in 1996, 2000, 2006, and 2009. The 2009 reauthorization, called the Ryan White HIV/AIDS Treatment Extension Act of 2009, continues the program through FY 2013 and authorizes a 5% increase for each fiscal year. The reauthorization still grants funding priority to urban areas with the highest

TABLE 6.1

Ryan White Act, fiscal years 2010–12

	Fiscal year 2010 appropriation	Fiscal year 2011 continuing resolution	Fiscal year 2012 budget request	Fiscal year 2012 +/− Fiscal year 2010
BA	$2,287,179,000	$2,265,888,000	$2,375,587,000	+$88,408,000
ADAP (non add)	858,000,000	835,000,000	940,000,000	+82,000,000
MAI (non add)	146,055,000	153,358,000	161,026,000	+14,971,000
SPNS	25,000,000	25,000,000	25,000,000	—
Total funding	**$2,312,179,000**	**$2,290,888,000**	**$2,400,587,000**	**+$88,408,000**
FTE	72	50	50	−22

BA = Budget authorization. ADAP = AIDS Drug Assistance Program. MAI = Minority AIDS Initiative. SPNS = Special Projects of National Significance. FTE = Full-time equivalents.
Note: The amounts include funding for Special Projects of National Significance (SPNS) funded from Department Public Health Service (PHS) Act evaluation set-asides in fiscal year 2011 president's budget and proposed for fiscal year 2012.

SOURCE: "Ryan White HIV/AIDS Overview," in *FY 2012 Congressional Justification for the Health Resources and Services Administration (HRSA)*, Health Resources and Services Administration, 2011, http://www.hrsa.gov/about/budget/budgetjustification2012.pdf (accessed June 14, 2011)

number of people living with AIDS, while helping eligible metropolitan areas and midsized cities with emerging needs, which are called transitional grant areas.

The 2009 reauthorization requires planning councils to characterize not only the demographics of people with HIV/AIDS but also the population of people unaware of their HIV status. The councils must develop plans to identify people with HIV/AIDS who do not know their status and to assist these people in obtaining health care services. The councils must also work to eliminate "barriers to routine testing and disparities in access to services for minorities and underserved communities."

The funds from the Ryan White HIV/AIDS Treatment Extension Act are appropriated using five formulas. Part A funds eligible metropolitan areas (EMAs) that are disproportionately affected by HIV/AIDS and transitional grant areas. Part B funds states to improve the quality, availability, and organization of HIV/AIDS health care and support services. Part C funds early intervention services and ambulatory care. Part D funds do not have to be used for primary care; instead, they may be used to help improve access to clinical trials and research. Part F funds encompass Special Projects of National Significance, which support the demonstration and evaluation of innovative models of HIV/AIDS care delivery for hard-to-reach populations as well as for AIDS Education and Training Centers, dental programs, and the Minority AIDS Initiative.

To qualify for Part A funds, EMAs must have more than 2,000 cumulative AIDS cases reported during the preceding five years and a population of at least 500,000. (The population provision does not apply to any EMA that was named and funded before FY 1997.) The U.S. Department of Health and Human Services' Health Resources and Services Administration explains in *Justification of Estimates for Appropriations Committee:*

Fiscal Year 2012 (February 2011, http://www.hrsa.gov/about/budget/budgetjustification2012.pdf) that in FY 2009 Parts A and B supported 2.5 million visits and 2.1 million visits, respectively, and that in FY 2012 they were expected to support 2.6 million visits and 2.2 million visits, respectively, for health care services—medical, dental, mental health, substance abuse, rehabilitative, and home health care. Table 6.1 is an overview of funding by the Ryan White HIV/AIDS Treatment Extension Act for FYs 2010, 2011, and 2012.

The 2009 reauthorization requires that Part A and B grantees who use code-based reporting to convert, over a period of three years, to name-based reporting. In FY 2013 only name-based data reporting will be acceptable.

Private Insurance and Medicaid

The financing of HIV/AIDS care is increasingly becoming the responsibility of Medicaid. The greater reliance on Medicaid funding is due in large part to the increase in the number of HIV/AIDS cases among injection drug users and poor people who are unlikely to be covered by private health insurance. In addition, many patients who once had private insurance through their workplace lost their coverage when the illness made them too sick to work, or they lost their job and job-related health benefits during the economic recession, forcing them to turn to Medicaid and other public programs.

Added to this list are those whose employment or economic status would normally ensure them insurance coverage, but who became virtually ineligible for private health insurance coverage once they tested positive for HIV. Others need assistance because some insurance companies consider HIV infection to be a preexisting condition, making it ineligible for payment of claims. Even insurance companies that do cover HIV treatment often impose caps, limiting coverage to relatively small dollar amounts.

The National Association of Health Underwriters explains in "Consumer Guide to Individual Health Insurance" (2011, http://www.nahu.org/consumer/individualinsurance.cfm) that in 2011 a person with HIV could be turned down for individual coverage by private insurers in most states. However, many states have developed ways to provide uninsurable people with access to individual health insurance coverage through high-risk pools. Passage of the 2010 health care reform legislation promises to resolve this problem. Beginning in 2014 private health insurance companies will be prohibited from discriminating against or denying people coverage because they have preexisting conditions.

Death Benefits

Since 1988 an industry has developed that offers dying AIDS patients the opportunity to collect a portion of their life insurance benefits before they die, either to pay for their treatment or to spend as they wish during their remaining time. These viatical (money for necessities given to a person dying or in danger of death) settlements are reached when an insured person sells his or her life insurance policy to an independent insurance company at a reduced or discounted price. This enables the patient to have some cash from the policy while he or she is still alive. After the patient dies, the company that bought the policy is paid the full death benefits. Regulators with the U.S. Securities and Exchange Commission are scrutinizing some practices they believe may victimize AIDS patients.

Some larger companies, such as Prudential, offer policyholders more than 90% of their policy payouts,

but only with a physician's certification that they have less than six months to live. Smaller companies usually pay 50% to 80% of the benefit payable at death, although they will pay benefits to people who still have up to five years to live. The longer the policyholders are expected to live, the less the cash disbursement they receive.

Most insurers will not write new life insurance policies for people known to have AIDS. Those that do offer life insurance policies to people infected with HIV or people with AIDS often have stringent requirements and limited benefits. For example, some policies for AIDS patients stipulate that should death occur due to illness during the first two or three years of coverage, then the benefits paid are simply a return of premiums paid plus an annual interest rate. Others offer an initial two- or three-year incremental period; after that initial period full benefits are paid whether death occurs due to accident or to illness.

TREATMENT RESEARCH

Medical and pharmaceutical research to develop and conduct clinical trials of antiretroviral drugs is expensive. According to the National Institutes of Health (NIH), just over $2.9 billion was allocated for AIDS research in FY 2008 and just under $3.2 billion was budgeted for FY 2012. Table 6.2 shows budget allocations by the type of activity funded between FYs 2008 and 2012.

Decisions about how much is spent to research a particular disease are not based solely on how many people develop the disease or die from it. Rightly or wrongly, economists base the societal value of an individual on his or her earning potential and productivity—the

TABLE 6.2

Budget allocation by activity, fiscal years 2008–12

[Dollars in thousands]

Area of emphasis	Fiscal year 2008 actual	Fiscal year 2009 actual	Fiscal year 2010 actual	Fiscal year 2011 CR	Fiscal year 2012 PB*	Dollar change
HIV microbicides	$115,495	$128,670	$143,162	$143,162	$146,741	$3,579
Vaccines	556,139	560,956	534,972	534,972	551,021	16,049
Behavioral and social science	412,502	434,305	429,313	429,339	443,440	14,127
Therapeutics						
Treatment as prevention	74,521	84,775	67,734	68,521	70,005	
Drug discovery, development, and treatment	623,940	585,786	617,257	616,695	630,047	
Total, therapeutics	**698,461**	**670,561**	**684,991**	**685,216**	**700,052**	**15,061**
Etiology and pathogenesis	703,874	729,991	744,649	744,649	762,226	17,577
Natural history and epidemiology	227,900	247,914	275,098	275,098	280,600	5,502
Training, infrastructure, and capacity building	171,706	198,028	216,329	216,329	218,051	1,722
Information dissemination	42,268	48,868	56,832	56,832	57,400	568
Total	**2,928,345**	**3,019,293**	**3,085,346**	**3,085,597**	**3,159,531**	**74,185**

*Includes approximately $27 million to be provided to the Office of the Assistant Secretary of Health (OASH) in support of the National HIV/AIDS Strategy.
CR = Continuing resolution. PB = President's budget. HIV = Human immunodeficiency virus.

SOURCE: "Budget Authority by Activity," in *Office of AIDS Research Trans-NIH AIDS Research Budget*, U.S. Department of Health and Human Services, National Institutes of Health, 2011, http://www.oar.nih.gov/budget/pdf/fy12justification.pdf (accessed June 14, 2011)

ability to contribute to society as a worker. The bulk of the people who die from heart disease, stroke, and cancer are older adults. Many have retired from the workforce and their potential economic productivity is often minimal. This economic measure of present and future financial productivity should not be misinterpreted as a casting-off of older adults; instead, it is simply an economic measure of present and future financial productivity.

In contrast, AIDS patients are usually much younger and, until recently, often died young—in their 20s, 30s, and 40s. Until they develop AIDS, the potential productivity of these people, measured in economic terms, is high. The number of work years lost when they die is considerable. Using this economic equation to determine how disease research should be funded, it may be considered economically wise to invest more money to research AIDS because the losses, measured in potential work years rather than in lives, are so much greater.

The primary goals of HIV/AIDS therapy are to prolong life and improve its quality. Even though during the early days of AIDS research a cure for the disease was envisioned, few researchers at the turn of the 21st century realistically expected any one drug to cure HIV infection in all people. The bottom-line objective became making the virus less deadly by foiling its efforts to reproduce within the body.

A major obstacle to the discovery of such treatments is the cost of drug research and development. Pharmaceutical manufacturers spend millions of dollars researching and developing new medicines. According to the Pharmaceutical Research and Manufacturers of America (PhRMA), since 1992 U.S. pharmaceutical companies have consistently spent more money each year on research and development (R&D) activities than the NIH has spent on its annual budget. For example, PhRMA reports in *2011 Profile Pharmaceutical Industry* (March 2011, http://www.phrma.org/sites/default/files/159/phrma_profile_2011_final.pdf) that in 2010 the estimated total pharmaceutical R&D budget was $67.4 billion. By contrast, the Department of Health and Human Services states in "Fiscal Year 2010 Budget in Brief: National Institutes of Health" (June 4, 2009, http://www.hhs.gov/asrt/ob/docbudget/2010budgetinbriefh.html) that the entire NIH budget (research and other activities) was $31 billion. Furthermore, private-sector spending has been outpacing government spending since 1995.

PhRMA explains in *2011 Profile Pharmaceutical Industry* that a pharmaceutical manufacturer must cover the cost not only of R&D for the approximately two out of 10 drugs that succeed but also for many of the drugs—eight out of 10—that fail to make it to the marketplace. Because of this cost, once a new drug receives FDA approval, its manufacturer ordinarily holds a patent or gains exclusivity rights, which guarantee that it will be

the sole marketer for a specified time (usually from three to 20 years) to recoup its investment. During this time the drug is priced much higher than if other manufacturers were allowed to compete by producing generic versions of the same drug. In contrast to the original manufacturer, the generic manufacturer does not have to pay for the successes and failures that occurred in the drug development pathway or pursue the complicated, time-consuming process of seeking FDA approval. The producer of generic drugs has the formula and must simply manufacture the drugs properly. Because of the lower cost of the generic drug after the original patent or exclusivity period has expired, competition among pharmaceutical manufacturers generally lowers the price. HIV/AIDS drugs are granted seven years of exclusivity under legislation that is aimed at encouraging research and promoting development of new treatments.

PhRMA also describes HIV/AIDS drug development as not only improving peoples' lives but also as saving money. In *2011 Profile Pharmaceutical Industry*, PhRMA asserts that in 1985 multiple hospitalizations resulted in the U.S. Army spending a staggering $500,000 to treat each patient with AIDS. The advent of antiretroviral drugs reduced the rate of hospitalization for HIV/AIDS by 32% despite the overall 28% increase in the number of people with HIV, which was largely attributable to increased survival (people with HIV live about 15 years longer than they did during the 1980s).

The issue of patent protection for HIV/AIDS drugs is understandably contentious. Pharmaceutical manufacturers and others argue that patent protection is necessary to allow for the financial investments necessary to breed innovation. However, to those directly affected by HIV/AIDS and those governments or health care systems that provide care, the enormous costs can be infuriating, especially with the knowledge that generic drugs carrying a lower price tag are possible. The need for less expensive HIV/AIDS drugs is especially urgent in the developing world.

In "Medicines Patent Pool Aims to Increase Access to HIV Drugs in Developing Countries" (March 10, 2011, http://www.ip-watch.org/weblog/2011/03/10/medicines-patent-pool-aims-to-increase-access-to-hiv-drugs-in-developing-countries/), Tavengwa Runyowa asserts that UNITAID, an organization that was founded to help offset the increasing costs of HIV/AIDS, malaria, and tuberculosis treatment, created the Medicines Patent Pool in 2010. Runyowa explains that "the pool operates a scheme in which pharmaceutical patent holders voluntarily licence their drugs to generic manufacturers who then produce more affordable versions for patients in poorer countries." Besides increasing access to established medication, the Medicines Patent Pool hopes to stimulate R&D in pediatric HIV medications and in drug formulations that can withstand heat for use in areas where refrigeration is unavailable.

FDA-APPROVED DRUGS

The first drug thought to delay symptoms was ZDV. Even though initially promising, ZDV's effects were found to be temporary at best. Several other drugs worked using the same mechanism of action as ZDV—exclusion of HIV from the host chromosome. A newer class of drugs called protease inhibitors (PIs) appears to keep HIV already in the host cells from reproducing. PIs block the ability of HIV to mature and infect new cells by suppressing a protein enzyme of the virus, called protease, which is crucial to the progression of HIV. Roy M. Gulick et al. indicate in the landmark study "Treatment with Indinavir, Zidovudine, and Lamivudine in Adults with Human Immunodeficiency Virus Infection and Prior Antiretroviral Therapy" (*New England Journal of Medicine*, vol. 337, no. 11, September 11, 1997) that a combination of indinavir, zidovudine, and lamivudine reduces the viral load and CD4 cell count. In the researchers' study, the changes in the viral load and the CD4 cell count lasted for as long as 52 weeks and the drug regimen was generally well tolerated.

Even if the effectiveness of PIs proves to be transient, they improve patients' prospects simply by creating more roadblocks for HIV, which mutates so rapidly that it becomes resistant to most drugs when the drugs are used alone. Even if a cure is never found, new and better drugs used in various combinations have helped transform HIV infection from a certain death sentence to a chronic but manageable disease, much like diabetes.

The cost, however, is high. Robert Steinbrook indicates in "HIV Infection—A New Drug and New Costs" (*New England Journal of Medicine*, vol. 348, no. 22, May 2003) that by 2003 the cost of many PIs rose to between $10,000 and $12,000 for a year's supply. AVERT, an international AIDS charity, observes in "Reducing the Price of HIV/AIDS Treatment" (2011, http://www.avert.org/generic.htm) that at a cost of $10,000 to $15,000 per person per year, "these antiretroviral drugs [are] far too expensive for the majority of people infected with HIV in resource poor countries."

In *Curing HIV: What It Means and Why It Must Be Done* (September 2008, http://www.projectinform.org/), Martin Delaney observes that lifetime treatment costs are high. He calculates an annual cost of treatment as $16,000 and multiplies it by 50 years, because treatment is lifelong, for a lifetime total of $800,000 in drug treatment costs alone. Delaney's estimates do not even consider cost increases over time.

Types of Antiretroviral Agents

The FDA notes in "Antiretroviral Drugs Used in the Treatment of HIV Infection" (August 15, 2011, http://www.fda.gov/ForConsumers/byAudience/ForPatientAdvocates/HIVandAIDSActivities/ucm118915.htm) that it approves seven classes of antiretroviral agents for the treatment of HIV/AIDS.

PROTEASE INHIBITORS. As of August 2011, the FDA had approved the following PIs:

- Amprenavir
- Tipranavir
- Indinavir
- Saquinavir (no longer marketed)
- Saquinavir mesylate
- Lopinavir and ritonavir
- Fosamprenavir calcium
- Ritonavir
- Darunavir
- Atazanavir sulfate
- Nelfinavir mesylate

NUCLEOSIDE REVERSE TRANSCRIPTASE INHIBITORS. Nucleoside reverse transcriptase inhibitors (NRTIs) were among the first compounds shown to be effective against viral infections. Research during the 1970s led to the development of the drug acyclovir, which is still being used to treat herpes infections. The first four anti-HIV drugs to be approved—ZDV, didanosine, dideoxycytosine, and stavudine—were nucleoside analogs.

As their name implies, NRTIs exert their action based on their three-dimensional structure, which mimics the structure of the nucleoside building blocks of deoxyribonucleic acid (DNA). By becoming incorporated into the DNA as the molecule is replicated, the analogs can preserve the structure of DNA but make it impossible for the HIV to use its reverse transcriptase to hijack the host replication machinery to make new viral copies.

As of August 2011, the following NRTIs had received FDA approval for use with HIV/AIDS:

- Lamivudine and zidovudine
- Emtricitabine
- Lamivudine
- Abacavir and lamivudine
- Zalcitabine, dideoxycytidine (no longer marketed)
- ZDV, azidothymidine
- Abacavir, zidovudine, and lamivudine
- Tenofovir disoproxil fumarate and emtricitabine
- Enteric coated didanosine
- Tenofovir disoproxil fumarate
- Stavudine
- Abacavir sulfate

NONNUCLEOSIDE REVERSE TRANSCRIPTASE INHIBITORS. Another class of antiretroviral drugs that were approved during the late 1990s is nonnucleoside reverse transcriptase inhibitors (NNRTIs). NNRTI compounds slow down the process of the reverse transcriptase enzyme that allows the virus to become part of the infected cell's nucleus. The compounds accomplish this by binding to the viral enzyme, which blocks the ability of the enzyme to function.

As of August 2011, there were six NNRTIs approved for use by the FDA:

- Rilpivirine
- Etravirine
- Delavirdine
- Efavirenz
- Nevirapine (immediate release)
- Nevirapine (extended release)

MULTICLASS COMBINATION PRODUCTS. The FDA approves another class of HIV medications that consist of combinations of specific drugs. As of August 2011, there were two combinations approved for use:

- Efavirenz, emtricitabine, and tenofovir disoproxil fumarate
- Emtricitabine, rilpivirine, and tenofovir disoproxil fumarate

OTHER APPROVED DRUGS. As of August 2011, the FDA also approved the fusion inhibitor drug enfuvirtide, which interferes with the fusion of HIV with the host cell membrane; the entry inhibitor drug maraviroc, which binds CCR5, an essential co-receptor for most HIV strains, and blocks them from entering T cells; and the HIV integrase strand inhibitor drug raltegravir, which acts against an enzyme that HIV uses to integrate its viral material into the host's chromosomes.

Aggressive Treatment

With new drugs in the anti-HIV/AIDS arsenal, many people with HIV/AIDS who had given up hope of effective treatment returned to clinics and doctors' offices. Even though treatment guidelines previously promoted early intervention with ZDV, recommended treatment now combines PIs with other antiretroviral drugs. Treatment recommendations change rapidly in response to the development of new drugs and clinical trials indicating the effectiveness of different combinations of antiretroviral drugs. Researchers are acting quickly to develop new mixtures of the recently approved and older drugs. Because HIV mutates to resist any drug it faces, including all PIs, researchers find that varying the combination of drugs prescribed can "fool" the virus before it has time to mutate.

Near the end of the first decade of the 21st century thinking about the timing of treatment of people infected with HIV but without symptoms was beginning to change. Mari M. Kitahata et al. indicate in "Effect of Early versus Deferred Antiretroviral Therapy for HIV on Survival" (*New England Journal of Medicine*, vol. 360, no. 18, April 30, 2009) that starting HIV treatment before the patient's immune system is too badly compromised can dramatically improve survival. The researchers find that, compared to patients who started treatment early, those who delayed therapy increased their odds of dying by either 69% or 94%, depending on the patient's initial CD4 blood cell count.

Patients undergoing therapy with new drugs or drug combinations must be highly disciplined. For instance, indinavir must be taken on an empty stomach, every eight hours, not less than two hours before or after a meal, and with large amounts of water to prevent the development of kidney stones. Patients must also be careful to never skip doses of indinavir, otherwise HIV will quickly grow immune to its effect. (Indinavir has been found to generate cross-resistance, meaning it makes patients resistant to other PIs.) Saquinavir mesylate must be taken in large doses. Ritonavir must be carefully prescribed and administered because it interacts negatively with some antifungals and antibiotics used by AIDS patients. Because there are many minor and serious risks that are associated with use of these drugs, patients must be closely monitored.

When effective AIDS drugs were introduced, patients sometimes had to wake up during the middle of the night to take pills, and some treatment regimens consisted of as many as 50 or 60 pills administered several times a day. Even with intense pressure to simplify treatment regimens, pharmaceutical companies remained skeptical about an effective once-a-day pill despite the consensus opinion that it would help more people start, and stick with, treatment. Even as recently as 2005, many combined HIV/AIDS medication regimens were administered two to three times per day. Once-a-day regimens were sought after, but were not available until 2006.

Once-a-Day AIDS Treatment

In July 2006 the FDA approved the first once-a-day AIDS treatment, a combination of efavirenz, tenofovir disoproxil fumarate, and emtricitabine. Even though this once-a-day drug combination reduces the number of pills a patient must take and as a result improves adherence to treatment, it is probably not the sole drug an AIDS patient needs. Many patients also require additional prescription medications to support their immune system and help them resist infection. As of August 2011, this was the only once-a-day AIDS treatment that had been approved by the FDA. However, other types of once-a-day combinations were under development.

THE DISCOVERY OF AN HIV-RESISTANT GENE

In August 1996 scientists working independently at the Aaron Diamond AIDS Research Center in New York City and the Free University of Brussels, Belgium, announced that some white (Caucasian) people have genes that may protect them from HIV, regardless of how many times they are exposed to the virus. The researchers hope their findings will lead to new HIV/AIDS therapies or to the development of drugs or vaccines to prevent HIV infection.

The researchers discovered that a gene called CCR5 is associated with HIV resistance. The gene codes for a protein called CC chemokine receptor 5 (CCR5) that is located on the surface of host cells including macrophages, monocytes, and T cells. HIV exploits this protein by using it as a receptor to bind to, and subsequently infect, cells such as T cells. The CCR5 mutation blocks the manufacture of CCR5. Thus, HIV loses its surface target and cannot invade the immune system.

Subsequent studies conducted in the United States found that one out of 100 people inherits two copies of this gene—one from each parent—and is completely immune to HIV infection. One out of five people with only one copy of the CCR5 gene can become infected, but will remain healthy two to three years longer than those without the altered gene. This may be because these people have half as many CCR5 receptors as normal, which limits or slows the spread of the virus.

According to Michael Fischereder et al., in "CC Chemokine Receptor 5 and Renal-Transplant Survival" (*Lancet*, vol. 357, no. 9270, June 2, 2001), the gene is most common in white Americans (10% to 15% of the population). It is rarely found in African-Americans and almost never in Asian-Americans, perhaps reflecting the origins of the mutation.

Certain populations appear to be resistant to HIV because they lack or have a mutated form of the CCR5 receptor. Most populations that carry the mutant CCR5 gene come from Europe, and there are indications that the mutation arose only about 700 years ago. For a mutation to be sustained in a population at a rate of 10%, there must be some benefit bestowed by the mutation. It is likely nothing to do with HIV, because HIV did not appear until the late 20th century.

The exact nature of the selective pressure that caused the appearance of the CCR5 mutation is the subject of considerable debate. The prevailing theory has been that the selective pressure was the bubonic plague; however, new research suggests that smallpox may have been the trigger. Which of these, if either, is true remains to be determined.

Research is also under way to learn more about other genes such as CCR2 that, when expressed dominantly, appears to slow the progression of AIDS. Vijay Kumar

et al. confirm in "Genetic Basis of HIV-1 Resistance and Susceptibility: An Approach to Understand Correlation between Human Genes and HIV-1 Infection" (*Indian Journal of Experimental Biology*, vol. 44, no. 9, September 2006) that site-specific mutations in these genes determine the susceptibility or resistance to HIV-1 infection and AIDS. Researchers hope that the study of host genes in relation to HIV-1 infection may speed the development of drug therapies to prevent or cure HIV-1 infection effectively.

OTHER RESEARCH LOOKS FOR PROTECTION AGAINST HIV INFECTION

A Natural Barrier to HIV

Olivier Schwartz of the Pasteur Institute identifies in "Langerhans Cells Lap up HIV-1" (*Nature Medicine*, vol. 13, no. 3, March 2007) a protein that acts as a natural barrier to HIV infection. The protein is called langerin, because it is produced by Langerhans cells, which form a network in the skin and mucosa (the membrane lining the vagina) and were previously thought to promote the spread of HIV. Instead, the Langerhans cells, which line the human genital tract, contain a protein that eats viruses. Langerin scavenges for viruses in the surrounding environment and thereby helps prevent infection. Langerhans cells do not become infected by HIV-1 because they have langerin on their surfaces. It appears that HIV infection occurs when levels of invading HIV are high or if langerin activity is especially weak. In either of these instances, Langerhans cells can become overwhelmed by the virus and infected.

In "Elevated Elafin/Trappin-2 in the Female Genital Tract Is Associated with Protection against HIV Acquisition" (*AIDS*, vol. 23, no. 13, August 24, 2009), Shehzad M. Iqbal et al. identify the protein elafin/trappin-2 as a novel innate immune factor that is strongly associated with HIV resistance. This innate immune factor was found in the mucosal secretions from the genital tracts of HIV-resistant women who are sex workers. Discovery of this factor enhances understanding of natural immunity to HIV infection.

Researchers are also looking at so-called elite suppressors, a small fraction (0.5%) of people who are infected with HIV that appear able to control infection without antiretroviral drugs. Erin H. Graf et al. find in "Elite Suppressors Harbor Low Levels of Integrated HIV DNA and High Levels of 2-LTR Circular HIV DNA Compared to HIV+ Patients on and off HAART" (*PLoS Pathogens*, vol. 7, no. 2, February 2011) that elite suppressors have much lower levels of HIV integrated into their immune cells than do HIV-infected people treated with antiretroviral drugs. This finding is believed to reflect the fact that elite suppressors mount a more effective immune response to HIV—meaning that their T cells more effectively combat the virus. The researchers posit that a vaccine that helps to generate killer T cells comparable to those in active elite suppressors might help others to more effectively combat infection.

Morning-After Treatment

HIV is classified as a communicable sexually transmitted disease in the United States. Some physicians prescribe the drugs that are used to treat established infections as "morning-after" pills in an attempt to prevent the transmission of the virus after risky sexual encounters. As of 2011, there was no scientific consensus on the validity of this approach, and the medications were not licensed for this use. Because some forms of HIV are halted by prompt use of the drugs, some doctors believe it is a worthwhile approach. Taryn Young et al. describe the results of a review of the medical literature on PEP in "Antiretroviral Post-exposure Prophylaxis (PEP) for Occupational HIV Exposure" (*Cochrane Database of Systematic Reviews*, no. 1, January 24, 2007) and conclude that "there is no direct evidence to support the use of multi-drug antiretroviral regimens following occupational exposure to HIV. However, due to the success of combination therapies in treating HIV-infected individuals, a combination of antiretroviral drugs should be used for PEP."

This "off-label" use of potent PIs in an attempt to prevent the spread of HIV is controversial. All the drugs that are used in the treatment of HIV have side effects, some of which may be potentially life threatening. PIs may cause high blood sugar and diabetes, lipodytrophy (problems with fat metabolism that can result in dangerously high cholesterol levels), and liver problems. Furthermore, some researchers fear that if people believe morning-after treatment will prevent HIV infection, they may stop taking precautions, such as using condoms, to prevent exposure to HIV. Others feel that the treatment is not appropriate as a preventive measure for people who are exposed to ongoing risk, such as relationships where only one partner is infected, because the drugs are too toxic. Other methods, such as the continued use of condoms, would be much safer.

Finally, postexposure treatment is expensive. The costs of two or three drugs taken for a month, plus laboratory tests and visits to the doctor, may cost more than $1,000. Of course, this is a fraction of the cost for lifetime treatment of HIV infection and certainly money well spent if it prevents a person from acquiring the virus.

In "Antiretroviral Therapy for Prevention of HIV Transmission in HIV-Discordant Couples" (*Cochrane Database of Systemic Review*, May 11, 2011), a meta-analysis of seven studies, Andrew Anglemyer et al. find that antiretroviral drugs may prevent the transmission of HIV from an infected person to an uninfected sexual partner by suppressing viral replication. In couples in which the infected partner was taking antiretroviral drugs, the unin-

fected partner had more than five times the lower risk of becoming infected than in couples where the infected partner was not receiving antiretroviral treatment.

Charlie Sayer et al. suggest in "Will I? Won't I? Why Do Men Who Have Sex with Men Present for Post-exposure Prophylaxis for Sexual Exposures?" (*Sexually Transmitted Infections*, vol. 85, no. 3, June 2008) that morning-after treatment has the potential to save lives. The drugs themselves will save some lives, and the offer of treatment will bring people who are at high risk for acquiring HIV into environments where they can get counseling and care. In San Francisco postexposure treatment is offered to victims of rape as a matter of course. Some doctors feel that if the treatment does not work to prevent the disease, it may work to at least treat it as early as possible. Even though there is disagreement about the effectiveness and wisdom of widespread use of postexposure treatment, nearly all researchers and health care providers agree that for sexually active people the best prevention is the use of condoms.

Topical Drugs to Block HIV Infection

In recent years there have been many efforts to develop topical microbicides—preparations to prevent HIV infection. Anita B. Garg, Jeremy Nuttall, and Joseph Romano report in "The Future of HIV Microbicides: Challenges and Opportunities" (*Antiviral Chemistry and Chemotherapy*, vol. 19, no. 4, 2009) that as of 2009 a safe and effective microbicide had not yet been identified; however, ongoing clinical trials of "vaginal gels containing non-specific compounds" had met with some success. One of the potential drawbacks of these gels is that they must be applied close to the time of sexual intercourse to be optimally effective.

THE PROMISE OF GENE THERAPY

In 2011 researchers reported progress using genetic engineering techniques to create HIV-resistant blood cells. This effort was inspired by the apparent cure of Timothy Rae Brown after he received a transplant of blood stem cells in 2007 to treat the leukemia (cancer of the blood cells) he had in addition to his AIDS diagnosis. Brown's physician, Gero Huetter, knew that the best chance of curing the leukemia was with a blood stem cell transplant, so he searched for a donor who was not only a tissue match for Brown but was also among the 1% of people with gene mutations that confer resistance to HIV. In preparation for the transplant, Brown was given chemotherapy and radiation treatment to destroy his immune system so that he would not reject the donor blood stem cells. Remarkably, four years after the procedure Brown was still disease free—there was no evidence of HIV in his body and he no longer required antiretroviral drug treatment. Even though this treatment is not feasible for everyone with HIV/AIDS—because it is physically grueling, involves considerable risk, and is prohibitively expensive—it offers tantalizing clues about new approaches for HIV/AIDS treatment.

IN SEARCH OF A VACCINE

Some pharmaceutical companies claim that the high costs of R&D and the relatively low return on their investments (because the period of patent protection is limited to seven years) leave little financial incentive to develop new HIV/AIDS drugs. The development of such drugs is, for better or worse, an economically driven, rather than strictly humanitarian, enterprise. Similarly, the companies allege that they have little economic motivation to research and develop HIV vaccines. In February 1996 Anthony S. Fauci (1940–), the head of the National Institute for Allergies and Infectious Diseases (NIAID), issued guidelines to promote cooperation between the government and private industry. The plan's goal was to overcome the alleged unfavorable market forces that have caused some companies to abandon research of potential HIV vaccines.

Such vaccine efforts continue. In the press release "HVTN 505 HIV Vaccine Study Begins Enrolling Volunteers" (August 24, 2009, http://www.niaid.nih.gov/news/newsreleases/2009/pages/hvtn505.aspx), the NIAID and the international HIV Vaccine Trials Network announced in 2009 the enrollment in HVTN 505, an exploratory HIV vaccine clinical study. In 2011 the study was under way in 12 cities and involved approximately 1,350 HIV-negative men aged 18 to 45 years. Half of the study participants received the investigational vaccine regimen and the other half were given placebo (an inactive substance that does not contain a drug) injections. The investigational vaccine consists of a series of three immunizations with a recombinant DNA-based vaccine over the course of eight weeks followed by a single immunization in week 24 with a recombinant vaccine that uses a weakened adenovirus as a carrier.

According to ClinicalTrials.gov (2011, http://www.clinicaltrials.gov/ct2/results?term=HIV+vaccine), a service of the NIH, as of August 2011 there were 555 studies researching various aspects of HIV vaccines. Of these, 123 were actively seeking new volunteers to serve as study subjects.

The design of the vaccines under trial varies. Some vaccines use a weakened and medically safe version of viruses as a delivery vehicle to carry various HIV genes into the human participants. The hope is that antibody production of the HIV-critical proteins encoded by these genes will occur and that this production will offer protection from HIV infection. Other vaccines use a DNA plasmid to ferry HIV genes into the human participants; the aim again is to stimulate antibody production.

There are experimental design challenges and ethical considerations involved in vaccine trials using human

FIGURE 6.1

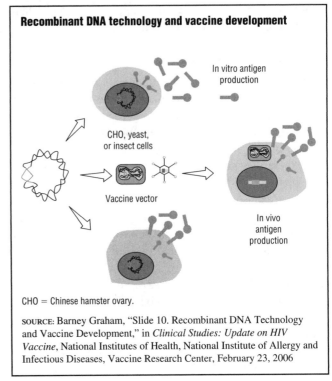

Recombinant DNA technology and vaccine development

In vitro antigen production

CHO, yeast, or insect cells

Vaccine vector

In vivo antigen production

CHO = Chinese hamster ovary.

SOURCE: Barney Graham, "Slide 10. Recombinant DNA Technology and Vaccine Development," in *Clinical Studies: Update on HIV Vaccine*, National Institutes of Health, National Institute of Allergy and Infectious Diseases, Vaccine Research Center, February 23, 2006

volunteers. Vaccines may be made using recombinant DNA technology—DNA that has been altered by joining genetic material from two different sources. Figure 6.1 shows how recombinant DNA is used to develop vaccines. Even though some recombinant technology uses live attenuated virus (virus that is genetically altered so it is less virulent), this is not feasible with HIV because it would be unwise to create any risk of infection. The challenges are to elicit cell-mediated immune responses against HIV and the need for a balanced immune response consisting of not only cellular immunity but also a broad and strong antibody response that can prevent infection with HIV. Concerning ethical considerations, most volunteers for a vaccine have behaviors that put them at risk for contracting HIV. Some may mistakenly believe that participating in the clinical trial of an experimental vaccine—which may be a vaccine or a placebo—protects them and, with a false sense of security, they may resume high-risk behaviors.

Despite optimistic projections during the early 1990s that a vaccine would be found in a few years, a considerable number of promising experimental HIV vaccines have proven ineffective against strains of HIV taken from infected people. Researchers reported developing antibodies that worked successfully against HIV grown in test tubes, but in every case they failed when used against HIV in human beings. As of August 2011, none of the candidate vaccines had shown sufficient promise in clinical trials to warrant its approval, manufacture, and widespread use.

The First Large-Scale Human Vaccine Trials

In "F.D.A. Authorizes First Full Testing for H.I.V. Vaccine" (*New York Times*, June 4, 1998), Lawrence K. Altman reports that in 1998 the FDA granted permission to VaxGen to conduct the first full-scale test of a vaccine to prevent HIV infection. The VaxGen vaccine—a genetically engineered molecule called AIDSvax—had been found "safe in tests involving 1,200 uninfected volunteers beginning in March 1992 and induced production of antibodies in more than 99 percent of the vaccinated participants." The 1998 test involved 5,000 volunteers in 40 clinics throughout the United States and Canada and 2,500 volunteers in 16 clinics in Thailand.

AIDSvax is made from part of HIV's outer coat, specifically a molecule called gp120. The molecule functions in the attachment of the virus to host cells. The vaccine does not contain the intact virus, only the gp120 protein from two strains of HIV. (Previous vaccines used one strain.) The two strains of the vaccine that were tested in North America were made with strains common in North America. The vaccine used in Thailand contained strains common to that part of the world. Participants in the North American study were men who have sex with men and uninfected partners of HIV-positive people. In Thailand, volunteers were uninfected injection drug users. Two-thirds of the North American volunteers were given the vaccine, and the rest received a placebo. In Thailand, half the group received the vaccine and half were given a placebo. The four-year trial ended in 2002.

The trial results were reported in February 2003. David R. Baker explains in "Vaccine Has No Impact, AIDSVAX's Failure a Blow to Treatment" (*San Francisco Chronicle*, November 13, 2003) that AIDSvax was determined to be a failure, as the comparison of those who received the vaccine versus those receiving a placebo demonstrated a slight reduction in new HIV infections in the vaccine population. Surprisingly, Asian-Americans and African-Americans who received the vaccine displayed a lower rate of infection than their racial counterparts who received the placebo. Considerable debate has arisen concerning these latter observations. Was this a statistical fluke? Or did AIDSvax display demographically specific protection, and if so, why?

Even though health officials and AIDS activists are hopeful, scientists are divided over when and which experimental vaccines should be approved for full-scale testing. Some favor trying any promising vaccine, whereas others advise waiting until the vaccine is completely understood before testing it. The results of the AIDSvax trial could sway this argument toward the latter camp.

One potential problem with AIDSvax, and perhaps a partial explanation of the poor overall results, is that previous tests indicated that it boosted only one part of the immune system—the component of the immune system that is responsible for antibody production. It is generally believed that a truly effective anti-HIV vaccine must boost another part of the immune system: the killer T cells that destroy virus-infected cells. Some experts consider the vaccine a long shot, but others point out that a failed vaccine does not mean that the experiment failed. Negative results can teach researchers what not to do in the future.

In 2011 another vaccine trial reported disappointing results. According to Glenda E. Gray et al., in "Safety and Efficacy of the HVTN 503/Phambili Study of a Clade-B-Based HIV-1 Vaccine in South Africa: A Double-Blind, Randomised, Placebo-Controlled Test-of-Concept Phase 2b Study" (*Lancet Infectious Diseases*, vol. 11, no. 7, July 2011), researchers conducted a clinical trial in South Africa with a vaccine that was designed to elicit T-cell-mediated immune responses capable of providing complete or partial protection from HIV-1 infection or a decrease in viral load after acquisition. When the researchers compiled the results following the completion of the trial, they determined that the vaccine failed to accomplish either of these objectives. Gray et al. opine that there are lessons to be learned from such trials, noting that "this is now the third study in human beings that has failed after initial successful data from studies in non-human primates, highlighting once again that human HIV-1 vaccines should not be based simply on non-human primate models. We should still strive for innovative strategies that prevent HIV, despite the success of antiretroviral drugs in those for whom they are available. It would not be surprising if further prophylactic studies yielded new mechanistic and therapeutic insights outside the remit of the initial endpoints, ultimately enabling the eradication of HIV."

Vaccine Research Center

In 2000 the Dale and Betty Bumpers Vaccine Research Center (VRC; http://www.niaid.nih.gov/about/organization/vrc/Pages/default.aspx) opened on the NIH campus in Bethesda, Maryland. The facility brings together private companies and federal agencies to research, develop, and produce vaccines. The VRC is not exclusively devoted to HIV research and works to develop vaccines for other diseases.

Johannes F. Scheid et al. report in "Broad Diversity of Neutralizing Antibodies Isolated from Memory B Cells in HIV-Infected Individuals" (*Nature*, vol. 458, no. 7238, April 2, 2009) that they made progress in the development of an AIDS vaccine. The researchers looked at HIV patients who progress very slowly to AIDS because they have a range of neutralizing antibodies that identify and attack the virus. The researchers isolated 433 neutralizing antibodies from the blood of these slow-to-progress HIV patients and uncovered how the antibodies disarm the virus.

In 2011 a study that was directed by NIAID researchers uncovered another genetic mechanism of protection that may be helpful in the design of an HIV vaccine for humans. The researchers administered to monkeys a vaccine made from DNA that encodes immunodeficiency virus proteins, followed by a booster vaccine containing an inactivated cold virus (adenovirus) and immunodeficiency virus proteins to help protect monkeys from simian immunodeficiency virus (the monkey analog of HIV). Norman L. Letvin et al. find in "Immune and Genetic Correlates of Vaccine Protection against Mucosal Infection by SIV in Monkeys" (*Science Translational Medicine*, vol. 3, no. 81, May 4, 2011) that neutralizing antibodies are a key component of the immune response needed to prevent HIV infection. This finding may help future vaccine development efforts.

Most researchers are optimistic that an effective vaccine will be developed, but many believe that perfecting a vaccine will take years. Researchers at the VRC believe that more than one vaccine formulation, or a vaccine that works two ways—to boost immunity provided by T cells and to produce antibodies to attach to HIV and mark it for destruction—may be necessary to provide complete protection.

On March 31, 2011, the VRC celebrated its 10th anniversary by recounting the progress that has been made in the search for a safe, effective HIV vaccine. In "30 Years of HIV/AIDS: A Personal Journey" (May 31, 2011, http://www.niaid.nih.gov/news/events/meetings/2011hivaids/Pages/default.aspx), a statement to commemorate the 30th anniversary of the first reported cases of HIV infection, Fauci recounted the early years of AIDS, when none of his patients survived; the increasing awareness of the global proportions and demographics of the epidemic; the discovery of HIV as the cause of AIDS; the development of lifesaving antiretroviral medications; and ongoing efforts to find new ways to prevent, treat, and cure HIV infection.

In September 2009 the World Health Organization and the Joint United Nations Program on HIV/AIDS heralded the report of promising results of an experimental vaccine that combines two previously unsuccessful ones. A study involving more than 16,000 volunteers in Thailand found that the combination vaccine reduced the risk of becoming infected with AIDS by about one-third of the volunteers. According to the article "A World First: Vaccine Helps Prevent HIV Infection" (Associated Press, September 24, 2009), Fauci said the results of the study gave him "'cautious optimism about the possibility of improving this result' and developing a more effective AIDS vaccine."

In a statement that was issued to commemorate HIV Vaccine Awareness Day, May 18, 2011, Fauci (http://www.nih.gov/news/health/may2011/niaid-11.htm) reflected that the 2009 trial in Thailand "demonstrated for the first time that a vaccine could safely prevent HIV infection in a modest proportion of study participants." He observed that the data from the trial were informing researchers' efforts to improve the efficacy (the ability of an intervention to produce the intended diagnostic or therapeutic effect in optimal circumstances) of this vaccine candidate. Fauci explained that, "in most individuals, only a small number of HIV particles—often just one—are responsible for establishing a sexually transmitted HIV infection. These researchers are identifying the unique qualities of these infection-causing forms of the virus to help other scientists design vaccines that target the specific HIV variants that penetrate the body's defenses."

CHAPTER 7
PEOPLE WITH HIV/AIDS

Large numbers of people are afflicted with HIV/AIDS in the United States. An increasing proportion of the population lives with HIV infection. At the end of the first decade of the 21st century more Americans than ever before are likely to know someone who is affected by HIV or AIDS. Even people who live in remote geographic areas and do not believe they are personally at risk of acquiring HIV are aware of the epidemic from ongoing public health education campaigns, reports in the media, school health programs, and health and social service agencies, all of which are dedicated to improving community awareness of HIV/AIDS.

PUBLIC FIGURES WITH HIV/AIDS

Perhaps one of the most famous HIV-infected people in the world is Earvin Johnson Jr. (1959–), better known as Magic Johnson, an internationally known former basketball player for the Los Angeles Lakers. When Johnson announced his HIV infection in November 1991, the world was shocked. He had no idea he was infected until he received the results of a routine physical examination for life insurance. Johnson freely admitted that before his marriage he had unprotected sexual contact with many women. He had no idea who transmitted the virus to him. The possibility exists that, however unknowingly, he passed the virus on to one or more subsequent sexual partners, who in turn, passed it on to others.

To many, Johnson became a hero for his courage and immediate public acknowledgment of his HIV status. He became an HIV/AIDS spokesperson and began working in prevention programs. In 1991 he started the Magic Johnson Foundation, which seeks to fund and establish community-based education and social and health programs (including HIV/AIDS awareness) in inner-city communities. He has given millions of dollars in grants to these causes. Johnson was even named to the President's Commission on AIDS, from which he eventually resigned, frustrated with the lack of progress in HIV/AIDS efforts by the administration of George H. W. Bush (1924–).

Despite his active, well-publicized efforts to increase awareness and prevention of HIV/AIDS, some people considered Johnson anything but a hero because his highly visible, promiscuous lifestyle sent the wrong message to the millions of young people who admired him.

In September 1992, 10 months after Johnson announced his retirement from professional basketball, he indicated that he was returning to basketball on a limited basis. He played on the U.S. "Dream Team" during the 1992 Summer Olympics, assisting the team in its successful bid for a gold medal. Johnson benched himself at the start of the 1993–94 season, when he cut himself in a preseason game, terrifying some of his fellow players. Some players feared infection, whereas others worried that they should not play against Johnson with full force; after all, he was a man with a fatal disease. Johnson retired again but then returned for the end of the 1995–96 season, helping his team reach the play-offs. He retired for a third and final time after that season, but he continues to play basketball with the Magic Johnson All-Stars Team. He shows others, as one observer notes, that HIV infection is not a certain death sentence, but a condition with which one can live.

In 1992 the former tennis star Arthur Ashe (1943–1993) announced that he had become infected with HIV from a blood transfusion in the mid-1980s during a heart bypass operation. His was not a voluntary announcement, but one made necessary when the news media discovered his HIV infection and threatened to announce it before he did. Ashe was reluctant to make his condition public, fearing the effect on his five-year-old daughter. He maintained that because he did not have a public responsibility, he should have been allowed to maintain his privacy. He died of pneumonia, a complication of AIDS, in 1993.

The diver Greg Louganis (1960–), who competed in the 1976, 1984, and 1988 Olympic games, was diagnosed with HIV infection in 1988, before his competition in the 1988 games. During the games, Louganis hit his head on the diving board while competing. Even though his injury was not serious, it did result in an open wound—making Louganis concerned that his blood might have entered the pool. However, Louganis did not reveal his HIV status at the time. The Olympic gold medalist announced that he had HIV in 1995. Louganis now competes in dog agility competitions with his dogs, is a published author of two books, and began coaching athletes in diving in 2010. He advocates safe sexual practices, because he attributes his HIV infection to unsafe sexual behavior.

Other sports figures diagnosed with HIV infection include Rudy Galindo (1969–), an American figure skater who earned a bronze medal at the 1996 world championships, and Roy Simmons (1956–), an American athlete who played for the National Football League.

Another sports celebrity who succumbed to AIDS was the National Association for Stock Car Auto Racing (NASCAR) racecar driver Tim Richmond (1955–1989). During his heyday on the NASCAR race circuit in the 1980s, Richmond was one of the circuit's premier drivers. He was also well known for his expensive tastes and playboy lifestyle. Whether his lifestyle contributed to his illness is conjecture. Nonetheless, by the end of the 1986 racing season Richmond had become noticeably ill. He was diagnosed with AIDS that same year. He was able to race again in 1987, but soon thereafter his health deteriorated precipitously. During another attempted comeback in 1988, when his illness was still unpublicized, Richmond faced the hostility and innuendo of his fellow drivers, who, guessing the nature of the illness, speculated about his sexual orientation and the possibility of drug abuse. In response, Richmond filed a defamation of character lawsuit against NASCAR. He subsequently withdrew the lawsuit to avoid making his condition public. Richmond ultimately retired from competitive racing and lived in seclusion with his mother until his death. After his death, as news of his illness and the treatment he received from his fellow drivers and NASCAR became public, many people were outraged at the NASCAR organization, which as of August 2011 had not apologized.

Mary Fisher (1948–), a heterosexual and nondrug user who contracted HIV from her husband, stood before her peers during the 1992 Republican National Convention and announced that she was infected with HIV. A former television producer and assistant to President Gerald R. Ford (1913–2006), she said she considered her announcement part of her contribution to the fight against HIV/AIDS. The wealthy and well-educated Fisher was among the first women to publicly dispel the image that still comes to mind when many people think of HIV/ AIDS: homosexual, poor, drug addicted, and lacking access to support systems or adequate medical care and housing.

Fisher established the Mary Fisher Clinical AIDS Research and Education Fund at the University of Alabama, Birmingham, in 2000. She is an accomplished artist, public speaker, and author of four books. In 2006 Peter Piot (1949–), the former under secretary-general of the United Nations, appointed Fisher to a two-year term as a special representative of the Joint United Nations Program on HIV/ AIDS, which Piot directed.

The actor Anthony Perkins (1932–1992), who is best known for his role as Norman Bates in the classic Alfred Hitchcock (1899–1980) film *Psycho* (1960), also died of AIDS. Forever typecast by that performance, Perkins was in fact an accomplished film and stage actor. He was bisexual and had relationships with a number of men, including the dancer Rudolf Nureyev (1938–1993), who also died of AIDS. Shortly before his death in 1992, Perkins commented in a press release about a *National Enquirer* article that revealed his AIDS-positive status by saying, "I have learned more about love, selflessness, and human understanding from the people I have met in this great adventure in the world of AIDS than I ever did in the cutthroat, competitive world in which I spent my life." Perkins's widow, Berry Berenson (1948–2001), was one of the passengers on American Airlines Flight 11, which was hijacked and crashed into the World Trade Center on September 11, 2001.

Another movie star who succumbed to AIDS was Rock Hudson (1925–1985). Indeed, Hudson was the first major U.S. celebrity known to have died from AIDS. His death was especially noteworthy, given his status during the 1950s as the quintessential rugged, all-American male. Despite his many movie roles as a leading man opposite many beautiful actresses, Hudson was homosexual, a fact that was covered up by movie studios. His 1955 marriage to the studio employee Phyllis Gates (1925–2006), which ended in divorce in 1958, is thought to have been a studio-orchestrated attempt to cover up his sexual orientation. Hudson died at the age of 59.

The African-American rap star Eazy-E (c. 1963–1995) rose to fame as one of the members of the group N.W.A. (Niggaz with Attitude), based in Compton, California. Using money obtained from illegal drug sales, Eazy-E founded Ruthless Records. Soon after, he recruited Ice Cube (1969–), Dr. Dre (1965–), MC Ren (1969–), DJ Yella (1967–), and Arabian Prince (1965–) to form N.W.A. Following the dissolution of N.W.A., Eazy-E went on to have a successful solo career. In 1995 he entered the hospital for treatment of what he thought was asthma. However, he was diagnosed with AIDS and died soon after. Eazy-E is now regarded as one of the influential founders of the style of music known as gangsta rap. Every year, the city of Compton celebrates his life by observing Eazy-E Day.

Another music icon who died of AIDS was Freddie Mercury (1946–1991), the lead vocalist of the British rock band Queen. His more than three-octave vocal range and operatic compositional approach to rock resulted in classic hits such as "Bohemian Rhapsody," "Somebody to Love," and "We Are the Champions." The video made for the 1975 release of "Bohemian Rhapsody" is considered by some music insiders to be one of the decisive influences that spurred the popularity of music videos. Mercury was well known for his extravagance and bisexuality. His diagnosis and deteriorating physical condition were kept private. Indeed, his eventual announcement that he had AIDS was made only one day before his death in 1991.

Elizabeth Glaser (1947–1994), the wife of the actor Paul Michael Glaser (1943–), was motivated to cofound the Pediatric AIDS Foundation in 1988 (now called the Elizabeth Glaser Pediatric AIDS Foundation), following the discovery that she and her children, Ariel (1981–1988) and Jake (1984–), were all infected with HIV. She originally contracted the virus from contaminated blood that was administered during pregnancy, but she was unaware of her illness until much later, already having unwittingly passed it to her children. In the ensuing years she became a vocal AIDS activist. The foundation that is her legacy contributes more than $1 million annually to pediatric AIDS research. Ariel died at the age of seven, and Elizabeth died in 1994. Because Jake has a mutation of the CCR5 gene that delays onset by restricting the virus's ability to enter white blood cells, he remains symptom free and no longer takes HIV medication. He and Paul continue to raise money and AIDS awareness through Elizabeth's foundation.

Finally, in a list of examples that is by no means complete, the prolific and influential science-fiction author Isaac Asimov (1920–1992) contracted HIV from infected blood that was given to him in a transfusion during heart bypass surgery in 1983. He died in 1992 of heart and renal failure that were complications of AIDS.

OLDER PEOPLE WITH HIV/AIDS

In "AIDS among Persons Aged Greater Than or Equal to 50 Years—United States, 1991–1996" (*Morbidity and Mortality Weekly Report*, vol. 47, no. 2, January 23, 1998), the Centers for Disease Control and Prevention (CDC) reports that most older people infected with HIV early in the epidemic were typically infected through contaminated blood or blood products. Through 1989 only 1% of HIV/ AIDS cases of people aged 13 to 49 years was due to contaminated blood. However, during this same period 6% of cases of people aged 50 to 59 years, 28% of cases of people aged 60 to 69 years, and 64% of cases of those aged 70 years and older resulted from contaminated blood or blood products.

In 1985 changes introduced to improve the safety of the nation's blood supply, including routine screening of blood donations for HIV, sharply reduced the risk of contracting the virus from contaminated blood or blood products. Subsequently, the proportion of people aged 50 years and older who acquired HIV from other types of exposure increased. Even though male-to-male sexual contact and injection drug use remain the primary means by which HIV is transmitted among all age groups in the United States, heterosexual transmission of HIV is steadily increasing in people more than 50 years old.

HIV/AIDS Cases among People Aged 45 Years and Older

The CDC notes in "HIV/AIDS among Persons Aged 50 and Older" (February 2008, http://www.cdc.gov/Hiv/topics/over50/resources/factsheets/pdf/over50.pdf) that in 2005, 15% of new HIV/AIDS cases reported in the United States occurred in people over the age of 50 years. Nearly a quarter (24%) of people living with HIV/AIDS were over the age of 50 years, up from 17% in 2001. The proportion of adults over the age of 50 years with HIV/ AIDS is expected to increase as HIV-infected people of all ages live longer as a result of effective drug therapy and other advances in medical treatment.

Through 2009 an estimated 276,108 cases of AIDS in people over the age of 45 years had been reported. (See Table 3.1 in Chapter 3.) Of these reported cases, 126,380 (46% of the cumulative total) were among people aged 45 to 49 years, 72,327 (26%) were among people aged 50 to 54 years, 39,025 (14%) were among people aged 55 to 59 years, 20,633 (8%) were among people aged 60 to 64 years, and 17,743 (6%) were among people aged 65 years and older.

HIV Testing for Those over 50

Many older adults do not seek routine screening for HIV infection because they do not believe they are at risk of acquiring HIV. Figure 7.1 shows that in 2010 the lowest rates of testing among adults over the age of 18 years were among people aged 65 years and older—just 13.3% of older adults had ever been tested for HIV, compared to well over half of those aged 25 to 34 years and 35 to 44 years and more than one-third of people aged 45 to 64 years. Among women over the age of 50 years, the absence of the risk of pregnancy may lead to a false sense of security and the mistaken belief that they are at less risk for sexually transmitted diseases, including HIV. HIV-infected people aged 50 years and older may not be tested promptly for HIV infection. As a result, opportunities to start these patients on therapies to slow the progression of the disease are often lost. The failure to test or the late testing of older patients may be because:

- Physicians are less apt to look for HIV in people of this age group.

- Some opportunistic AIDS illnesses that occur in older people, such as encephalopathy (any of various

FIGURE 7.1

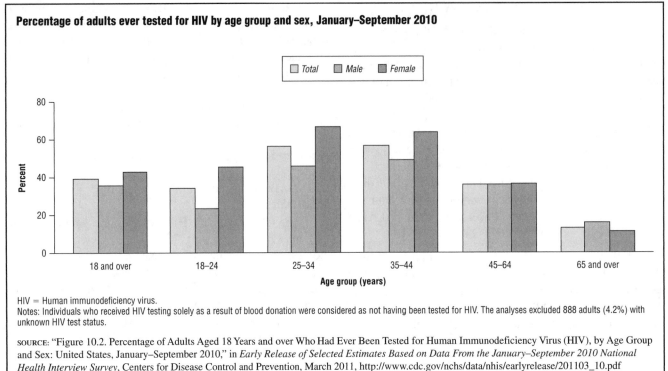

Percentage of adults ever tested for HIV by age group and sex, January–September 2010

HIV = Human immunodeficiency virus.
Notes: Individuals who received HIV testing solely as a result of blood donation were considered as not having been tested for HIV. The analyses excluded 888 adults (4.2%) with unknown HIV test status.

SOURCE: "Figure 10.2. Percentage of Adults Aged 18 Years and over Who Had Ever Been Tested for Human Immunodeficiency Virus (HIV), by Age Group and Sex: United States, January–September 2010," in *Early Release of Selected Estimates Based on Data From the January–September 2010 National Health Interview Survey*, Centers for Disease Control and Prevention, March 2011, http://www.cdc.gov/nchs/data/nhis/earlyrelease/201103_10.pdf (accessed June 16, 2011)

diseases of the brain) and wasting disease, have similar symptoms to other diseases that are associated with aging, such as Alzheimer's disease (a progressive form of dementia that is characterized by impairment of memory and intellectual functions), depression, and malignancies.

It is vitally important to overcome older adults' reluctance to seek testing and other delays to diagnosis because research shows that age speeds the progression of HIV to AIDS and blunts CD4 response to highly active antiretroviral therapy. Equally important is continuing the research to improve the treatment of HIV-infected older adults and the development of effective education programs to prevent infection in this population.

LIVING WITH HIV/AIDS

To gain a more complete view of the impact of HIV/AIDS, it is important to understand the psychosocial and emotional consequences of diagnosis with a potentially fatal disease.

A Frightening Diagnosis

In the introduction to *When Someone Close Has AIDS: Acquired Immunodeficiency Syndrome* (1989), Lewis L. Judd, the former director of the National Institute of Mental Health, writes about the meaning of the diagnosis of AIDS. It means not only a shortened life but also one that is "marred by chronic fatigue, loss of appetite and weight,

frequent hospitalizations, AIDS dementia, and debilitating bouts of illness from unusual infections." The person who is diagnosed with HIV/AIDS often also feels anger, confusion, depression, isolation, and hopelessness, which can affect those around him or her who are often unprepared for the suffering they witness.

Judd explains that people who are diagnosed with HIV/AIDS need support and reassurance from friends and relatives that they will not be abandoned or isolated. He also recommends that those around HIV/AIDS patients encourage them to pursue hobbies, work as long as they can, and engage in social activities. Judd warns that caring for someone with AIDS is physically and emotionally exhausting and calls for inner strength, as well as the caregivers' coming to terms with their own feelings about the illness.

At the beginning of the second decade of the 21st century, Judd's advice is still sound. Even though HIV is no longer a certain death sentence, its diagnosis may still elicit feelings of fear, confusion, depression, and anger. Furthermore, researchers have identified another reason that people who are diagnosed with HIV infection require additional emotional support: there is an association between psychosocial stress and HIV disease progression. Yoichi Chida and Kavita Vedhara report in "Adverse Psychosocial Factors Predict Poorer Prognosis in HIV Disease: A Meta-analytic Review of Prospective Investigations" (*Brain, Behavior, and Immunity*, vol. 23, no. 4, May 2009) the results of a review of 36 articles describing the association between psychosocial factors such as personality types, coping styles, psychological distress, and HIV disease progression. The researchers find a strong relationship between adverse psychosocial factors such as difficulty coping with stress and HIV disease progression.

The 2011 release of *Aging with HIV: A Gay Man's Guide* by James Masten and James Schmidtberger offers guidance to the growing numbers of men who are living with HIV/AIDS. Masten and Schmidtberger address many of the issues that are related to aging with HIV/AIDS. They outline strategies for maintaining physical and emotional health and well-being and approaches to help men break unhealthy habits. They also offer examples of coping strategies that have worked for men, many of whom are surprised to have lived to midlife and old age and never dreamed they would have to plan for a future.

Coping with Discrimination

Unlike people who are diagnosed with other terminal or catastrophic illnesses such as cancer or multiple sclerosis, people with HIV/AIDS often confront the social isolation and discrimination that accompany a stigmatized status. Many people continue to mistakenly characterize HIV/AIDS as exclusively a disease of homosexual men and drug users and condemn HIV-infected people for inflicting themselves with the condition. Some still believe that AIDS is divine retribution for an "immoral lifestyle." The fear of unfavorable judgment keeps many infected individuals from disclosing their HIV infection to others, even friends and family. Others simply do not want the pity that is often extended to people with potentially fatal conditions. Still others worry that friends and family, fearing infection, will abandon them.

Under the Americans with Disabilities Act (ADA) of 1990, people infected with HIV and those diagnosed with AIDS are considered disabled and as such are subject to the antidiscrimination provisions of this landmark legislation. As a result, employers may not ask job applicants if they are HIV infected or have AIDS, nor can they require an HIV test of prospective employees. The only exceptions to this provision are those employers who can demonstrate that such questions or testing are job-related and absolutely necessary for the employer to conduct business.

More important, the ADA requires employers to make "reasonable accommodations" for disabled employees. Reasonable accommodation is an adjustment to a job or modification of the responsibilities or work environment that will enable the worker with a disability to gain equal employment opportunity. Examples include flexible work schedules to allow for medical appointments, treatments, and counseling and the provision of additional unpaid leave.

PRESIDENT PROCLAIMS JUNE 2011 AS LESBIAN, GAY, BISEXUAL, AND TRANSGENDER PRIDE MONTH. On May 31, 2011, President Barack Obama (1961–; http://www .whitehouse.gov/the-press-office/2011/05/31/presidential-proclamation-lesbian-gay-bisexual-and-transgender-pride-mon) issued a proclamation naming June 2011 as Lesbian, Gay, Bisexual, and Transgender (LGBT) Pride Month. He acknowledged the contributions of LGBT Americans and lauded their efforts to spur the nation to respond to the HIV/AIDS epidemic and their role in broadening the United States' response to HIV/AIDS worldwide. President Obama said, "Though we have made strides in combating this devastating disease, more work remains to be done, and I am committed to expanding access to HIV/AIDS prevention and care. Last year, I announced the first comprehensive National HIV/AIDS Strategy for the United States. This strategy focuses on combinations of evidence-based approaches to decrease new HIV infections in high risk communities, improve care for people living with HIV/AIDS, and reduce health disparities."

THE STIGMA OF AIDS. In "A Comparison of HIV Stigma and Discrimination in Five International Sites: The Influence of Care and Treatment Resources in High Prevalence Settings" (*Social Science and Medicine*, vol. 68, no. 12, June 2009), a study designed to examine HIV stigma and discrimination in five high prevalence settings, Suzanne Maman et al. observe that the factors that contribute to HIV stigma and discrimination include the fear of transmission, the fear of suffering and death, and the burden of caring for people with AIDS.

According to Maman et al., the family, access to antiretroviral drugs, and other resources offered some protection against HIV stigma and discrimination. Variation in the availability of health and social services designed to lessen the impact of HIV/AIDS helps explain differences in HIV stigma and discrimination across the settings. The researchers opine that "increasing access to treatment and care resources may function to lower HIV stigma, however, providing services is not enough." They also assert that it is necessary to develop "effective strategies to reduce HIV stigma as treatment and care resources are scaled up in the settings that are most heavily impacted by the HIV epidemic."

Three decades after the first diagnosis of AIDS and widespread public health and community education efforts to inform people about HIV infection and prevent the spread of HIV, ignorance and misunderstanding of HIV/AIDS persist. Health educators and HIV/AIDS activists stress the importance of intensified, ongoing education to destigmatize people who are affected by HIV/AIDS and prevent discrimination. Reducing the stigma that is associated with HIV/AIDS may also encourage individuals to get tested and, for those who are infected, begin treatment as soon as possible.

Because stigma, even among personnel who work with people with HIV/AIDS, persists, efforts to reduce it continue. The HIV/AIDS Stigma Program, which is funded by the Health Resource and Services Administration's HIV/AIDS Bureau, offers training programs that explore the stigma associated with HIV/AIDS. The programs, which are made available to staff employed by agencies and organizations funded by the Ryan White Comprehensive AIDS Resources Emergency Act of 1990, focus on:

- Defining stigma and its origins in society.

- The impact of stigma on an individual's decision-making process and how it deters him or her from seeking HIV testing and counseling services.

- How stigma affects access to care and disclosure of HIV-positive status.

Dealing with Emotions

Not unexpectedly, anger and depression are natural and common reactions to discovering that one is infected with HIV. Experts stress the importance of recognizing and expressing anger and depression; however, if these feelings become all consuming, they can prevent health- and life-improving actions. Many people with HIV/AIDS admit that sharing feelings with friends and family members and participating in support groups ease anguish and help generate more positive attitudes and actions.

Many HIV/AIDS sufferers report that the most difficult thing they had to do after being diagnosed with HIV was to inform people in their present or recent past whom they might have exposed to the virus. If the patient is unable to do this, a physician or public health official can notify present or former sexual partners without revealing the infected person's name.

Early Medication Improves Outlook and Protects against Spread of HIV

The earlier people learn of their infection, the earlier they can begin medical treatment to suppress the virus's destructive growth, delay the onset of AIDS symptoms, and extend life. Along with antiretroviral drugs there are medications that fight the life-threatening opportunistic infections that eventually may afflict people who are HIV infected. Even though these drugs cannot cure HIV infection, they have been shown to keep HIV/AIDS patients healthy and symptom free for increasingly longer periods.

In 2011 the results of an international study definitively concluded that prompt treatment of HIV infection, before a person develops symptoms, dramatically reduces the risk that the person with HIV will transmit the virus to a sexual partner. According to the article "Early HIV Therapy Protects against Virus Spread" (Associated Press, May 12, 2011), the study followed 1,763 couples in which one partner was HIV infected and the other was not. The study participants were from Botswana, Brazil, India, Kenya, Malawi, South Africa, Thailand, the United States, and Zimbabwe. Half of the couples received early treatment of the infected partner and the other half waited until the infected partner's CD4 cell count fell below 250 per cubic millimeter of blood or until symptoms appeared. Among the untreated couples, 28 previously uninfected partners were infected. Among the treated couples, just one previously uninfected person became infected. Anthony S. Fauci (1940–), the head of the National Institute for Allergies and Infectious Diseases, said the study's finding "promises to change practice worldwide."

Practicing Good Health Habits

Experts advise HIV-infected people to exercise and maintain a balanced diet with sufficient lean protein. Not only does exercise improve overall fitness and generate a sense of well-being but also it releases endorphins, which are natural substances produced by the brain that boost immunity, reduce stress, and elevate mood. People with HIV/AIDS are advised to avoid smoking, excessive alcohol consumption, and using illegal drugs, all of which can act to depress the immune system.

HOUSING PROBLEMS

The difficulty of finding affordable and appropriate housing can be an acute crisis for people living with HIV/AIDS. HIV-infected people need more than just a safe shelter that provides protection and comfort; they may also require a base from which to receive services, care, and support. Adherence to complicated medical regimens is challenging for many HIV-infected people, but for some homeless people it is nearly impossible.

Some individuals are homeless when they acquire the HIV infection, whereas others lose their home when they are no longer able to hold jobs or cannot afford to pay for health care and housing costs. The National AIDS Housing Coalition (NAHC) indicates in the fact sheet "Breaking the Link between Homelessness and HIV" (February 2011, http://www.nationalaidshousing.org/PDF/Factsheets-Homelessness.pdf) that:

- Housing status is a key factor affecting access to care and health behaviors among people with HIV/AIDS—housing assistance reduces HIV health risk behaviors, improves health outcomes, and reduces use of costly emergency and inpatient hospital services.

- Housing remains one of the greatest unmet needs of Americans with HIV/AIDS—at least half of all people with HIV/AIDS experience housing instability or homelessness.

- Even though about 500,000 households affected by HIV/AIDS will require some form of housing assistance during the course of their illness, the federal program Housing Opportunities for Persons with AIDS (HOPWA) serves less than 60,000 households per year.

In the fact sheet "Housing Is HIV Prevention" (February 2011, http://www.nationalaidshousing.org/PDF/Factsheets-Prevention.pdf), the NAHC describes the relationship between HIV risk and housing instability and homelessness. The more than 140,000 people with HIV/AIDS who are homeless or unstably housed are two to six times more likely to report recent illegal drug use and to have shared needles or engaged in high-risk sex. Homeless women were up to five times more likely to report drug use and high-risk sexual practices, many of which were attributable to coercion, abuse, victimization, and physical violence. In contrast, at-risk youth with stable housing were significantly more likely to practice safe sex and reported fewer sex partners.

According to the NAHC, in the fact sheet "Housing Is Cost-Effective HIV Prevention and Care" (February 2011, http://nationalaidshousing.org/PDF/Factsheets-Cost%20Effective.pdf), housing for people with HIV/AIDS not only saves lives but also saves money. The NAHC observes that housing assistance improves health outcomes, reduces utilization of emergency and other costly health services such as hospitalization by 57%, and reduces involvement with the criminal justice system. Each new HIV infection that is prevented saves an estimated $300,000 in lifetime health care costs.

SUICIDE

Depression is a common psychiatric problem among patients who are seriously ill with HIV/AIDS. Even though this is a normal grief response, the combination of alienation, hopelessness, guilt, and lack of self-esteem can lead some to contemplate and plan for suicide in search of lost dignity and control. Others counter that the real dignity is in seeing the disease to the end. Those who encourage people with HIV/AIDS to "stick it out" often see the disease as becoming increasingly manageable with drugs and improved treatment techniques.

Several factors make HIV/AIDS patients more likely to commit suicide. They may feel they are certain to die sooner than they expected and worry that their deaths will be prolonged and emotionally and physically painful. They may also be despondent about the prospects of losing their job, their insurance, or their home. Furthermore, they may be ostracized from society. Researchers find that factors that have a considerable impact on the quality of life include security, family, love, pleasurable activity, and freedom from pain, suffering, and debilitating disease. AIDS patients may lose all of these, or they may be consumed by the fear of losing vital capacities and freedoms. For some, suicide seems like a reasonable alternative; it offers an end to pain and suffering, insecurity, self-pity, dependency, and hopelessness.

William Breitbart et al. examine in "Impact of Treatment for Depression on Desire for Hastened Death in Patients with Advanced AIDS" (*Psychosomatics*, vol. 51, no. 2, March 2010) the impact of treatment for depression on advanced AIDS patients who expressed a desire for hastened death. The researchers interviewed 372 patients shortly after they were admitted to a palliative care unit (palliative care focuses on symptom relief rather than on cure) and reinterviewed them monthly for two months. Patients who were identified as depressed were treated with antidepressant medication and reinterviewed weekly. Breitbart et al. find that the desire for death was highly associated with depression and that it decreased dramatically in patients who responded to antidepressant treatment. In contrast, patients whose depression did not improve with treatment had little or no change in their desire for hastened death. Even though relief from symptoms of depression was not significantly associated with the use of antidepressant medication, patients receiving antidepressant drugs had the largest decreases in the desire for hastened death.

According to Pablo Aldaz et al., in "Mortality by Causes in HIV-Infected Adults: Comparison with the General Population" (*BMC Public Health*, May 11, 2011), people with HIV infection have higher mortality (deaths) than uninfected people of the same age and sex for many causes of death including suicide. The researchers analyzed deaths among HIV-infected people aged 20 to 59 years between 1999 and 2006 and compared mortality from the same causes in the general population. Aldaz et al. conclude that "in agreement with other studies, we found a high mortality from suicide among HIV-infected persons."

Highly active antiretroviral therapy has resulted in people aging with HIV. David E. Vance, Linda Moneyham, and Kenneth F. Far of the University of Alabama, Birmingham, note in "Suicidal Ideation in Adults Aging with HIV: Neurological and Cognitive Considerations" (*Journal of Psychosocial Nursing*, vol. 46, no. 11, November 2008) that older adults with HIV are more vulnerable to cognitive declines (impaired thinking and reasoning) than are older adults who are not infected. The researchers posit that stressors such as coping with neurological or cognitive changes that are associated with aging with HIV may result in increased levels of depression and thoughts of suicide.

The Physician's Role

During the 1990s there were heated debates, voter initiatives, and court decisions about the legalization of physician-assisted suicide. As of August 2011, only two states—Oregon (in 1994) and Washington (in 2008)—had legalized physician-assisted suicide. Oregon and Washington voters determined that the right to end one's own life is intensely personal and should not be forbidden by law. (Even though attempts and acts of suicide are no longer subject to criminal prosecution in the United States, aiding a suicide is considered a criminal offense.)

Both the public and physicians themselves are divided about the issue of physician-assisted suicide. People who support the practice believe that doctors should make their skills available to patients to end anguish and suffering. Those who oppose physician-assisted suicide argue that better end-of-life care—effective pain management, emotional and spiritual support, and widespread education to reduce anxiety about dying—may reduce the frequency of requests for physician-assisted suicide. Opponents also fear that the legal right to assist suicide can be misused or abused and that such abuses might victimize already vulnerable populations.

Some of opponents' worst fears about the practice of euthanasia are confirmed by Diane Martindale in "A Culture of Death" (*Scientific American*, vol. 292, no. 6, June 2005). Martindale describes the research of Russel Ogden, a former Canadian graduate student in criminology who interviewed 17 people—social workers, physicians, counselors, nurses, and two priests—about their efforts to help AIDS patients kill themselves. Ogden found that half of the assisted suicides were botched and ultimately resulted in increased suffering and even failed attempts. However, this did not prompt Ogden to renounce the practice of assisted suicide. Instead, he asserted that "without medical supervision and formal regulations, euthanasia is happening in horrific circumstances, similar to back-alley abortions."

The June 2011 death of Jack Kevorkian (1928–2011), the outspoken advocate of assisted suicide who spent eight years in prison for helping ailing patients to end their lives, reignited public debate about this controversial issue. According to Lydia Saad of the Gallup Organization, in *Doctor-Assisted Suicide Is Moral Issue Dividing Americans Most* (May 31, 2011, http://www.gallup.com/poll/147842/Doctor-Assisted-Suicide-Moral-Issue-Dividing-Americans.aspx), a poll that was conducted just prior to Kevorkian's death found Americans divided about the moral acceptability of physician-assisted suicide. Forty-five percent of poll respondents deemed it morally acceptable and 48% said it is morally wrong. Public opinion about this issue has not changed significantly since 2001. (See Figure 7.2.)

FIGURE 7.2

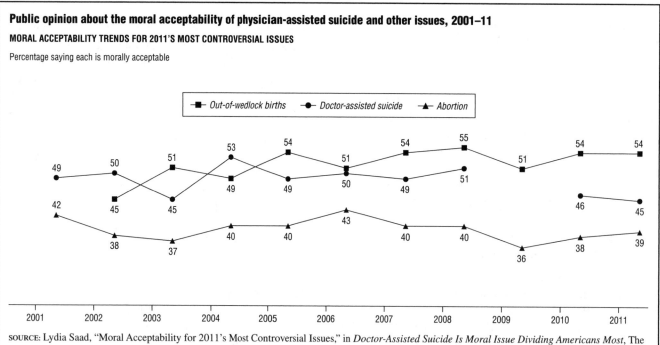

Public opinion about the moral acceptability of physician-assisted suicide and other issues, 2001–11

MORAL ACCEPTABILITY TRENDS FOR 2011'S MOST CONTROVERSIAL ISSUES

Percentage saying each is morally acceptable

SOURCE: Lydia Saad, "Moral Acceptability for 2011's Most Controversial Issues," in *Doctor-Assisted Suicide Is Moral Issue Dividing Americans Most*, The Gallup Organization, May 31, 2011, http://www.gallup.com/poll/147842/Doctor-Assisted-Suicide-Moral-Issue-Dividing-Americans.aspx (accessed June 16, 2011). Copyright © 2011 by The Gallup Organization. Reproduced by permission of the Gallup Organization.

CHAPTER 8
TESTING, PREVENTION, AND EDUCATION

HIV TESTING
Voluntary, Not Mandatory

Few issues about the HIV/AIDS epidemic have prompted more controversy than the use of antibody tests to identify people who are infected with HIV. Soon after the enzyme-linked immunosorbent assay test was developed and licensed in 1985, many public health officials supported testing in an attempt to change "undesirable" behaviors that were determining the course of the epidemic (such as unsafe male-to-male sexual contact and injection drug use). Those who favored testing claimed that if a person knew he or she was HIV positive, the infected person would change his or her behavior. Others argued that aggressive public health education and thoughtful counseling would be more productive strategies to achieve the desired results, even if people did not know their HIV status.

During the early years of the epidemic, health care officials in the public and private sectors refrained from advocating mandatory testing; instead, they focused on HIV testing that would be performed by physicians for patients they considered to be at risk for infection. In 1990 the House of Delegates of the American Medical Association (AMA) voted to declare HIV/AIDS a sexually transmitted disease (STD). This designation allowed physicians more freedom to decide the conditions under which HIV testing should take place.

During the late 1980s, when the research community announced that HIV-infected, symptom-free people could receive early intervention with azidothymidine (now called zidovudine [ZDV]) to slow the effects of the illness and delay the onset of *Pneumocystis carinii* pneumonia, the debate took another turn. Gay rights advocates, such as the Gay Men's Health Crisis Center in New York, began to encourage those who were at risk for HIV infection to get tested rather than discouraging testing, as they had previously done. In June 1997 the Gay Men's

Health Crisis Center (http://www.gmhc.org/) opened its own testing facility in the Michael Palm Treatment Center. This service was still available in 2011 as part of the range of care and support services offered. The center also offered a 12-week "harm reduction program" that was designed to curb risky behaviors such as substance abuse and unprotected sex. The intent of the program was to encourage people to change their risky behavior in a supportive atmosphere of care.

Another controversy surrounding testing concerns reporting HIV-positive patients by name. Every state is required to report AIDS cases. As of 2011, all 50 states and six dependent areas (American Samoa, Guam, the Northern Mariana Islands, Palau, Puerto Rico, and the U.S. Virgin Islands) had implemented HIV case surveillance using the same confidential system for name-based case reporting for both HIV infection and AIDS. Table 8.1 shows the states and dependent areas using name-based case reporting and the years they initiated this practice.

Critics, including the American Civil Liberties Union, assail name reporting as an invasion of privacy that carries social and economic risks. They claim that any benefit that would result from reporting names could not override the negative consequences (such as ostracism and the potential loss of jobs and health insurance) of being classified as infected. They add that name reporting discourages those at risk for HIV from coming forward to seek testing and timely treatment.

Name-based reporting will necessarily become the norm by 2013 because the Ryan White HIV/AIDS Treatment Extension Act of 2009, the largest federally funded program for people with HIV/AIDS, requires grantees to convert to name-based reporting by fiscal year 2013 or risk loss of funding.

As the name-reporting debate subsides, with the overwhelming majority of states acquiescing to federal

TABLE 8.1

HIV diagnoses by state and U.S. dependent areas, 2009

Area of residence (date confidential name-based HIV infection reporting initiated)	No.[b]	Estimated[a] No.	Rate
Alabama (January 1988)	690	788	16.7
Alaska (February 1999)	21	22	3.2
Arizona (January 1987)	653	786	11.9
Arkansas (July 1989)	214	294	10.2
California (April 2006)	4,886	—	—
Colorado (November 1985)	391	421	8.4
Connecticut (January 2005)	366	508	14.4
Delaware (February 2006)	168	—	—
District of Columbia (November 2006)	713	—	—
Florida (July 1997)	5,775	6,120	33.0
Georgia (December 2003)	2,073	3,229	32.9
Hawaii (March 2008)	70	—	—
Idaho (June 1986)	42	49	3.2
Illinois (January 2006)	1,708	2,029	15.7
Indiana (July 1988)	483	531	8.3
Iowa (July 1998)	125	139	4.6
Kansas (July 1999)	150	161	5.7
Kentucky (October 2004)	361	393	9.1
Louisiana (February 1993)	1,247	1,295	28.8
Maine (January 2006)	57	80	6.1
Maryland (April 2007)	1,400	—	—
Massachusetts (January 2007)	484	—	—
Michigan (April 1992)	827	1,001	10.0
Minnesota (October 1985)	393	419	8.0
Mississippi (August 1988)	559	630	21.3
Missouri (October 1987)	547	599	10.0
Montana (September 2006)	30	—	—
Nebraska (September 1995)	105	113	6.3
Nevada (February 1992)	386	418	15.8
New Hampshire (January 2005)	43	58	4.3
New Jersey (January 1992)	1,252	1,986	22.8
New Mexico (January 1998)	170	184	9.2
New York (June 2000)	4,649	5,765	29.5
North Carolina (February 1990)	1,719	1,844	19.7
North Dakota (January 1988)	14	15	2.3
Ohio (June 1990)	1,144	1,374	11.9
Oklahoma (June 1988)	297	403	10.9
Oregon (April 2006)	235	—	—
Pennsylvania (October 2002)[c]	1,736	1,829	14.5
Rhode Island (July 2006)	123	—	—
South Carolina (February 1986)	789	906	19.9
South Dakota (January 1988)	23	28	3.5
Tennessee (January 1992)	999	1,080	17.2
Texas (January 1999)	4,291	4,563	18.4
Utah (April 1989)	125	140	5.0
Vermont (April 2008)	11	—	—
Virginia (July 1989)	997	1,359	17.2
Washington (March 2006)	557	—	—
West Virginia (January 1989)	80	93	5.1
Wisconsin (November 1985)	305	334	5.9
Wyoming (June 1989)	19	21	3.8
Subtotal	**44,502**	**42,011**	**17.4**

Area of residence (date confidential name-based HIV infection reporting initiated)	No.[b]	Estimated[a] No.	Rate
U.S. dependent areas			
American Samoa (August 2001)	0	0	0.0
Guam (March 2000)	3	4	2.2
Northern Mariana Islands (October 2001)	1	0	0.0
Puerto Rico (January 2003)	671	909	22.9
U.S. Virgin Islands (December 1998)	25	35	31.4
Subtotal	**700**	**948**	**21.7**
Total[d]	**45,202**	**42,959**	**17.4**

Note: Data include persons with a diagnosis of HIV infection regardless of stage of disease at diagnosis.

[a]Includes data from areas with confidential name-based HIV infection reporting since at least January 2006. Estimated numbers resulted from statistical adjustment that accounted for reporting delays, but not for incomplete reporting. Rates are per 100,000 population.

[b]Includes data from areas with confidential name-based HIV infection reporting as of December 2008.

[c]Pennsylvania implemented confidential name-based HIV infection reporting in October 2002 in all areas except Philadelphia, where confidential name-based HIV infection reporting was not implemented until October 2005.

[d]Because column totals for estimated numbers were calculated independently of the values for the subpopulations, the values in each column may not sum to the column total.

SOURCE: "Table 19. Diagnoses of HIV Infection, by Area of Residence, 2009—United States and 5 U.S. Dependent Areas," in "Diagnoses of HIV Infection and AIDS in 'the United States and Dependent Areas, 2009," *HIV Surveillance Report, 2009*, vol. 21, Centers for Disease Control and Prevention, February 2011, http://www.cdc.gov/hiv/surveillance/resources/reports/2009report/pdf/table19.pdf (accessed June 15, 2011)

Rates of HIV Testing among Men Who Have Sex with Men

In 2003 the CDC, in cooperation with state and local health departments, launched the National HIV Behavioral Surveillance System (NHBS). The NHBS considers people at risk for HIV infection and surveys the three populations at highest risk for HIV in the United States—men who have sex with men (MSM), injection drug users (IDUs), and high-risk heterosexuals—and collects information from them.

The most recent data that have been analyzed are from 7,271 MSM in 21 cities with high prevalence of AIDS. Alexandra M. Oster et al. of the CDC indicate in "HIV Testing among Men Who Have Sex with Men—21 Cities, United States, 2008" (*Morbidity and Mortality Weekly Report*, vol. 60, no. 21, June 3, 2011) that nearly two-thirds (61%) reported having an HIV test in the 12 months preceding the survey. Table 8.2 shows that a higher proportion of younger men and those with higher educational attainment and income had been tested in the 12 months prior to the survey.

Of the 7,271 survey participants, 9% (680) were HIV infected. Among the HIV-infected participants, 16% had never been tested for HIV and 29% had been tested in the six months prior to the survey. (See Figure 8.1.) Oster et al. observe that in view of the 7% prevalence of HIV infection among MSM who had not been diagnosed and

requirements, there is widespread agreement that testing is most effective if followed by counseling that completely explains the results and their consequences. Furthermore, Bernard M. Branson et al. of the CDC note in "Revised Recommendations for HIV Testing of Adults, Adolescents, and Pregnant Women in Health-Care Settings" (*Morbidity and Mortality Weekly Report*, vol. 55, RR-14, September 22, 2006) that the CDC's 2006 revision of HIV testing guidelines call for routine testing for everyone aged 13 to 64 years seen at a physician's office or medical clinic. Routine HIV tests in physicians' offices and clinics no longer require the pretest counseling that was a requisite part of all HIV testing before the revised guidelines.

TABLE 8.2

Most recent HIV test among MSM by selected characteristics, 2008

| | | Timing of most recent HIV test | | | | | |
| | | Never tested | | Tested >12 months ago | | Tested ≤12 months ago | |
Characteristic	Total No.	No.	(%)	No.	(%)	No.	(%)
Race/ethnicity							
Asian/Native Hawaiian/Pacific Islander	233	22	(9)	70	(30)	140	(60)
Black, non-Hispanic	1,674	241	(14)	417	(25)	1,014	(61)
Hispanic	1,850	205	(11)	523	(28)	1,118	(60)
White, non-Hispanic	3,163	244	(8)	943	(30)	1,961	(62)
Other[a]	346	33	(10)	97	(28)	216	(62)
Age group (years)							
18–19	416	102	(25)	47	(11)	264	(63)
20–24	1,411	205	(15)	249	(18)	956	(68)
25–29	1,434	127	(9)	357	(25)	949	(66)
30–39	1,975	138	(7)	604	(31)	1,226	(62)
40–49	1,402	111	(8)	540	(39)	746	(53)
≥50	633	62	(10)	254	(40)	312	(49)
Education							
Less than high school diploma	462	103	(22)	133	(29)	220	(48)
High school diploma or equivalent	1,694	265	(16)	459	(27)	963	(57)
Some college or technical college	2,379	237	(10)	674	(28)	1,464	(62)
College or higher education	2,736	140	(5)	785	(29)	1,806	(66)
Annual household income							
≤$19,999	2,082	322	(16)	581	(28)	1,169	(56)
$20,000–$39,999	1,875	196	(11)	498	(27)	1,178	(63)
$40,000–$74,999	1,801	142	(8)	515	(29)	1,139	(63)
≥$75,000	1,408	71	(5)	438	(31)	896	(64)
Health insurance							
None	2,508	317	(13)	754	(30)	1,426	(57)
Public	707	98	(14)	189	(27)	417	(59)
Private	3,894	314	(8)	1,072	(28)	2,501	(64)
Other/multiple	64	2	(3)	11	(17)	50	(78)
No. of male sex partners during the past 12 months							
1	1,854	257	(14)	580	(31)	1,010	(54)
2	1,185	153	(13)	345	(29)	683	(58)
3	940	100	(11)	263	(28)	576	(61)
≥4	3,292	235	(7)	863	(26)	2,184	(66)
Methamphetamine use during the past 12 months							
Yes	516	39	(8)	154	(30)	320	(62)
No	6,754	706	(11)	1,897	(28)	4,132	(61)
Drug use before or during sex during the past 12 months							
Yes	1,009	109	(11)	294	(29)	600	(59)
No	6,258	636	(10)	1,757	(28)	3,849	(62)
Most recent partner had concurrent partners							
Definitely yes	1,630	158	(10)	480	(29)	986	(61)
Probably yes	1,866	149	(8)	560	(30)	1,153	(62)
Probably no	1,219	124	(10)	335	(28)	758	(62)
Definitely no	1,924	223	(12)	479	(25)	1,217	(63)
Reports one or more high-risk behaviors[b]							
Yes	5,864	554	(9)	1,622	(28)	3,672	(63)
No	1,407	191	(14)	429	(31)	781	(56)

had been tested for HIV during the 12 months preceding the survey that sexually active MSM might benefit from more frequent testing—as often as every three to six months.

Contact Tracing/Partner Notification

A by-product of testing is contact tracing, or partner notification. When individuals test positive for HIV, health officials ask them to provide, with the promise of anonymity, the names of those with whom they have had sexual contact or shared needles. The CDC asks counselors to inform contacts if the patient is reluctant to do so and strongly endorses contact-tracing programs, but results vary. States struggling under the strain of many HIV/AIDS cases continue to support programs that encourage the infected people to notify partners on their own. Contact-tracing programs in states with fewer HIV/AIDS cases are more likely to contact partners. Many

TABLE 8.2

Most recent HIV test among MSM by selected characteristics, 2008 [CONTINUED]

| | | Timing of most recent HIV test | | | | | |
| | | Never tested | | Tested >12 months ago | | Tested ≤12 months ago | |
Characteristic	Total No.	No.	(%)	No.	(%)	No.	(%)
Unprotected anal intercourse during the past 12 months							
Yes	4,016	362	(9)	1,104	(28)	2,541	(63)
No	3,248	382	(12)	946	(29)	1,907	(59)
Total	7,271	745	(10)	2,051	(28)	4,453	(61)

Note: Numbers might not add to total because of missing data. HIV = Human immunodeficiency virus. MSM = Men who have sex with men.
[a]Includes persons who indicated American Indian/Alaska Native, multiple races, or other race.
[b]High-risk behavior defined as the following: more than one male sex partner during the past 12 months, methamphetamine use during the past 12 months, drug use before or during sex at most recent sex, or most recent partner definitely or probably had concurrent partners.

SOURCE: Alexandra M. Oster et al., "Table 1. Timing of Most Recent Human Immunodeficiency Virus (HIV) Test among Men Who Have Sex with Men (MSM) Not Previously Diagnosed with HIV Infection, by Selected Characteristics and Risk Behaviors—National HIV Behavioral Surveillance System, 21 Cities, United States, 2008," in "HIV Testing among Men Who Have Sex with Men—21 Cities, United States, 2008," *Morbidity and Mortality Weekly Report*, vol. 60, no. 21, June 3, 2011, http://www.cdc.gov/mmwr/pdf/wk/mm6021.pdf (accessed June 16, 2011).

FIGURE 8.1

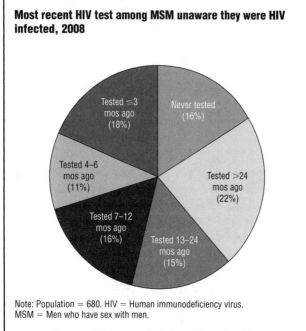

Most recent HIV test among MSM unaware they were HIV infected, 2008

Note: Population = 680. HIV = Human immunodeficiency virus. MSM = Men who have sex with men.

SOURCE: Alexandra M. Oster et al., "Figure. Time since Most Recent Human Immunodeficiency Virus (HIV) Test among Men Who Have Sex with Men Who Were Unaware They Were HIV-Infected—National HIV Behavioral Surveillance System, 21 Cities, United States, 2008," in "HIV Testing among Men Who Have Sex with Men—21 Cities, United States, 2008," *Morbidity and Mortality Weekly Report*, vol. 60, no. 21, June 3, 2011, http://www.cdc.gov/mmwr/pdf/wk/mm6021.pdf (accessed June 16, 2011).

patients who are HIV infected or have AIDS fear that promises of confidentiality will be broken; others fear retribution from those they may have infected.

In "A Systematic Review of HIV Partner Counseling and Referral Services: Client and Provider Attitudes, Preferences, Practices, and Experiences" (*Sexually Transmitted Diseases*, vol. 33, no. 5, May 2006), Warren F. Passin et al.

report on their research to improve understanding of client and provider attitudes about, and experiences with, partner notification. They also seek to identify potential negative effects of HIV partner notification on clients such as physical, emotional, or sexual abuse or ending of the relationship with the primary partner as a result of participating in partner notification. The researchers find that clients were willing to self-notify partners and participate in provider notification, and few reported negative effects. In terms of preferences, more clients were willing to provide partner information to a physician (64%) or social worker (62%) than to health department personnel (48%) or a member from the gay community (45%). Passin et al. attribute these preferences to a desire to work with familiar and trusted providers as opposed to seeking assistance from unfamiliar sources or providers whom many clients suspect will not maintain strict confidentiality.

The majority (68% to 98%) of health care providers also favored HIV partner notification, but they did not always refer clients to HIV partner notification programs. Passin et al. conclude, "Considering that clients have positive attitudes toward self- and provider referral, local HIV prevention programs need to ensure that all HIV-positive clients are offered partner notification services. Additional research is needed to assess the potential risks of notifying partners and to identify effective techniques to improve client and provider participation."

ETHICAL, LEGAL, AND MORAL DILEMMAS OF PARTNER NOTIFICATION. Worldwide, there is increasing emphasis on partner notification as a strategy with the potential not only to prevent HIV transmission to partners at risk but also to promote early diagnosis and prompt treatment for those found to be infected. Barnabas N. Njozing et al. of Umeå University assert in "'If the Patients Decide Not to Tell What Can We Do?'—TB/HIV Counsellors' Dilemma on Partner Notification for HIV" (*BMC International Health* and *Human Rights*, vol. 11, June 3, 2011) that counselors are often frustrated by HIV-positive patients' reluctance to voluntarily notify their sexual partners. The researchers interviewed counselors to identify the issues surrounding confidentiality and partner notification.

Njozing et al. find that all counselors encouraged voluntary notification but that counselors responded differently to people who refused to voluntarily notify their partners of their HIV status. One group believed in absolute respect of patients' autonomy and that it is not the counselors' responsibility to inform partners at risk without the patients' consent. The researchers note that legal counsel endorsed this position. A second group of counselors acknowledged the importance of respecting patients' autonomy, but also felt a responsibility for their partners' safety. They used strategies such as couples counseling as well as continuous reminders of the benefits of disclosure to encourage reluctant patients.

A third group of counselors wanted solutions that inform sexual partners who are at risk of HIV infection and legal protection for counselors. Njozing et al. state that this group believed "upholding confidentiality in absolute terms was morally wrong, and patients who refused to inform their partners about their status were selfish by not considering the health and wellbeing of their partners." Some of these counselors admitted that as a last resort they occasionally threatened patients to pressure them to inform partners. These counselors were very conflicted about their roles in terms of respecting patient confidentiality and informing sexual partners. They explained that this conflict was exacerbated when they were acquainted with the patients' sexual partners.

A fourth group of counselors felt that HIV/AIDS should be treated as any other chronic disease and advocated routine HIV testing and partner notification. Their goal is to destigmatize and normalize the diagnosis of HIV so that it is a medical condition like any other, for which diagnosis and disclosure are conducted based on medical necessity rather than on legal or ethical bases.

INTERNET-BASED PARTNER NOTIFICATION. Because research indicates that a substantial number of new HIV cases and STDs are acquired by MSM who meet new sexual partners on the Internet, health professionals wondered if the same medium could be used to convey information to men, such as in e-mails informing them that they had sex with someone infected with an STD and providing links about the STD and where to get tested for it. In "HIV and STD Status among MSM and Attitudes about Internet Partner Notification for STD Exposure" (*Sexually Transmitted Diseases*, vol. 35, no. 2, February 2008), Matthew J. Mimiaga et al. consider the acceptability and perceived utility of Internet-based partner notification of STD exposure for MSM by HIV status. The researchers find broad acceptance—more than 92% of those surveyed—of Internet partner notification by at-risk MSM, independent of HIV status. The MSM interviewed also expressed a willingness to receive or initiate partner notification-related e-mail.

Rapid Testing

The CDC indicates in "HIV Surveillance—United States, 1981–2008" (*Morbidity and Mortality Weekly Report*, vol. 60, no. 21, June 3, 2011) that in 2008, 20.1% of people living with HIV were undiagnosed and unaware of their infection. In view of this high percentage, researchers and public health professionals continue to seek more and better ways to increase the number of people who are aware of their HIV status. One way to increase access to HIV testing is through rapid testing, which may be readily performed in a variety of settings such as correctional facilities, military battlefield operations, and worksites where occupational exposures may occur.

Several rapid HIV antibody tests have been approved by the U.S. Food and Drug Administration (FDA) for use in the United States. Table 2.6 in Chapter 2 lists the FDA-approved rapid HIV screening tests and provides their features and prices. The tests contain test strips with HIV antigens. If the blood or sputum they come in contact with contains HIV antibodies, then the antibodies bind to the antigens and a reagent in the test kit creates a color change. The tests are interpreted visually and, like conventional HIV enzyme immunoassays, they are screening tests that require additional testing by a Western blot or immunofluorescent assay to confirm a positive response.

Because rapid HIV testing informs clients with reactive test results that it is highly likely that they are HIV positive, compared to receiving no test result information at the conclusion of a visit where a conventional HIV test specimen is drawn, it is vitally important for health care workers to explain the meaning of preliminary positive results. Counseling for patients who receive rapid HIV testing is somewhat different from conventional testing and involves determining how prepared clients are to receive test results in the same session.

As of 2011, the sale of rapid HIV tests was restricted to clinical laboratories where workers who administer the tests have reviewed and use the instructional materials provided with the tests. The FDA also requires that people tested with the rapid tests receive the informative pamphlet provided with the test.

Home Testing

Home HIV tests were developed during the mid-1980s but were opposed by the FDA and some HIV/AIDS organizations and health care agencies. The FDA was concerned about telephone counseling for those who tested positive, the accuracy of the tests, and confidentiality. In 1996 the FDA reversed its position, deciding that despite the limitations of home testing, the benefits outweigh the risks.

Public health officials explain that many people are afraid of obtaining testing at a physician's office or public clinic because of the associated stigma. Some drug companies suggest that an HIV-antibody test that can be performed at home may be the only way some of these people will learn their HIV status, and argue that more people will then enter treatment and take precautions to prevent spreading the infection.

Some home tests use saliva, which does not require a needle stick, and others use blood samples. When blood is tested, the patient draws a few drops of blood from a fingertip, places it on filter paper, and mails the paper to a company laboratory, which performs the standard HIV assay. If the results are positive, a confirmation test is performed. An HIV test kit called the Home Access Express HIV-1 Test System, manufactured by Home Access Health Corporation, which was approved by the FDA in 1996, was the only HIV home test kit approved by the agency as of 2011. Seven days (or sooner if express service is requested) after Home Access Health receives the test kit, results and counseling are available by calling a 24-hour toll-free number and giving an identification code. Home Access claims an accuracy rate of 99.9%.

Critics of home testing suggest that news of HIV infection is not as easy to accept as the results of other in-home tests, such as those for pregnancy and cholesterol. They claim that most people cannot properly prepare themselves for the news that they have a life-threatening disease. They advocate the expansion of current testing sites to include mobile vans, sports clubs, and other places that are not exclusively associated with HIV testing, but where in-person counseling can be provided.

Military Practices

The U.S. Department of Defense (DOD) regularly screens all members of the armed services as well as those seeking to join for HIV. The DOD states in "Department of Defense: Instruction" (October 17, 2006, http://www.dtic .mil/whs/directives/corres/pdf/648501p.pdf) that its policy is to "deny eligibility for Military Service to individuals with serologic evidence of HIV infection for appointment, enlistment, pre-appointment, or initial entry training for Military Service." Biannual HIV testing is required of all personnel on active duty, as well as of all members of the reserves and National Guard. In 1995, after two months of debate in Congress, federal legislators scrapped a discharge provision that would have forced the DOD to dismiss members of the military within six months of testing positive for HIV. Along with HIV infection, a number of chronic conditions, including cancer, asthma, diabetes, heart disease, or complications of pregnancy, place troops on limited assignment, precluding them from overseas service or combat.

In the article "HIV: A Question of Readiness for Militaries around the World" (USMedicine.com, May 2009), Richard Shaffer, the director of the DOD HIV/ AIDS Prevention Program, reports that the HIV infection rate across the military is about 0.3 per 1,000 individuals. Besides ensuring the health of U.S. military personnel, the program assists militaries worldwide to prevent HIV transmission in their personnel.

Pregnant Women and Newborns

The issue of testing newborns has placed the rights of mothers at odds with those of their newborns. States have kept HIV test results anonymous to preserve a mother's right to privacy. Civil libertarians (those that actively support the strengthening and protecting of individual rights and freedoms) and some groups that represent women, gays, and lesbians support anonymous testing, claiming that attaching names to test results would start local, state, and federal governments down the "slippery slope" of mandatory testing of adults. They also raise further privacy concerns, contending that once names are known, there is no guarantee they will not fall into the hands of employers, insurance companies, and others who might discriminate on the basis of HIV status.

On the contrary, proponents of disclosure claim newborns who test HIV positive could be denied adequate medical care because their parents are unaware of their status. M. Blake Caldwell et al. of the CDC explain in "1994 Revised Classification System for Human Immunodeficiency Virus Infection in Children Less Than 13 Years of Age" (*Morbidity and Mortality Weekly Report*, vol. 43, RR-12, September 30, 1994) that 15% to 30% of the babies who test positive for HIV immediately after birth actually develop the disease. However, if their mothers breastfeed, some may contract the infection from their mother's breast milk.

In May 1996 the U.S. House of Representatives and the U.S. Senate passed bills that would cut off federal money for HIV/AIDS treatment to states that failed to comply with the new disclosure requirements. President Bill Clinton (1946–) signed the Ryan White Comprehensive AIDS Resources Emergency Act Amendments, which required mandatory testing of newborns if too few pregnant women agreed to voluntary testing. In June 1996 New York became the first state to mandate that health officials tell parents the results of HIV tests that the state routinely performs on all newborns. Before June 1996 parents in New York did not receive results unless they requested them, as was still the case in many states in 2011.

NEW JERSEY LEGISLATION MANDATES TESTING OF PREGNANT WOMEN AND SOME NEWBORNS. In June 2007 New Jersey lawmakers approved a bill requiring pregnant women and some newborns—infants born to mothers who have tested positive or those whose HIV status is unknown at the time of birth—to be tested for HIV. The law requires that pregnant women be tested twice for HIV, once early and once late during the pregnancy, unless the mother specifically requests not to be tested.

Supporters of this legislation contend that the requirement for testing will save children's lives. Detractors argue that all infants of HIV-infected mothers test positive for HIV antibodies because they inherit their mother's antibodies. This initial positive result does not necessarily mean the infant is infected. Because it takes several months for the mother's antibodies to clear from the infant, it may be more prudent to test infants when they are between three and six months old to determine their HIV status. According to the Kaiser Family Foundation, in "New Jersey Legislature Approves Bill Requiring Pregnant Women, Some Infants to Receive HIV Tests" (June 25, 2007, http://www.kaiser healthnews.org/daily-reports/2007/june/25/dr00045784.aspx? referrer=search), the American Civil Liberties Union and women's health advocacy groups assert that the legislation "deprives women of authority to make medical decisions."

Even though the CDC recommends routine opt-out HIV screening of all pregnant women and newborn testing if the mother's HIV status is unknown, state policies vary. The National HIV/AIDS Clinicians' Consultation Center at the University of California, San Francisco, reports in *Compendium of State HIV Testing Laws—Perinatal Quick Reference Guide: Guide to States' Perinatal HIV Testing Laws for Clinicians* (http://www.nccc.ucsf.edu/docs/Perinatal_QRG.pdf) that as of April 2011, 20 states, the District of Columbia, and Puerto Rico had no specific provisions regarding prenatal testing. The balance of the states had provisions for prenatal testing. Ten states had opt-out HIV testing—it is part of routine prenatal care and pregnant women are tested unless they refuse or "opt-out." The remaining 40 states had opt-in HIV testing of pregnant women—an HIV test is not part of routine prenatal care and pregnant women must specifically request or "opt-in" to receive an HIV test.

Health Care Workers

There has been a continuing debate over whether health care workers should be required to obtain HIV tests. As of 2011, there was no law requiring health care workers to submit to HIV testing, although many employers require it as a condition of employment. They cannot, however, discriminate against health care workers on the basis of their HIV status because like other employees, they are covered by the Americans with Disabilities Act of 1990, the federal law that prohibits discrimination against individuals with disabilities.

According to the CDC, in "Are Health Care Workers at Risk of Getting HIV on the Job?" (March 25, 2010,

http://www.cdc.gov/hiv/resources/qa/transmission.htm), the risk of health care workers becoming infected with HIV on the job is very low, especially if they follow prudent safety measures known as universal precautions, which include the use of gloves, goggles, and masks to prevent HIV and other bloodborne infections. The largest risk is posed by accidental needle-stick injuries, but even this risk is less than 1%.

Furthermore, Mitchell J. Schwaber reports in "Investigation of Patients Treated by an HIV-Infected Cardiothoracic Surgeon—Israel, 2007" (*Morbidity and Mortality Weekly Report*, vol. 57, no. 53, January 9, 2009) about an investigation of HIV transmission from a heart surgeon to the surgeon's patients, which found no transmission from the infected surgeon to patients. Schwaber confirms that HIV transmission from health care worker to patient is rare. Reports such as this support the premise that when universal precautions are taken, HIV-infected health care workers pose negligible risk to their patients, especially when they are being treated, because blood infectivity of HIV carriers has been shown to vary as a function of the viral load, which can now be reduced to undetectable levels using antiretroviral drugs.

Testing Policies in U.S. Prisons

Guidelines for the testing of inmates for HIV exist in all 50 states, in the District of Columbia, and in the regulations of the Federal Bureau of Prisons. However, the timing of testing varies. The CDC finds in *HIV Testing Implementation Guidance for Correctional Settings* (January 2009, http://www.cdc.gov/hiv/topics/testing/resources/guidelines/correctional-settings/pdf/Correctional_Settings_Guidelines.pdf) that in 2006 less than half of the state prison systems and few jails routinely provided prisoners with HIV testing on entry, while in custody, or before release. Federal prisons and 45 states tested inmates if they had HIV-related symptoms, and federal prisons and 43 states tested inmates on request. Just 16 states and the federal system tested inmates who were considered to belong to high-risk populations.

The CDC recommends universal opt-out HIV screening in correctional facilities. It states that "voluntary HIV testing is as cost-effective as other screening programs in health care settings in which HIV prevalence is as low as 0.1%. Since many incarcerated populations have a prevalence of diagnosed HIV infection >1%, HIV screening in prisons and jails is a highly cost-effective public health strategy." The CDC acknowledges that some systems face logistical, security, and financial constraints that require alternative options. For these types of situations, the CDC advises several alternative approaches including risk-based screening that routinely offers HIV screening to inmates with HIV risk characteristics such as IDUs, MSM, or inmates diagnosed with another STD.

PREVENTION

Critics Fault Programs' Focus and Funding

The objective of HIV prevention programs is to reduce the number of new cases to as close to zero as possible. All prevention efforts are based on the belief that individuals can be educated in a way that will lead to changes in behavior, which will help bring an end to the spread of HIV/AIDS. However, many AIDS advocacy groups have long been critical of the ways the CDC has communicated this message. In 1987 CDC officials chose to emphasize the universality of AIDS, instead of focusing efforts on those most at risk: MSM and IDUs. According to AIDS advocates, this strategy misdirected the spending of available prevention dollars during the first decade of the epidemic. In 2011, even though the number of infected people outside of these two groups was growing, HIV/AIDS was still largely a threat to MSM, IDUs, their partners, and their children. Most women with HIV/AIDS were IDUs or were sex partners of IDUs.

Key Objectives of Prevention Programs

The 2011 National HIV Prevention Conference (http://2011nhpc.org/conference_purpose.asp) was held in Atlanta, Georgia, in August 2011. More than 3,000 attendees focused on key objectives of prevention programs:

- Reducing the number of people who become HIV infected

- Expanding access to health care and other support services and improving the health of people living with HIV

- Reducing health disparities in terms of education, prevention, testing, and access to timely treatment to reduce HIV incidence

- Disseminating knowledge about effective HIV prevention research, practices, and policies to clinicians and practitioners

- Creating new alliances and working relationships between all stakeholders—HIV researchers, prevention and health care providers, policy makers, advocacy groups, and people affected by HIV

CDC Prevention Activities

The CDC's HIV prevention strategy, as described in "CDC Responds to HIV/AIDS" (April 1, 2011, http://www.cdc.gov/hiv/aboutDHAP.htm#strategy), aims to reduce the incidence and prevalence of HIV infection as well as the morbidity (illnesses) and mortality (deaths) that result from HIV infection by working with communities and other partners. The agency's efforts focus on four areas:

- Incorporating HIV testing as a routine part of care in traditional medical settings

- Implementing new models for diagnosing HIV infection outside of medical settings

- Preventing new infections by working with people diagnosed with HIV and their partners

- Screening and treating expectant mothers to further decrease mother-to-child HIV transmission

The prevention strategy capitalizes on new rapid test technologies, interventions that bring people unaware of their HIV status to HIV testing, and behavioral interventions that provide prevention skills to people living with HIV. To carry out its strategy, the CDC works in conjunction with governmental and nongovernmental partners to implement, evaluate, and further develop and strengthen effective HIV prevention efforts nationwide. Along with direct programs and service, the CDC provides financial and technical support for:

- Disease surveillance

- HIV antibody counseling, testing, and referral services

- Street and community outreach

- Risk-reduction counseling

- Prevention case management

- Prevention and treatment of other STDs

- Public information and education

- School-based AIDS education

- International research studies

- Technology transfer systems

- Organizational capacity building

- Program-relevant epidemiological, sociobehavioral, and evaluation research

CDC health education and disease prevention efforts continue to emphasize that the most reliable ways to avoid HIV infection or virus transmission are by abstaining from sexual intercourse; maintaining a mutually monogamous, long-term relationship with a partner who is uninfected; and/or refraining from sharing needles and syringes in drug use. Even though seemingly logical, critics contend that the CDC's emphasis on abstinence burdens people with an unrealistic expectation. Critics also point to the insistence on abstinence policies as a condition of U.S. government assistance for other countries' health programs to be an ill-advised foreign policy intrusion.

According to the Kaiser Family Foundation, in the fact sheet "U.S. Federal Funding for HIV/AIDS: The President's FY 2012 Budget Request" (March 2011, http://www.kff.org/hivaids/upload/7029-07.pdf), for fiscal year 2012 the CDC was allocated $997 million for domestic HIV/AIDS prevention activities conducted by the National Center for HIV/AIDS, Viral Hepatitis, STD, and TB Prevention, a 10% increase ($93 million) from fiscal year 2011.

EDUCATING YOUTH

In "Basic Statistics" (August 11, 2011, http://www.cdc.gov/hiv/topics/surveillance/basic.htm), the CDC estimates that in 2009, 12,188 new cases of HIV infection and 5,571 new cases of AIDS were reported for people aged 20 to 29 years. With an average incubation period of 10 years, it is likely that most of these young people were infected while they were teenagers. Because some people begin having sexual relationships and using injection drugs at earlier ages, many health officials fear the number of HIV-positive young people will grow.

Most states offer prevention programs for students in public schools. However, youths who are not in school may not have ready access to such programs. Many homeless shelters and local health departments employ roving counselors who seek out these young people to offer prevention information and direct them to health and social service agencies.

Sexual Health Education

Many education programs offer students sufficient information about STDs and HIV/AIDS, but only high-quality education affects behavior. In "Sex and HIV Education Programs: Their Impact on Sexual Behaviors of Young People throughout the World" (*Journal of Adolescent Health*, vol. 40, no. 3, March 2007), Douglas B. Kirby, B. A. Laris, and Lori A. Rolleri look at 83 studies that measure the impact of HIV and sex education programs on sexual behavior of young people under the age of 25 years worldwide. The researchers find that about two-thirds of the programs significantly improved one or more sexual behaviors. The programs acted by delaying or decreasing sexual behaviors or by increasing condom and contraceptive use. The characteristics of effective programs include:

- Focus on curricula, clear statements about health and behavioral goals, a clear picture of the risks of unprotected sex, and ways to avoid it

- Focus on specific behaviors (psychosocial risk factors and protective factors) that produce or hamper achieving these health goals and identification of challenging situations

- Provision of a safe social environment for participants

- Use of instructionally sound teaching methods that personalize the information and effectively engage participants

- Addressing topics in a logical sequence using approaches and materials that are consistent with the participants' culture, age, and sexual experience

The provision of comprehensive sex education remains controversial in 2011. Some people do not agree that information about sexual health or decisions should be offered in public schools, preferring that parents instill their own values in their children. However, others point out that some parents never talk to their children about sex and drugs and that school may be the only place a child can get reliable information. According to the Guttmacher Institute, in "State Policies in Brief: Sex and STI/HIV Education" (August 10, 2011, http://www.guttmacher.org/statecenter/spibs/spib_SE.pdf), 33 states and the District of Columbia required HIV/AIDS prevention education in 2011. Twenty states and the District of Columbia required HIV education and sex education, and 13 only required HIV education. Twenty-two states and the District of Columbia required schools to notify parents that HIV education or sex education will be provided to students. Even though laws vary from state to state, and some allow local school districts to decide on curricula, many of these states have one or more mandates determining the material that may be taught in the programs. The mandates range from requiring age-appropriate materials, to teaching comprehensive sex education programs (advocating contraceptive and condom use), to providing programs in which abstinence from premarital sex is presented as the only 100% effective means of preventing HIV/AIDS. The Guttmacher Institute notes that in 2011 only 13 states required the information that is taught be medically accurate.

Federal funding for abstinence-only educational programs was initiated in 1998. Proponents of these programs claim they change attitudes about casual sex by reducing both teen pregnancies and rates of STDs. They also maintain that teaching students about contraceptive and condom use condones, or even encourages, unsafe sexual behavior. Critics of these programs argue that there is no reliable evidence that abstinence-only programs are effective. In addition, they contend that for the five out of 10 teens aged 15 to 19 years who do choose to have sex, lack of knowledge about contraception and condom use will only result in continued teen pregnancies, STDs, and HIV infections.

The U.S. Department of Health and Human Services concludes in *Review of Comprehensive Sex Education Curricula* (May 2007) that abstinence-only education is ineffective. The review finds that students given abstinence-only education were no more likely to abstain from sex, that those who had sex did so with a similar number of partners as those who had not received abstinence-only education, and that students first had sex at the same age, independent of the type of education they had received.

In his fiscal year 2010 budget, President Barack Obama (1961–) eliminated federal funding for abstinence-only education. However, Rob Stein notes in "Health Bill Restores $250 Million in Abstinence-Education Funds" (*Washington Post*, March 27, 2010) that the health care reform legislation passed in 2010 restored $250 million over five years for states to provide programs that are intended to prevent pregnancy and STDs by focusing exclusively on abstinence only. Critics of abstinence-only education are disheartened by continued funding of such programs in view of the dearth of evidence of their efficacy (the ability of an intervention to produce the intended diagnostic or therapeutic effect in optimal circumstances).

CONDOM USE

In June 2000 a workshop organized by the National Institutes of Health in collaboration with the CDC, the FDA, and the U.S. Agency for International Development evaluated published evidence on the effectiveness of latex male condoms in preventing STDs, including HIV. In the fact sheet "Male Latex Condoms and Sexually Transmitted Diseases" (April 11, 2011, http://www.cdc.gov/condomeffectiveness/latex.htm), the CDC indicates that studies provide compelling evidence that latex condoms are highly effective in protecting against HIV infection when used properly for every act of intercourse. However, the agency warns that "the most reliable ways to avoid transmission of sexually transmitted diseases (STDs), including human immunodeficiency virus (HIV), are to abstain from sexual activity or to be in a long-term mutually monogamous relationship with an uninfected partner."

The CDC analysis of data from Youth Risk Behavior Surveys conducted between 1991 and 2009 finds that U.S. high school students are engaging in fewer HIV-related risk behaviors—decreasing percentages of students reported being sexually active and having had sexual intercourse with four or more people in their life. Condom use increased between 1991 and 2003, but since then has leveled off. (See Table 5.6 in Chapter 5.) Condom use among sexually active students rose from 46.2% in 1991 to 61.1% in 2009.

Other Forms of Protection

In 1993 the FDA approved Reality, a female condom that serves as a mechanical barrier to viruses. The condom is designed for women to protect themselves from STDs, including HIV. It is made of polyurethane (a resin made of two different compounds used in elastic fibers, cushions, and various molded products) and is unlikely to rip or tear. The condom is prelubricated and is intended for use during only one sex act.

The use of female condoms is low. Rebecca Bowers cites in "Status Report on the Female Condom: What Will Increase Use in the U.S.?" (AIDS Alert, vol. 23, no. 3, March 2008) the findings of a New York State study—that 69% of women had heard about female condoms but just 2.6% had used one. Bowers describes the development of a new generation of female condoms, which because they may be more comfortable and easier to use, may be better accepted and more widely used. She observes that there is still no commercially available product other than the female condom that women can use to protect themselves from HIV/AIDS.

CIRCUMCISION MAY SLOW THE SPREAD OF HIV

According to the press release "WHO and UNAIDS Announce Recommendations from Expert Consultation on Male Circumcision for HIV Prevention" (March 28, 2007, http://www.who.int/hiv/mediacentre/news68/en/index.html), in 2007 the World Health Organization (WHO) and the United Nations Joint Program on HIV/AIDS recommended circumcision as a strategy to prevent heterosexually acquired HIV infection in men. Circumcision, the surgical removal of the foreskin from the penis, has long been thought to reduce men's susceptibility to HIV infection because the skin cells in the foreskin are especially vulnerable to the virus. Kevin De Cock, the former director of the WHO HIV/AIDS Department, asserts that "countries with high rates of heterosexual HIV infection and low rates of male circumcision now have an additional intervention which can reduce the risk of HIV infection in heterosexual men. Scaling up male circumcision in such countries will result in immediate benefit to individuals. However, it will be a number of years before we can expect to see an impact on the epidemic from such investment."

According to the article "Circumcision Key to Curbing AIDS Spread" (Associated Press, July 24, 2007), Robert Bailey of the University of Illinois urges government endorsement of circumcision to slow the spread of HIV. Exhorting international agencies to increase funding for circumcision in countries hardest hit by the epidemic, Bailey contends that "circumcision could drive the epidemic to a declining state toward extinction.... We must make safe, affordable, voluntary circumcision available now."

Research conducted in Kenya, South Africa, and Uganda demonstrates that circumcision reduces HIV incidence. In "Can Routine Neonatal Circumcision Help Prevent Human Immunodeficiency Virus Transmission in the United States?" (American Journal of Men's Health, vol. 3, no. 1, March 2009), Xiao Xu et al. of the University of Michigan question whether it would be beneficial to implement routine circumcision of newborn males in the United States for HIV prevention. More than half of male newborns in the United States are circumcised at birth. Xu et al. call for "comprehensive cost-effectiveness analysis considering the various elements of HIV transmission in the context of the United States" to determine potential cost, benefit, and risks of recommending universal circumcision as an HIV prevention strategy.

In "Male Circumcision for Prevention of Homosexual Acquisition of HIV in Men" (Cochrane Database of Systematic Reviews, no. 6, June 15, 2011), an exhaustive review of the relevant medical literature that included 21 studies of 71,693 subjects, Charles Shey Wiysonge et al.

conclude that "current evidence suggests that male circumcision may be protective among MSM who practice primarily insertive anal sex, but the role of male circumcision overall in the prevention of HIV and other sexually transmitted infections among MSM remains to be determined. Therefore, there is not enough evidence to recommend male circumcision for HIV prevention among MSM at present." The researchers call for completion of a randomized controlled trial, the most rigorous type of clinical research, to definitively determine whether male circumcision protects against HIV transmission.

IMPROVING PREVENTION SERVICES

Cynthia M. Lyles et al. of the CDC discuss in "Best-Evidence Interventions: Findings from a Systematic Review of HIV Behavioral Interventions for US Populations at High Risk, 2000–2004" (*American Journal of Public Health*, vol. 97, no. 1, January 2007) the results of a CDC evaluation of behavioral intervention programs to reduce HIV risk. The researchers considered approximately 100 interventions in an effort to identify "best practices" and "best evidence" of efficacy in reducing HIV-related risk behaviors, STDs, or HIV incidence.

Lyles et al. identify 18 behavioral interventions as demonstrating the best evidence of efficacy. These interventions were based on behavioral change theories or models, most often social cognitive theory or social learning theory. These theories posit that human behavior is the product of a dynamic interplay of personal, behavioral, and environmental influences. The researchers use a variety of strategies and approaches to change behaviors, including providing consequences (in the form of rewards or punishments for specific behaviors) and learning by observation of others. Social cognitive theory proposes that people are most likely to model the behaviors of someone with whom they strongly identify. Both theories have been used successfully to help people develop new health-supporting skills.

Even though the content of the effective interventions varied, all included learning and practicing skills such as condom use and relaxation techniques as well as interpersonal, communication, and decision-making skills. Most of the effective interventions targeted populations that are disproportionately affected by the HIV/AIDS epidemic and in urgent need of effective prevention programs. Some best-evidence interventions focused on African-American or Hispanic heterosexual women at risk for HIV infection and two targeted African-American youths at high risk. Others aimed to prevent infection in minority drug users and one focused on female IDUs. Still other best-evidence interventions served people living with HIV. In "Best-Evidence Risk Reduction Interventions" (April 18, 2011, http://www.cdc.gov/hiv/topics/research/prs/best-evidence-intervention.htm#completelist), the CDC identifies a list of 42

best-evidence interventions (programs that are considered to provide the strongest scientific evidence of efficacy) and the target populations they aim to serve.

SYRINGE EXCHANGE PROGRAMS

IDUs often share the syringes they use to inject drugs into their body. When an HIV-positive IDU uses a syringe, he or she may contaminate it with HIV-positive blood that can then spread the disease to other IDUs who use that syringe. Syringe exchange programs (SEPs) attempt to prevent the spread of HIV in this manner by encouraging IDUs to bring in their used, unsafe syringes and exchange them for new, safe syringes. The reasoning behind these programs is that if people are going to use drugs, at least an effort can be made to make sure they do not contract HIV because of it. Proponents of these programs point out that the spread of HIV among IDUs threatens everyone, as people who contract HIV through drug use can then pass it on to their sexual partners and children.

Despite these arguments, SEPs are highly controversial due to their connection to drug use. Some opponents see them as helping IDUs avoid the consequences of their actions, or even providing them with the means to continue their illegal activities. In April 1998, after much debate, the Clinton administration decided not to lift a nine-year-old ban on federal financing for programs to distribute clean needles to drug addicts. This meant that state and local governments that received federal block grants for HIV/AIDS prevention were not permitted to use this money for SEPs. Public health experts and advocates for people with HIV/AIDS criticized the decision. Later in 1998 Congress considered even more restrictive legislation that would ban indirect federal funding (such as funding for counseling, medical care, or funds dispersed by city or state) to needle exchange agencies. Regardless, in 2000 five U.S. health groups (including the AMA and the American Pharmaceutical Association) spoke out in favor of SEPs and advised state leaders to coordinate efforts to make clean needles easily available to IDUs.

In "Syringe Exchange Programs—United States, 2008" (*Morbidity and Mortality Weekly Report*, vol. 59, no. 45, November 19, 2010), the CDC summarizes a survey of SEP activities in the United States. The survey was conducted in March 2009 by the Beth Israel Medical Center (BIMC) in New York City, with the North American Syringe Exchange Network (NASEN). Questionnaires were mailed to the directors of all 184 SEPs in the United States that were members of the NASEN. (Previous surveys contacted SEPs between 1994 and 2007.) The BIMC contacted SEP directors and conducted telephone interviews based on the questionnaires. The directors responded to questions about the number of syringes exchanged in 2008 through program operations and services.

TABLE 8.3

Number of syringes exchanged by syringe exchange programs, by program size, 2008

Syringe exchange program size	No. of syringes exchanged per syringe exchange program	No. of syringe exchange programs	Total no.of syringes exchanged	% of total syringes exchanged
Small	<10,000	20	67,593	0.2
Medium	10,000–55,000	33	982,317	3.4
Large	55,001–499,999	54	9,894,182	34.1
Very large	≥500,000	15	18,113,914	62.3
Total		**122***	**29,058,006**	**100.0**

*One of 123 programs responding to the survey did not track the number of syringes exchanged in 2008.

SOURCE: "Table 2. Number of Syringes Exchanged by Syringe Exchange Programs (SEPs), by Program Size—United States, 2008," in "Syringe Exchange Programs— United States, 2008," *Morbidity and Mortality Weekly Report*, vol. 59, no. 45, November 19, 2010, http://www.cdc.gov/mmwr/pdf/wk/mm5945.pdf (accessed June 16, 2011)

Of the 184 SEPs, 123 (67%) participated in the survey. The SEPs operated in 98 cities in 29 states/territories and in the District of Columbia. A majority of the SEPs were located in six states: California (30), Washington (16), Wisconsin (14), New York (11), and Connecticut and Illinois (5 each).

In 2008, 123 SEPs exchanged nearly 29.1 million syringes. (See Table 8.3.) The 15 largest SEPs (those that traded 500,000 or more syringes) exchanged over 18.1 million (62.3% of all replaced syringes).

Besides exchanged syringes, most of the SEPs provided other public health and social services. Nearly all the SEPs provided alcohol pads (100%), male condoms (98%), and referrals to substance-abuse treatment (89%). (See Table 8.4.) Other on-site health care services provided by some of the SEPs included counseling and testing for HIV (87%) and hepatitis C (65%). Table 8.4 lists the kinds of prevention, screening, supplies, referral, and education services that were offered by the SEPs between 2005 and 2008.

State Laws Governing SEPs Vary

The CDC reports in "Syringe Exchange Programs— United States, 2008" that in 2008, 120 of the nation's 184 SEPs reported budgets totaling $21.3 million, of which 79% of funding was from state and local governments. The Kaiser Family Foundation reports in "Sterile Syringe Exchange Programs, 2011" (http://www.state healthfacts.org/comparetable.jsp?ind=566&cat=11) that in 2011 there were 221 SEPs operating in 33 states and the District of Columbia. The foundation notes the variation in legislation governing SEPs. For example, in Arizona, Colorado, Georgia, Indiana, Michigan, Minnesota, Montana, New York, North Carolina, Oklahoma, and Texas, SEPs operated without specific legislation authorizing them. In contrast, California, Connecticut, Delaware, the District of Columbia, Hawaii, Maine, Maryland, Massachusetts, New Hampshire, New Jersey, New Mexico, Rhode Island, Vermont, and Washington had state

laws that authorize SEPs. There were no SEPs operating in Alabama, Arkansas, Idaho, Iowa, Kansas, Kentucky, Mississippi, Nevada, New Hampshire, North Dakota, South Carolina, South Dakota, Tennessee, Utah, Virginia, West Virginia, and Wyoming.

Helping IDUs Saves Lives

Scott Burris of Temple University observes in "Overview of Syringe Access Interventions" (January 2009, http://saprp.org/knowledgeassets/knowledge_detail .cfm?KAID=15) that because IDU with unsterile needles and syringes remains a major source of HIV infection in the United States, accounting for approximately one-third of AIDS cases, "the US Public Health Service deems one-time-only use of sterile syringes to be essential to reducing rates of transmission among injection drug users (IDUs)." Burris also notes that "despite substantial evidence that expanded syringe access benefits public health without causing other harms, state laws on syringe distribution and possession, law enforcement practices, and actions by the US Congress that limit federal funding for SEPs may be inhibiting the potential of syringe access programs to prevent HIV."

In "Spatial Access to Syringe Exchange Programs and Pharmacies Selling Over-the-Counter Syringes as Predictors of Drug Injectors' Use of Sterile Syringes" (*American Journal of Public Health*, vol. 101, no. 6, June 2011), Hannah L. Cooper et al. look at relationships between access to SEPs and pharmacies selling over-the-counter syringes and the behaviors of 4,003 IDUs in New York City between 1995 and 2006. The researchers find that greater access to SEPs and pharmacies that sell syringes over-the-counter improved IDUs' abilities to engage in risk reduction practices that reduce the likelihood and frequency of both HIV and hepatitis C virus transmission.

PHYSICIANS SUPPORT ACCESS TO STERILE SYRINGES FOR IDUS. In many states syringe prescription laws effectively block access to sterile syringes for IDUs. Pharmacists

TABLE 8.4

Services provided by syringe exchange programs (SEPs), 2005–08

	Survey year (No. of SEPs)							
	2005 (sample size = 118)		2006 (sample size = 150)		2007 (sample size = 131)		2008 (sample size = 123)	
Supplies and services	No.	(%)	No.	(%)	No.	(%)	No.	(%)
Prevention supplies								
Male condoms	115	(97)	148	(99)	130	(99)	121	(98)
Female condoms	98	(83)	115	(77)	112	(85)	97	(79)
Alcohol pads	117	(99)	148	(99)	131	(100)	123	(100)
Bleach	82	(69)	89	(59)	77	(59)	69	(56)
On-site medical screenings and services								
HIV counseling and testing	96	(81)	126	(84)	115	(88)	107	(87)
Hepatitis C counseling and testing	66	(56)	94	(63)	72	(55)	80	(65)
Hepatitis B counseling and testing	44	(37)	71	(47)	30	(23)	30	(24)
Hepatitis A counseling and testing	28	(24)	57	(38)	22	(17)	22	(18)
Hepatitis B vaccination	46	(39)	77	(51)	58	(44)	60	(49)
Hepatitis A vaccination	43	(36)	74	(49)	59	(45)	58	(47)
Sexually transmitted disease (STD) screening	57	(48)	75	(50)	64	(49)	67	(55)
Tuberculosis screening	33	(28)	39	(26)	31	(24)	38	(31)
On-site medical care	34	(29)	50	(33)	43	(33)	47	(38)
Referrals								
Substance-abuse treatment	102	(86)	133	(89)	120	(92)	110	(89)
Education								
HIV/AIDS prevention/STD prevention	116	(98)	139	(93)	124	(95)	118	(96)
Hepatitis A, B, and C prevention	114	(97)	148	(99)	127	(97)	119	(97)
Safer injection practice	113	(96)	129	(86)	126	(96)	116	(94)
Abscess care/vein care	107	(91)	141	(94)	123	(94)	113	(92)
Male condom use	112	(95)	145	(97)	125	(95)	120	(98)
Female condom use	97	(82)	119	(79)	104	(79)	91	(74)

HIV = Human immunodeficiency virus.
STD = Sexually transmitted disease.

SOURCE: "Table 3. Services And Supplies Provided by Syringe Exchange Programs (SEPs)—United States, 2005–2008," in "Syringe Exchange Programs—United States, 2008," *Morbidity and Mortality Weekly Report*, vol. 59, no. 45, November 19, 2010, http://www.cdc.gov/mmwr/pdf/wk/mm5945.pdf (accessed June 16, 2011)

may be reluctant to sell syringes to suspected IDUs, and police may take possession of syringes or arrest IDUs who cannot demonstrate a medical need, other than injection drug use of illegal drugs, for the syringes they possess. These barriers could be eliminated by physician prescription of syringes.

Grace E. Macalino et al. conducted the first national survey of physicians to determine their willingness to prescribe syringes for IDUs and reported the results in "A National Physician Survey on Prescribing Syringes as an HIV Prevention Measure" (*Substance Abuse Treatment, Prevention, and Policy*, vol. 4, June 8, 2009). The researchers find that despite the fact that physicians have, in general, never actually prescribed syringes to IDUs, most would consider doing so. Macalino et al. conclude, "The physicians in our study were generally amenable to participating in syringe prescription programs, but physician willingness to act can be supported by better communication of what constitutes evidence-based practice, alleviation of legal concerns, and explicit validation by peers and professional organizations. Requiring substance abuse as a subject in medical training and continuing medical education would also promote better care for IDUs."

Legal Barriers to Federal Funding of SEPs

Despite the preponderance of evidence from myriad sources that SEPs are effective strategies for the prevention of HIV transmission, the federal government, as well as most local and state governments, have not made them legal. They argue that taxpayers should not finance illicit drug use. Since 1988 Congress has passed at least six laws that contain provisions that specifically prohibit or restrict the use of federal funds for SEPs and activities. The Comprehensive Alcohol Abuse, Drug Abuse, and Mental Health Amendments Act of 1988 requires states, as a condition for receiving block grant funds, to agree that funds will not be used "to carry out any program of distributing sterile needles for the hypodermic injection of any illegal drug or bleach for the purpose of cleansing needles for such hypodermic injection."

However, the Community AIDS and Hepatitis Prevention Act was introduced in January 2009. The bill aimed to lift the ban on federal funding for SEPs and allow local communities to make their own choices of how to spend federal funds. The bill was referred to the House Energy and Commerce Committee, where it died. President Obama expressed support for lifting the ban on federal funding, but as of August 2011, his administration had yet to take action on this issue.

SEP advocates were heartened by a February 2011 determination by Regina Benjamin (1956–), the U.S. surgeon general. In "Determination That a Demonstration Needle Exchange Program Would be Effective in Reducing Drug Abuse and the Risk of Acquired Immune Deficiency Syndrome Infection among Intravenous Drug Users" (*Federal Register*, vol. 76, no. 36, February 23, 2011), Benjamin opines that SEPs "would be effective in reducing drug abuse and the risk of infection with the etiologic agent for acquired immune deficiency syndrome" and that the scientific evidence supporting the health benefits of SEPs fulfills "the statutory requirement permitting the expenditure of Substance Abuse Prevention and Treatment (SAPT) Block Grant funds."

CHAPTER 9
HIV AND AIDS WORLDWIDE

This new fourth decade of the epidemic should be one of moving towards efficient, focused and scaled-up programmes to accelerate progress for Results. Results. Results.

—Michel Sidibé, Joint United Nations Program on HIV/AIDS Executive Director and Under Secretary-General of the United Nations, *Global Report: UNAIDS Report on the Global AIDS Epidemic, 2010* (2010)

SCOPE OF THE PROBLEM

Few factors have changed global demographics as inalterably as the HIV/AIDS pandemic (worldwide epidemic). According to the Joint United Nations Program on HIV/AIDS (UNAIDS), in *Global Report: UNAIDS Report on the Global AIDS Epidemic, 2010* (2010, http://www.unaids.org/globalreport/documents/20101123_GlobalReport_full_en.pdf), an estimated 33.3 million people were living with HIV in 2009. Even though more than 5 million people were receiving HIV treatment in 2009, this number was just 35% of the people who needed treatment, according to the World Health Organization's (WHO) 2010 guidelines. An estimated 10 million people living with HIV remained untreated.

The number of new HIV infections reported each year continues to decline from a peak of about 3.2 million in 1997 to about 2.6 million in 2009. The decline in HIV incidence is attributable not only to the efficacy (the ability of an intervention to produce the intended diagnostic or therapeutic effect in optimal circumstances) of HIV prevention activities but also to the natural course of HIV epidemics. The prevalence of HIV in a population does not increase indefinitely, because at some point the population is saturated. Generally, after the initial spread of HIV there is likely to be a decrease in the incidence of infection, which results in a decrease in prevalence.

The HIV/AIDS pandemic is actually many separate epidemics, each with its own distinctive origin and shaped by specific geography and populations. Each epidemic involves different risk behaviors and practices, such as unprotected sex with multiple partners or sharing injection drug equipment. According to UNAIDS, some countries have made tremendous strides in expanding and ensuring access to treatment. It also notes that there has been progress in advancing HIV prevention programs—new HIV infections are declining in many countries that have been hardest hit by the epidemic and some of the big epidemics in sub-Saharan Africa have stabilized or are beginning to decline.

However, the epidemics are not subsiding everywhere. In countries in eastern Europe and Central Asia—Armenia, Bangladesh, Georgia, Kazakhstan, Kyrgyzstan, the Philippines, and Tajikistan—the incidence of HIV rose by more than 25% between 2001 and 2009. Nearly 90% of newly reported HIV infections in eastern Europe were in the Russian Federation and Ukraine, which both had an HIV prevalence of at least 1%.

UNAIDS indicates that women continue to account for more than half (52%) of all people living with HIV infection. The estimated number of children living with HIV was 2.5 million in 2009. Outside of sub-Saharan Africa, HIV disproportionately affects injection drug users (IDUs), men who have sex with men (MSM), and sex workers.

Global Trends and Projections

Even though public health programs have made impressive progress in eliminating and controlling many infectious diseases, UNAIDS explains in *Global Report: UNAIDS Report on the Global AIDS Epidemic, 2010* that while fewer people are becoming HIV infected and fewer are dying from AIDS, HIV/AIDS remains a global health problem of unprecedented dimensions.

In "Projections of Global Mortality and Burden of Disease from 2002 to 2030" (*PLoS Medicine*, vol. 3, no. 11, November 2006), Colin D. Mathers and Dejan Loncar develop three forecasts of future health trends: baseline, optimistic, and pessimistic projections. In the baseline forecast, which assumes that antiretroviral drug use rises to 80% of the population in all regions by 2012, the researchers project that global HIV/AIDS deaths will rise to 6.5 million in 2030. In the optimistic projection, which assumes heightened prevention activities, there will be 3.7 million HIV/AIDS deaths in 2030. In the pessimistic projection, which assumes that antiretroviral therapy will reach 60% by 2012 in all regions except Latin America, where it reaches 70% in 2013, 6.6 million deaths will occur in 2030. In the baseline projection, HIV/AIDS is the third-leading cause of death worldwide in 2030.

John Bongaarts, François Pelletier, and Patrick Gerland examine in *Poverty, Gender, and Youth: Global Trends in AIDS Mortality* (2009, http://www.popcouncil.org/pdfs/wp/pgy/016.pdf) past trends and future projections of AIDS mortality worldwide. The researchers explain that the HIV/AIDS epidemics began at different times in different regions—earlier in the United States and Uganda and later in the Russian Federation and South Africa—but that the prevalence patterns are similar. The epidemics began by spreading slowly, then entered periods of rapid expansion, and then plateaued during the 1990s and the first decade of the 21st century. Bongaarts, Pelletier, and Gerland observe that the natural course of the epidemics plateaued when the virus had infected the vulnerable populations as completely as possible and that the initial wave of infections was followed by a wave of AIDS deaths (prior to the advent of antiretroviral therapy). These deaths removed HIV-infected people from the population, which contributed to plateaus or declines in HIV prevalence rates. The researchers also believe that a reduction in high-risk behaviors in many countries including Kenya, Malawi, Thailand, Uganda, and Zimbabwe has contributed to stable and declining infection levels.

Bongaarts, Pelletier, and Gerland estimate that there were 24 million AIDS deaths between 1980 and 2007. They predict that absent intensified and more effective prevention strategies and interventions, by 2030 approximately 75 million deaths will be attributable to AIDS worldwide.

PATTERNS OF INFECTION

Globally, HIV/AIDS is primarily a sexually transmitted disease (STD) that is transmitted through unprotected sexual intercourse between men and women or MSM. Like some other STDs, HIV infection can also be spread through blood, blood products, donated organs, semen, or vaginal fluids and perinatally from a pregnant mother to her unborn child. The majority of worldwide cumulative (over the entire time that statistics have been kept) HIV infections in adults are estimated to have been transmitted through heterosexual intercourse, although the relative proportion of infections resulting from heterosexual con-

tact as opposed to MSM varies greatly in different parts of the world.

More than 90% of children with HIV acquired the virus during pregnancy, birth, or breastfeeding. The balance were infected by contaminated injections, transfusion with infected blood, sexual abuse, or sexual intercourse.

HIV-1 and HIV-2

Kevin Peterson et al. explain in "Antiretroviral Therapy for HIV-2 Infection: Recommendations for Management in Low-Resource Settings" (*AIDS Research and Treatment*, February 9, 2011) that two types of HIV have been recognized and identified: HIV-1, the predominant worldwide virus, and HIV-2. HIV-2 has much lower rates of progression and infectivity than does HIV-1, and the majority of people that become infected are likely to be long-term nonprogressors (people who become infected but do not develop AIDS). HIV-2 also responds differently to antiretroviral drugs and is frequently resistant to two of the major classes of antiretroviral drugs—the fusion inhibitors and the nonnucleoside reverse transcriptase inhibitors—that are the standard treatment for HIV-1.

HIV-1 and HIV-2 also show an extraordinary difference in global distribution. In North and South America HIV-1 has reached pandemic proportions among certain risk groups, primarily through MSM and IDU. Some African and Asian countries have also experienced extensive heterosexual transmission of HIV-1. HIV-2 is largely restricted to West Africa, where it is mostly attributable to heterosexual transmission and accounts for a third of the HIV prevalence cases. Other countries with sizeable populations infected with HIV-2 are European countries with colonial links to West Africa, such as France, Portugal, and the United Kingdom, as well as other countries with previous Portuguese ties, such as Angola, Brazil, India, and Mozambique.

DIFFERENCES IN EPIDEMIOLOGY, INCIDENCE, AND TRANSMISSION. The epidemiological characteristics (factors such as distribution, incidence, and prevalence that determine the presence, extent, or absence of a disease) of HIV-2 are different from those of HIV-1. Perhaps reflecting these differences, the international spread of HIV-2 is quite limited. During the early course of infection, people with HIV-2 are less infectious than those with HIV-1. This is due to the low levels of the virus isolated from the blood of immunodeficient people with HIV-2. Over time, as an individual's immunodeficiency progresses, HIV-2 probably becomes more infectious, but this more infectious period is relatively shorter than for HIV-1 and tends to occur in older individuals.

According to Elizabeth Pádua et al., in "Assessment of Mother-to-Child HIV-1 and HIV-2 Transmission: An AIDS Reference Laboratory Collaborative Study" (*HIV Medicine*, vol. 10, no. 3, March 2009), multiple studies demonstrate evidence that HIV-2 is not frequently transmitted from mother to child. Even though the mechanics of perinatal transmission are not completely understood, advanced immunodeficiency of the mother is certainly a risk factor. Low levels of the virus are not sufficient to transmit to the baby, and higher levels of virus infection in women past childbearing years may explain why perinatal transmission is less frequent. This is the most likely explanation for the observation that HIV-2 infection is so rare in children.

Interactions and HIV Transmission

One of the major concerns of public health officials worldwide is the possible interaction between HIV and other infections. The same risky behaviors that expose individuals to potential HIV infection also expose them to other STDs, such as gonorrhea, syphilis, and chancroid (a genital ulcer). Considerable data suggest that STDs, particularly herpes simplex, chancroid, and syphilis (which all cause ulcerative lesions), promote the transmission of HIV.

In "Herpes Simplex Virus Type 2: Epidemiology and Management Options in Developing Countries" (*Postgraduate Medical Journal*, vol. 84, no. 992, 2008), Gabriela Paz-Bailey et al. observe that genital herpes simplex virus type 2 is highly prevalent worldwide and is an increasingly important cause of genital ulcer disease, which in turn increases the risk of HIV transmission and acquisition. The researchers call for actions "to improve recognition of genital herpes, to prevent its spread and also to prevent its potential to promote HIV transmission in developing countries."

TUBERCULOSIS. HIV infection is recognized as the strongest known risk factor for the development of active tuberculosis (TB), because people with a latent TB infection are more apt to develop the disease once their immune system has been compromised by HIV. According to the WHO, in *Guidelines for Intensified Tuberculosis Case-Finding and Isoniazid Preventive Therapy for People Living with HIV in Resource-Constrained Settings* (2011, http://whqlibdoc.who .int/publications/2011/9789241500708_eng.pdf), people with HIV have 20 to 37 times the risk of developing TB as people without HIV infection. More than one-quarter of all deaths of people with HIV are attributable to TB.

UNAIDS confirms in *Global Report: UNAIDS Report on the Global AIDS Epidemic, 2010* that TB is a leading cause of death among people with HIV. In 2009 an estimated 380,000 deaths of people living with HIV were the result of TB. Sub-Saharan Africa is home to more than three-quarters of all people with HIV-related TB and in some countries nearly 80% of people with TB also are infected with HIV.

People infected with HIV who test tuberculin-positive are not only more likely to develop TB but also are likely to develop TB more rapidly than people without HIV infection. An even more disastrous consequence is that half of all people infected with both will develop contagious TB, which they could then spread to susceptible people, even those not infected with HIV.

The WHO 2011 guidelines offer recommendations that are intended to reduce TB in people living with HIV, their families, and their communities via a combination of screening for TB and preventive therapy. The guidelines advise screening all people with HIV for TB and treating those with positive test results prophylactically (to prevent the disease). Furthermore, they advise starting all HIV-infected people who also have active TB on antiretroviral therapy regardless of their CD4 cell counts.

UNAIDS explains in *Global Report: UNAIDS Report on the Global AIDS Epidemic, 2010* that TB is the most common opportunistic infection for people living with HIV (including those on antiretroviral drugs) and a leading cause of death in low- and middle-income countries. Africa is in the throes of the worst TB pandemic since the advent of widespread use of antibiotics. UNAIDS states that "in sub-Saharan Africa, which accounts for 78% of people with HIV-related TB . . . , the HIV prevalence among people with TB is as high as 80% in some countries." As many as half of children living with HIV in South Africa also have TB.

Highly Drug-Resistant Tuberculosis

In *HIV and Tuberculosis: Ensuring Universal Access and Protection of Human Rights* (March 2010, http://data.unaids .org/pub/ExternalDocument/2010/20100324_unaidsrghrtsis suepapertbhrts_en.pdf), UNAIDS observes that people living with HIV/AIDS are more likely to have multidrug-resistant tuberculosis (MDR-TB; this type of TB does not respond to two first-line anti-TB drugs—rifampicin and isoniazid) than people who are not HIV infected. Extensively drug-resistant tuberculosis (XDR-TB; this type of TB does not respond to first- and second-line anti-TB drug treatment) is associated with extremely high mortality rates in people with HIV/AIDS.

To a large extent, drug-resistant TB occurs in response to inadequate TB control, poor patient or clinician adherence to TB treatment regimens, poor-quality drugs, or a lack of drug supplies. People living with HIV are particularly vulnerable to developing drug-resistant TB because of their compromised immune system, which makes them more susceptible to infection and more likely to progress to active TB.

XDR-TB has occurred in other locales as well as sub-Saharan Africa. In "Emergence of *Mycobacterium tuberculosis* with Extensive Resistance to Second-Line Drugs—Worldwide, 2000–2004" (*Morbidity and Mortality Weekly Report*, vol. 55, no. 11, March 24, 2006), the WHO and the Centers for Disease Control and Prevention report that between 2000 and 2004, 2% of TB cultures performed at

25 reference laboratories met the criteria for XDR-TB and conclude that XDR-TB is present in all regions of the world. Because TB culture and drug sensitivity testing are not performed routinely in many developing countries, the number of people affected and the full extent of the pandemic cannot be accurately measured or projected.

UNAIDS observes that each year only about half of adults in South Africa with active TB are cured, which is a very low cure rate compared to other countries. Furthermore, disparities in access to health care and the quality of health care exacerbate the problem of drug-resistant TB in developing countries. MDR- and XDR-TB arose largely in response to inadequate care of poor and neglected populations. Inappropriate drug choices, drug doses, and duration of treatment, as well as an irregular supply of drugs, poorly trained personnel, and poor adherence to treatment, all act to increase the development and transmission of drug-resistant TB.

Geographic Differences

In North America and Europe during the 1980s and early 1990s, HIV was transmitted predominantly through unprotected sexual intercourse among MSM and through IDU with contaminated needles. During the late 1990s heterosexual intercourse and IDU became the prevailing modes of HIV transmission in North America and Europe.

In sub-Saharan Africa the overwhelming mode of transmission has been heterosexual intercourse. In this part of the world, transmission through MSM contact or through IDU is slight. Because many women have been infected, preventing perinatal transmission is increasingly important. UNAIDS reports in *Global Report: UNAIDS Report on the Global AIDS Epidemic, 2010* that the increasing numbers and percentages of HIV-infected pregnant women receiving antiretroviral drugs to prevent mother-to-child transmission of HIV has effectively reduced transmission. For example, there were just 370,000 HIV diagnoses attributable to perinatal transmission in 2009, down from 500,000 in 2001. In South Africa 90% of expectant mothers receive treatment to prevent transmission of HIV and as a result perinatal transmission has been dramatically reduced. In contrast, perinatal transmission remains high in Papua New Guinea, where almost 10% of all newly diagnosed cases are attributable to mother-to-child transmission.

The rates of MSM transmission in Latin America are similar to those of Europe and the United States, but IDU is less frequent, whereas heterosexual transmission is considerably higher. In South and Southeast Asia the rapid increase of HIV can be traced to shared contaminated injection equipment and heterosexual intercourse. According to UNAIDS, in *UNGASS Country Progress Report: P.R. China* (December 2007, http://www.unaids.org/), almost half of HIV-infected people living in China in 2007 were thought to have been infected as a result of

IDU and 40.6% acquired the disease via heterosexual intercourse. Similarly, the National AIDS Control Programme indicates in *Injecting Drug Use: Strategy Report for NACP IV Planning* (June 2011, http://nacoonline.org/) that even though most HIV infections in India are occurring because of unprotected heterosexual intercourse, contaminated injection drug equipment is also a significant risk factor for HIV infection in several states in India, such as Manipur, Punjab, and Tamil Nadu, where more than 15% of IDUs were HIV infected in 2008.

The highest national HIV infection levels in Asia continue to be found in Southeast Asia, where combinations of unsafe practices with sex workers and MSM, along with IDU, continue to fuel and maintain the epidemics. Even though the HIV infection rate has peaked and leveled off in other parts of the world, it is escalating in Indonesia, Pakistan, Vietnam, China, and Bangladesh, largely from heterosexual intercourse and through sex workers.

Unless otherwise noted, the following data and statistics, which describe the epidemics in various regions and countries, are drawn from UNAIDS reports. UNAIDS and the WHO provide the most recent and reliable estimates of HIV incidence and prevalence, generally from 2007 to 2009.

AFRICA
North Africa and the Middle East

Unreliable and often inadequate HIV surveillance systems complicate an accurate assessment of the patterns and trends of the epidemics in many countries in North Africa and the Middle East—especially among high-risk populations. Improved data collection and surveillance in some countries such as Algeria, Iran, Libya, and Morocco show that HIV epidemics do exist across the region and that an epidemic continues in the Sudan. In Algeria and Morocco the majority of reported HIV infections are attributable to unprotected sex, and women make up a growing proportion of people living with HIV. In *Global Report: UNAIDS Report on the Global AIDS Epidemic, 2010*, UNAIDS notes that an estimated 460,000 people were living with HIV in the region, including 75,000 newly infected in 2009.

UNAIDS also observes that the transmission of HIV is fueled significantly by sex workers and IDUs. In Iran 14% of male IDUs were thought to be HIV infected in 2007, and IDU is considered a major route of transmission in Algeria, Libya, Morocco, Syria, and Tunisia. In Egypt 6% of MSM and 1% of female sex workers were living with HIV in 2006. That same year an even higher percentage of female sex workers—from 2% to 4%—in Algeria, Morocco, and Yemen were thought to be living with HIV.

According to UNAIDS, at the close of 2009 an estimated 460,000 adults and children in North Africa and the Middle East were infected with HIV, 75,000 acquired the infection, and 24,000 deaths were due to AIDS-related illnesses. The largest epidemic in the region is in the Sudan, and surveys indicate that between 8% and 9% of the MSM population is infected with HIV. Historically, unreliable reporting and data, especially about high-risk populations, have made it challenging to accurately track and forecast the epidemics in many countries. However, recent efforts to improve surveillance reveal local epidemics in Algeria, Iran, Libya, and Morocco and a more generalized epidemic throughout the Sudan.

The HIV epidemic in the Sudan is attributable to heterosexual transmission of the virus. Here, as in other countries, an increasing number of women are acquiring the virus from husbands or boyfriends who became infected from IDU or paid sex. Besides MSM and female sex workers, UNAIDS identifies in *2010 UNGASS Report: North Sudan* (March 2010, http://www.unaids.org/en/dataanalysis/monitoringcountryprogress/2010progressreportssubmittedbycountries/sudan_2010_country_progress_report_en.pdf) several populations at risk—tea sellers, military personnel, youth in and out of school, and truck drivers—that should be targeted for prevention programs and interventions to change behaviors and reduce transmission risk.

Unparalleled Infection Rates

UNAIDS reports in *Global Report: UNAIDS Report on the Global AIDS Epidemic, 2010* that a staggering 22.5 million adults and children (more than two-thirds of the global HIV burden) in sub-Saharan Africa were living with HIV in 2009. The national prevalence rates (the number of cases of the disease present in a specified population at a given time) of HIV infection among adults vary widely. Swaziland has the highest HIV prevalence in the world—25.9% of adults were living with HIV in 2009. Some West African countries report relatively low rates of infection, whereas others in the southern portion of the continent experience much higher rates. Some of the HIV epidemics in this region have already peaked and are diminishing. In 22 countries including four with the largest epidemics—Ethiopia, South Africa, Zambia, and Zimbabwe—the HIV incidence rate fell by more than 25% between 2001 and 2009. In sub-Saharan Africa the number of new infections decreased from 2.2 million in 2001 to 1.8 million in 2009. In some countries, including Uganda and Rwanda, HIV prevalence has leveled off at about 7% and 3%, respectively.

SEVERAL MODES OF TRANSMISSION. Because heterosexual transmission is the predominant mode of transmission in Africa, men and women have been almost equally infected. However, UNAIDS finds in *Global Report: UNAIDS Report on the Global AIDS Epidemic, 2010* that in 2009 more women than men were infected with HIV, and they were also more likely to be the ones caring for others infected with HIV or suffering from AIDS. Approximately three-quarters of all HIV-infected women in the world live in sub-Saharan Africa.

According to UNAIDS, young women are disproportionately affected. For example, in Lesotho (a country completely surrounded by South Africa) almost 8% of young women aged 15 to 19 years and 3% of young men were living with HIV in 2009. In South Africa 21% of young women aged 20 to 24 years and 5% of young men were living with HIV.

Paid sex workers and their customers play a significant role in the spread of HIV in many countries. For example, in West, Central, and East Africa between 10% and 32% of new HIV infections were attributable to paid sex workers. In 12 African countries between 36% and 86% of couples had one member who was HIV infected.

IDU also contributes to the pandemic in eastern and southern Africa. In Mauritius, IDU was the major source of HIV infection, and it contributed to the epidemics in Kenya, Tanzania, and Zanzibar. MSM also fuels the pandemic in Africa. For example, in Cape Town, South Africa, and Mombasa, Kenya, more than 40% of MSM were HIV infected.

NEW INFECTIONS AMONG TEENS DECLINE. In *South African National HIV Prevalence, Incidence, Behaviour, and Communication Survey, 2008: A Turning Tide among Teenagers?* (June 2009, http://www.mrc.ac.za/pressreleases/2009/sanat.pdf), Olive Shisana et al. find that the number of new infections among teens and young adults are declining despite the fact that the percentages of adolescents and young adults that continue to have multiple sex partners has actually increased. The decline in HIV incidence is almost entirely attributable to increasing condom use—among males aged 15 to 24 years condom use rose from 57.1% in 2002 to 87.4% in 2008. More females aged 15 to 24 years also reported using condoms—from 46.1% in 2002 to 73.1% in 2008. Condom use among males aged 25 to 49 years doubled, and among females in the same age group it nearly tripled.

The increase in condom use is at least in part attributable to heightened awareness resulting from the intensive national HIV communication and education program that was conducted between 2005 and 2008. Approximately 90.2% of young people reported seeing or hearing about HIV/AIDS through this communication program, and 62.2% of older adults (aged 50 years and older) said they had been reached by the program. Despite the success of the national communication program, serious gaps in knowledge persist. The survey found that knowledge of how to prevent HIV infection actually declined among people aged 15 to 49 years, from 64.4% in 2005 to 44.8% in 2008.

PAYING THE PRICE FOR YEARS OF EVASION. Even though Kenya had experienced the ravages of AIDS for about a decade, the Kenyan parliament and cabinet did not debate the issue publicly until 1993. Physicians diagnosed the first AIDS cases in 1984, but the government did not issue national statistics until 1986, when it announced one AIDS-related death. The nation's president and vice president regularly warned the public in speeches to avoid infection, and national officials instructed district administrators, including local tribal chiefs, to encourage their people to practice safe sex and limit their partners, but there had been no official statement.

For many Kenyans, the government's belated commitment to dealing with HIV/AIDS came too late. UNAIDS reports in *Global Report: UNAIDS Report on the Global AIDS Epidemic, 2010* that even though there was a decline in the prevalence of HIV infection among adults from 14% during the mid-1990s to 5% in 2006 and fewer AIDS-related deaths, it may not be entirely attributable to prevention efforts and the observation of increased condom use and a smaller proportion of the population with multiple sex partners. Instead, the lower prevalence of HIV infection may reflect the saturation of the infection in the at-risk population, meaning that the peak of the epidemic may have passed or that deaths from AIDS have served to reduce HIV prevalence.

The Kenyan government's reticence and seeming inability to deal with the epidemic came as a surprise to many observers. Kenya has endured an economic decline that many blame on corruption and the collapse of global commodity prices. Nonetheless, Kenya is still one of Africa's wealthiest countries and has remained relatively stable since gaining its independence from Great Britain in 1963. Many observers thought that if any African country could cope with or even head off an HIV/AIDS epidemic, it would be Kenya.

However, Kenyan officials chose to downplay the threat, lest it frighten away the much-needed tourist dollars. Even though the country did not launch major prevention efforts until 2000, these relatively late efforts seem to have already made an impact on the epidemic in terms of reducing the prevalence of many, though not all, high-risk behaviors. One remaining challenge is that IDU appears to be fueling the country's HIV epidemic.

Besides the risk of IDU as a factor in the transmission of HIV, long-standing social and cultural practices also abet HIV transmission. For example, "wife inheritance," which was once a socially useful tradition, continues to contribute to the spread of HIV/AIDS. In western Kenya, when a woman is widowed, her former husband's family takes care of her and her children. For generations, a brother-in-law or male cousin took her in with his family. Initially, tradition frowned on his having sexual relations with the inherited wife. Eventually, the inheritors began to ignore this restriction and had sex with the widow. If the widow's former husband had died of AIDS, she was likely to be infected and could pass the virus on to her inheritor, who would pass it on to his wife, causing the disease to spread.

UGANDA'S EFFORTS TO REDUCE HIV INFECTION. Scientists think that about 30 years ago, during the early 1980s, truck drivers first spread HIV in Uganda's Rakai District, which lies along a Lake Victoria trade route to the capital city of Kampala. Because commercial sex is widely available along the trade route, HIV quickly spread throughout Uganda and all of Africa. At one time, Uganda had the world's highest HIV infection rates. At the turn of the 21st century, it was one of only two developing nations (Thailand is the other) where there was nationwide evidence of declining HIV rates in response to strong prevention programs. UNAIDS indicates in *Global Report: UNAIDS Report on the Global AIDS Epidemic, 2010* that these programs, which emphasized changes in sexual behavior, helped reduce the percentage of HIV infection among people aged 15 to 49 years.

Uganda was the first African country to respond powerfully to its HIV/AIDS epidemic. The government began by gathering religious and traditional leaders, along with representatives of other sectors of society, in an effort to reach agreement that the problem had to be confronted. Prevention efforts targeted specific populations or communities. For example, prevention programs that focused on safe sex practices and/or delaying sex were presented in schools. Community groups were formed to counsel and support those living with the virus. Condom use was heavily promoted.

Unlike Kenya, Uganda began an aggressive campaign against the spread of HIV/AIDS during the mid-1980s, when it had the highest number of recorded HIV cases in Africa. With virtually every family touched by HIV/AIDS, much of the cultural, religious, and psychological stigma disappeared in Uganda, where HIV infection rates began to decline. Despite a concerted prevention campaign, UNAIDS notes that the steady decline of Uganda's epidemic had stabilized at 6.5% in 2009. Even though education did prompt behavior changes that in turn resulted in lower HIV prevalence among pregnant women in Kampala and other cities from the early 1990s to the first decade of the 21st century, the decline was also due in part to increased AIDS mortality.

According to UNAIDS, a rise in multiple concurrent partnerships and a shift in the epidemic from people in casual relationships to those in long-term relationships has prevented the prevalence rate from declining further. In *UNGASS Country Progress Report: Uganda* (March 2010, http://www.unaids.org/en/dataanalysis/monitoringcountryprogress/2010progressreportssubmittedbycountries/uganda_2010_country_progress_report_en.pdf), UNAIDS reports that in 2009 about the same proportion of new HIV infections occurred in people in monogamous relationships (43%) as did among people with multiple partners (46%). Just 39% of people in need were receiving antiretroviral therapy in 2009 and just over half of pregnant women (52%) were receiving treatment to prevent transmission to their unborn children.

There have also been reports of higher than anticipated rates of HIV infection in adults seeking treatment for malaria in Uganda. (Malaria is a serious, infectious disease that is spread by mosquitoes and is most common in tropical climates.) Lisa M. Bebell et al. report in "HIV-1 Infection in Patients Referred for Malaria Blood Smears at Government Health Clinics in Uganda" (*Journal of Acquired Immune Deficiency Syndrome*, vol. 46, no. 5, December 15, 2007) that among Ugandans evaluated for suspected malaria, associations between malaria test results and HIV infection differed between children and adults. In children, HIV was more common among those with negative malaria blood smears, whereas in adults HIV infection was more common among those with positive blood smears. The researchers conclude that the diagnosis of malaria "is a warning sign for HIV infection in adults, because HIV infection likely diminishes acquired antimalarial immunity. In children, malaria is very common, and a negative malaria smear suggests other causes of fever, including HIV-related infections."

UNAIDS asserts that the challenges to managing the HIV/AIDS epidemic in Uganda include:

- Inadequate, uncoordinated data collection, documentation, and dissemination
- Lack of preventive services including testing, counseling, and treatment to prevent mother-to-child transmission
- Inadequate resources, personnel, and systems to effectively manage the logistics of a national HIV/AIDS response
- Limited funding to address the needs of orphans, children, families, and people living with HIV/AIDS

In "The Effects of an HIV Project on HIV and Non-HIV Services at Local Government Clinics in Urban Kampala" (*BMC International Health and Human Rights*, vol. 11, suppl. 1, March 9, 2011), Toru Matsubayashi et al. observe that there is "widespread consensus that weak health systems hamper the effective provision of HIV/AIDS services." The researchers examine the effects of an HIV/AIDS program that was funded by the President's Emergency Plan for AIDS Relief. Specifically, the program provided health care delivery to six government-run general clinics in Kampala. Besides analyzing the volume of services provided, the researchers interviewed patients to compare perceptions of the experiences of patients receiving HIV care and those receiving non-HIV care. More than 90% of all patients reported high levels of satisfaction with care. Matsubayashi et al. conclude that "when a collaboration is established to strengthen existing health systems, in addition to providing HIV/AIDS services in a setting in which other primary health care is being delivered, there are positive effects not only on HIV/AIDS services, but also on many other essential services," such as treatment for malaria and TB as well as pediatric care and immunization. They also note that "there was no evidence that the HIV program had any deleterious effects on health services offered at the clinics studied."

EUROPE

Western and Central Europe

HIV in western and central Europe is spread primarily through MSM. UNAIDS reports in *Global Report: UNAIDS Report on the Global AIDS Epidemic, 2010* that in 23 European countries the annual number of HIV diagnoses among MSM increased by 86% between 2000 and 2006. The number of people living with HIV in western and central Europe rose by 30% from an estimated 1.8 million in 2001 to 2.3 million in 2009. Because HIV is primarily transmitted via MSM, more men than women were living with HIV—women accounted for just 29% of this population in western and central Europe. Even though MSM accounted for just 1.6% of the population in France, they made up more than half of new HIV infections among men. In 2007 a record 3,160 new HIV cases were diagnosed in MSM in the United Kingdom.

THE UNITED KINGDOM. According to UNAIDS, in *UNGASS Country Progress Report: United Kingdom* (July 2010, http://www.unaids.org/en/dataanalysis/monitoringcountryprogress/2010progressreportssubmittedbycountries/unitedkingdom_2010_country_progress_report_en.pdf), at the close of 2008 an estimated 83,000 people were living with HIV/AIDS in the United Kingdom. Of this total, more than one-quarter (27%) of these were unaware of their infection status. Fifty percent of the 7,382 new HIV infections diagnosed in 2008 were attributable to heterosexual transmission and 42% were in MSM. Just 185 (2.5% of cases) were diagnosed as IDUs. The low prevalence of HIV in IDUs is attributable to the institution of needle exchange programs during the 1980s. Even though MSM continue to be the population at greatest risk of acquiring HIV in the United Kingdom, heterosexual transmission has increased, accounting for 58% of new diagnoses in 2008, while MSM accounted for 38%.

Since the mid-1990s AIDS diagnoses have declined significantly, from a peak of 1,882 in 1994 to 700 in 2008; likewise, AIDS deaths decreased during this same period, from 1,726 to 571. Rates of diagnosis of HIV in pregnant women have increased, from 70% in 1999 to 90% in 2008, and 95% of pregnant women received HIV testing.

THE NETHERLANDS. In "National Estimate of HIV Prevalence in the Netherlands: Comparison and Applicability of Different Estimation Tools" (*AIDS*, vol. 25, no. 2, January 14, 2011), Maaike G. van Veen et al. estimate that as of January 2008 there were 23,969 people living with HIV/AIDS in the Netherlands. Adult HIV prevalence was estimated at 0.2%, and 40% of people with HIV were undiagnosed.

UNAIDS reports in *UNGASS Country Progress Report: The Netherlands and the Netherlands Antilles* (February 2008, http://www.unaids.org/en/dataanalysis/monitoringcountryprogress/2010progressreportssubmittedbycountries/2008progressreportssubmittedbycountries/the_netherlands_2008_country_progress_report_en.pdf) that HIV transmission in the Netherlands is primarily via MSM. In 2006 MSM accounted for 59% of new cases of HIV infection, whereas heterosexual transmission accounted for 33% of new diagnoses. Transmission via IDU, blood products, and mother to child was low, with each accounting for less than 1% of cases.

SPAIN. Historically, Spain has had the highest number of HIV/AIDS cases per capita in the European Union. The Ministerio de Sanidad y Consumo Centro de Publicaciones indicates in *HIV and AIDS in Spain, 2001* (September 2002, http://www.isciii.es/htdocs/pdf/libroing.pdf) that the first case of HIV was reported in Spain in 1981; by the end of 2001, 110,000 to 150,000 people were living with HIV. According to the Ministerio de Sanidad y Consumo Centro de Publicaciones, in *Informe Nacional Sobre Los Progresos Realizados En La Aplicación Del UNGASS España Enero de 2008–Diciembre de 2009* (2010, http://www.unaids.org/en/dataanalysis/monitoringcountryprogress/2010progressreportssubmittedbycountries/spain_2010_country_progress_report_es.pdf), there were 78,654 new diagnoses of HIV infection, 1,600 AIDS deaths, and between 120,000 and 150,000 people living with HIV/AIDS at the end of 2009.

The article "Spain's War on AIDS Visits the Prado" (*New York Times*, August 27, 1997) explains that drug use in Spain began to increase during the 1970s and 1980s, after the long Francisco Franco (1892–1975) dictatorship ended. Isabel Noguer of the Health Ministry describes this period as a time of heavy heroin use, with addicts sharing infected needles. In 1997 IDUs still made up the highest risk group, whereas unprotected heterosexual relations was the next most common form of transmission. By 2003 HIV prevalence among IDUs declined in cities that had instituted effective long-standing harm-reduction programs. In *Global Report: UNAIDS Report on the Global AIDS Epidemic, 2010*, UNAIDS notes that in 2006 Spain was one of just eight countries that provided comprehensive harm reduction, which included needle and syringe exchange and treatment programs for IDUs in prisons.

J. M. Arroyo-Cobo chronicles in "Public Health Gains from Health in Prisons in Spain" (*Public Health*, vol. 124, no. 11, November 2010) the HIV epidemic in Spanish prisons and describes how the implementation of comprehensive harm reduction, including needle and syringe exchange and treatment programs, significantly reduced both the incidence and prevalence of HIV/AIDS.

Eastern Europe and Central Asia

The HIV pandemic did not reach eastern Europe until the mid-1990s. According to UNAIDS, in *Global Report: UNAIDS Report on the Global AIDS Epidemic, 2010*, in 2009 eastern Europe and Central Asia were the only regions where HIV prevalence continued to rise. In 1995 only 30,000 out of 450 million people were infected throughout all of eastern Europe; by 1997 about 190,000 adults were infected with HIV. The number of people living with HIV has nearly tripled, rising to 1.4 million between 2000 and 2009. Much of this increase is attributable to a sharp increase in HIV infections among people who injected drugs during the late 1990s and the first half of the first decade of the 21st century.

Ukraine and the Russian Federation have been the hardest hit countries in eastern Europe. In 2009 nearly 90% of all new HIV infections were in these two countries. Ukraine, where HIV diagnoses have doubled since 2001, has the highest prevalence of adults living with HIV—1.1% in the entire region. Other countries experienced skyrocketing HIV incidence rates between 2001 and 2009—increases in excess of 25% occurred in Armenia, Georgia, Kazakhstan, Kyrgyzstan, and Tajikistan.

Historically, IDU has been the primary source for the spread of the virus. According to UNAIDS, in 2009 about 25% of the 3.7 million IDUs in the region were living with HIV. The prevalence of HIV infection among IDUs in the Russian Federation was 37%—more than one-third of the 1.8 million IDUs in this country had HIV infections.

The region has also seen an increasing proportion of HIV infections in women. In 2009 an estimated 45% of people living with HIV in Ukraine were women, up from 37% in 1999. These cases most likely result from women infected by sex partners who were IDUs.

UNAIDS indicates that even though IDU is the "main mode of HIV transmission" in the region, there are few harm reduction programs in place, and there is very limited access to drug rehabilitation services. Furthermore, because possession of even small amounts of narcotics is harshly punished in many countries in eastern Europe, IDUs are understandably reluctant to participate in needle exchange programs.

ASIA

Asia could eventually overtake Africa as the continent most affected by HIV. The HIV/AIDS pandemic arrived in Asia much later than in the rest of the world.

Until the mid-1990s HIV/AIDS was uncommon, but because the average incubation period is approximately 10 years, more people are now beginning to die from the disease. UNAIDS estimates in *Global Report: UNAIDS Report on the Global AIDS Epidemic, 2010* that 4.9 million Asian adults and children were infected with HIV in 2009. About 360,000 people were newly diagnosed with the infection that year, and an estimated 300,000 deaths were attributed to AIDS.

Thailand

The spread of HIV in Thailand is unprecedented. Thailand's commercial sex industry is notorious, and travel packages based on the availability of sex workers in Thailand are common in Asia (as they are in other countries, including the United States). In the capital city of Bangkok, brothels are found in virtually every neighborhood. Cheewanan Lertpiriyasuwat, Tanarak Plipat, and Richard Jenkins find in "A Survey of Sexual Risk Behavior for HIV Infection in Nakhonsawan, Thailand, 2001" (*AIDS*, vol. 17, no. 13, September 5, 2003) that in 1990, 20% of all Thai men reported having paid for sex in the previous year. After a military coup in 1991, the transitional government instituted a comprehensive HIV/AIDS education program, which included a media campaign and condom distribution to brothels and massage parlors. Brothels that refused to use condoms were closed down. Even though the anti-HIV program came too late for those infected during the mid- to late 1980s, Thailand recorded a drop in new HIV infections until the late 1990s.

UNAIDS notes that in 2009 an estimated 530,000 adults and children in Thailand were living with HIV and approximately 28,000 died from AIDS-related illnesses. Despite a high prevalence of HIV among people aged 15 to 49 years (1.3%), the number of new HIV infections has been decreasing—largely in response to national prevention initiatives. However, the number of new HIV infections has not declined in all age groups—there have been increases reported among adolescents, pregnant women, and military recruits aged 20 to 24 years.

In "National Expansion of Antiretroviral Treatment in Thailand, 2000–2007: Program Scale-up and Patient Outcomes" (*Journal of Acquired Immune Deficiency Syndrome*, vol. 50, no. 5, April 15, 2009), Sanchai Chasombat et al. observe that before 2000 antiretroviral treatment in Thailand was only available in selected research facilities and private hospitals. Beginning in 2000 all government and some private and university hospitals provided treatment. The program was scaled up so that by the end of 2006 an estimated 115,994 patients had begun antiretroviral treatment. As treatment reached more HIV-infected people, the risk of death and AIDS-related death rates began to decline. The researchers conclude that the observed "treatment outcomes in Thai-

land are encouraging for other resource-limited countries that are also scaling up HIV treatment programs."

Human rights issues such as HIV-related stigma and discrimination continue to challenge the national response to HIV in Thailand. The Research Triangle Institute notes in "Human Rights at the Center of the HIV Response in Thailand" (February 14, 2011, http://www.rti.org/page.cfm ?objectid=2FC52265-5056-B100-0C286B36C344112B) that at a February 2011 conference aimed at incorporating human rights concerns into Thailand's new national HIV strategic plan for 2012–16, Sofia Gruskin, the director of the Program on International Health and Human Rights at the Harvard School of Public Health, underscored the importance of human rights, especially those of vulnerable populations such as women. Gruskin exhorted the development of national universal access to treatment goals that consider not only the total numbers of people receiving care but also "who is gaining access (and who is not), how they are gaining access, and over what period of time."

Other Southeast Asian Countries

In other parts of Southeast Asia data about the epidemics reveal different patterns.

Cambodia has been the hardest hit country in the region. However, there is evidence that the epidemic is subsiding. In *Global Report: UNAIDS Report on the Global AIDS Epidemic, 2010*, UNAIDS finds that in 2009 there were an estimated 63,000 adults and children living with HIV and 3,100 deaths attributable to AIDS. HIV prevalence in Cambodia is declining. UNAIDS indicates in "Cambodia: Country Situation" (July 2008, http://data .unaids.org/pub/FactSheet/2008/sa08_cam_en.pdf) that in June 2007 HIV prevalence among adolescents and young adults aged 15 to 49 years was 0.9%, down from 1.2% in 2003.

In 2005 Cambodia opened public antiretroviral clinics, so the rising percentages of HIV-infected people in treatment reflect increased access to treatment. Not surprisingly, treatment outcomes improved as well. For example, in "Impact of a Public Antiretroviral Program on TB/HIV Mortality: Banteay Meanchey, Cambodia" (*Southeast Asian Journal of Tropical Medicine and Public Health*, vol. 40, no. 1, January 2009), Benjamin Eng et al. compare treatment outcomes of HIV patients newly diagnosed with TB in 2004 (before clinics opened) with outcomes of HIV patients diagnosed in 2005 (after the public clinics opened). They state that "in 2004, 37% of HIV-infected tuberculosis patients died during TB treatment compared with 5% of HIV-uninfected tuberculosis patients. In 2005, 18% of HIV-infected tuberculosis patients died compared with 5% of HIV-uninfected tuberculosis patients."

Even though Cambodia has reduced its number of new HIV infections and more than nine out of 10 people in need of antiretroviral drugs are receiving them, Peter Moszynski notes in "Cambodia's AIDS Strategy Could Fail without Sustainable Financing" (*BMJ*, vol. 341, December 21, 2010) that these treatment programs are funded nearly entirely by foreign donors. He warns that this is not an optimal strategy for the country because donor funding is often uncertain. Moszynski also asserts that Cambodia must develop a more sustainable strategy to fund its HIV/AIDS programs.

India

At the International AIDS Conference held in Vancouver, Canada, in July 1996, a United Nations official reported that India had emerged as the country with the most people infected with HIV. This news came as a surprise to many of the conferees because HIV was not detected in India until 1986. According to UNAIDS, in *Global Report: UNAIDS Report on the Global AIDS Epidemic, 2010*, in 2009 approximately 2.4 million people in India were HIV positive, down from 2.5 million in 2001. Of this total, an estimated 880,000 were women. In 2009, 170,000 deaths were attributable to AIDS.

In *UNGASS Country Progress Report: India* (March 31, 2010, http://www.unaids.org/en/dataanalysis/monitoring countryprogress/2010progressreportssubmittedbycountries/ india_2010_country_progress_report_en.pdf), UNAIDS notes that the epidemic is declining in most states in India. Most HIV infections are attributable to unprotected heterosexual relationships, and there is also overlap of IDU and sex work. Researchers speculate that more than 90% of women with HIV acquired the virus from their regular partners, who were infected during paid sex.

Sex trafficking and female sex workers contribute to the epidemic in many states. In "History of Sex Trafficking, Recent Experiences of Violence, and HIV Vulnerability among Female Sex Workers in Coastal Andhra Pradesh, India" (*International Journal of Gynecology and Obstetrics*, vol. 142, no. 2, August 2011), Jhumka Gupta et al. examine associations between sex trafficking and recent violence experiences and HIV vulnerability among female sex workers in Andhra Pradesh. The researchers find that one out of five female sex workers met the United Nations definition of sex trafficking (exploitation and abuse of people for revenue through sex) and that these sex workers were at increased risk for both violence and HIV.

According to Puspen Ghosh et al., in "Factors Associated with HIV Infection among Indian Women" (*International Journal of STD and AIDS*, vol. 22, no. 3, March 2011), the most common risk factor for HIV transmission for women is an exclusive sexual relationship with their husband. The researchers analyzed data from the National Family Health Survey 2005–06 to identify other risk factors. They find that women at highest risk were those aged 26 to 35 years, were impoverished, and had more than one sexual partner during their lifetime. Women with a history of a genital sore (a marker for other sexually transmitted infections) were also at increased risk. Because most HIV transmission in women takes place within marriage, Ghosh et al. advocate targeting risk-reduction programs to this population, especially in view of their finding of a low percentage of condom use by married men with their wife and other sexual partners.

China

The first HIV case in China was identified in 1985, but the disease did not begin to spread until the early 1990s, when changes in the structure of the economy produced an increase in drug use and prostitution. The U.S. embassy in China indicates in *Flying Blind on a Growing Epidemic: AIDS in China* (September 15, 1997, http://www.csssm.org/English/e5.htm) that the government of China estimated in 1997 that between 100,000 and 300,000 people were living with HIV/AIDS. By the beginning of 1998 this estimate had doubled. UNAIDS notes in *Global Report: UNAIDS Report on the Global AIDS Epidemic, 2010* that in 2009 an estimated 740,000 people were living with HIV in China. That same year an estimated 26,000 deaths were attributed to AIDS.

As in other countries, HIV transmission and infection in China have migrated from the traditional high-risk populations—sex workers, IDUs, and the overlap of these populations—to the general population, and as a result the number of HIV infections in women is growing. According to UNAIDS, in *UNGASS Country Progress Report: P.R. China*, China's "HIV epidemic remains one of low prevalence overall, but with pockets of high infection among specific sub-populations and in some localities." Specifically, the organization notes that 40.6% of people living with HIV in 2007 were infected via heterosexual transmission.

UNAIDS observes that seven out of 10 (70%) HIV infections were in young adults aged 20 to 39 years in 2007 and that nearly the same percentage of AIDS cases (69.9%) and AIDS-related deaths (72%) occurred in people aged 20 to 49 years. The majority of people living with HIV were male (71.3%) and nearly two-thirds (60.6%) of AIDS cases at the close of 2007 were male. The principal mode of transmission is heterosexual contact, which was responsible for 44.7% of new infections in 2007, compared to MSM, which accounted for just 1.1% of new cases of infection.

According to UNAIDS, 9.3% of people living with HIV in 2007 were infected through infected blood products and 38.1% were infected through IDU. China's epidemic is fueled by three main factors: 40% of IDUs share needles, 60% of sex workers do not use condoms consistently, and 70% of MSM do not consistently practice safe sex.

Even though AIDS deaths have declined in China, some observers, such as Jane Qiu, in "Stigma of HIV Imperils Hard-Won Strides in Saving Lives" (*Science*, vol. 332, no. 6035, June 10, 2011), and Talha Khan Burki, in "Discrimination against People with HIV Persists in China" (*Lancet*, vol. 377, no. 9762, January 2011), are concerned that stigma about homosexuality and discrimination against people living with HIV may hamper China's efforts to further reduce the size of its epidemic. People with HIV are often barred from education and employment opportunities and may be demoted or forced to resign. Hospitals and universities frequently disclose workers' HIV test results to employers and policies regarding confidentiality and consent vary from one province to the next.

CENTRAL AND SOUTH AMERICA

In *Global Report: UNAIDS Report on the Global AIDS Epidemic, 2010*, UNAIDS indicates that the number of new HIV infections in Central and South America is on the decline. In 2009 there were an estimated 92,000 new cases of HIV, down from 99,000 in 2001, and approximately 1.4 million adults and children in Central and South America were living with HIV. One-third of all people living with HIV in the region are in Brazil. There were 58,000 AIDS-related deaths in 2009.

The majority of HIV/AIDS cases in Central and South America can be traced to MSM transmission. There are high rates of HIV prevalence—10% or higher—in 12 countries in the region. In five countries the incidence of HIV among MSM was an estimated 5.1%. Social stigma continues to challenge efforts to identify, educate, and prevent infection among MSM. The number of new cases of HIV in children remains low and appears to be decreasing. In 2009 there were 400 new HIV infections in children.

UNAIDS indicates that even though MSM remain the principal source of transmission, IDUs and sex workers continue to contribute to the pandemic in many countries. In "Efficacy of HIV Prevention Interventions in Latin American and Caribbean Nations, 1995–2008: A Meta-analysis" (*AIDS and Behavior*, vol. 14, no. 6, December 2010), Tania B. Huedo-Medina et al. analyze 37 HIV prevention interventions that were evaluated in Latin American and Caribbean nations. The researchers find that the most effective interventions were those that focused on high-risk populations, distributed condoms, provided at least three hours of instruction/content, and incorporated an understanding of sociocultural issues. Examples of sociocultural issues that act to enforce taboos and encourage high-risk behaviors are "machismo" or male pride, which is the belief that men should be dominant, have multiple sex partners, and engage in unprotected intercourse; "simpatia," which supports a traditional female role of sexual submission; and "familismo," traditional family values that may be at odds with condom use as well as homosexuality.

THE CARIBBEAN

The first suspected AIDS cases in the Caribbean appeared in Jamaica in 1982. UNAIDS indicates in *Global Report: UNAIDS Report on the Global AIDS Epidemic, 2010* that since then the epidemic has changed from a mostly homosexual phenomenon to a largely heterosexual one, attributable to unprotected sex between partners and sex workers.

UNAIDS notes that in 2009 an estimated 240,000 adults and children in the Caribbean were living with HIV and 17,000 had contracted the infection during that year. Even though these numbers reflect a decline in the region's pandemic that is at least in part attributable to behavior changes and improved access to antiretroviral drugs, AIDS remains a leading cause of death among people aged 15 to 44 years in the Caribbean and was responsible for 12,000 deaths in 2009.

The prevalence of HIV infection varied between countries in the Caribbean in 2009, from a high of 3.1% in the Bahamas to a low of 0.1% in Cuba. Like sub-Saharan Africa, the percentage of females living with HIV (53%) was higher than the percentage of males.

HIV infection was prevalent among female sex workers in 2009, including 4% in the Dominican Republic, 9% in Jamaica, and 27% in Guyana. Twenty percent of MSM in Trinidad and Tobago and 32% of MSM in Jamaica were living with HIV. IDU contributed to the epidemics in Puerto Rico and Bermuda. In Puerto Rico, about 40% of new HIV infections in men and 27% in women were attributable to IDU in 2006.

In "From Haiti, a Surprise: Good News about AIDS" (Associated Press, July 6, 2009), Jonathan M. Katz reports that among pregnant women HIV infection rates decreased from 6.2% in the mid-1990s to 3.1% in 2009. Katz observes that coordinated efforts, implemented by two nonprofit groups—Partners in Health and GHESKIO—to ensure widespread antiretroviral drug use, education, and increasing use of condoms as well as the closing of unregulated blood banks, helped stem Haiti's epidemic.

CONTROVERSIES

Even though great strides have been made in the treatment of HIV infection and AIDS and in raising public awareness about the nature of the disease and preventing its spread, several issues and controversies continue to hamper the unity of purpose that is required to effectively combat HIV/AIDS worldwide.

Among its goals, UNAIDS states in "HIV Treatment" (2011, http://www.unaids.org/en/strategygoalsby2015/hivtreatment/) that it hopes to achieve "universal access to antiretroviral therapy for people living with HIV who are eligible for treatment" by 2015. UNAIDS estimates that in

2010 there were 10 million people living with HIV who did not have access to needed treatment.

The Cost of Treatment in Developing Countries

Bruce R. Schackman et al. estimate in "The Lifetime Cost of Current Human Immunodeficiency Virus Care in the United States" (*Medical Care*, vol. 44, no. 11, November 2006) that the direct medical care cost for people with HIV, from their diagnosis until death, is an average of about $2,100 per month. The average projected life expectancy for people receiving optimal HIV treatment is 24.2 years, which yields a lifetime cost of $618,900 per person. Even in a wealthy country such as the United States, this is beyond the reach of most Americans. In the developing world, where the annual income may be only several hundred dollars, the cost of treatment can prove absolutely prohibitive without government subsidies for HIV treatment.

Cost of Drugs

The high price of HIV/AIDS drugs has been and continues to be a contentious issue. In the press release "UNAIDS/UNDP/WHO Concerned over Sustainability and Scale up of HIV Treatment" (March 15, 2011, http://www.unaids.org/en/resources/presscentre/pressre leaseandstatementarchive/2011/march/20110315prtrips/), UNAIDS observes that during the first decade of the 21st century the annual cost of antiretroviral drugs for low-income countries decreased by almost 99%—from more than $10,000 per person in 2000 to less than $116 in 2010 for the least expensive drug regimen recommended by the WHO. However, even this dramatic reduction is not sufficient to ensure access to HIV/AIDS treatment for people in developing and low-income countries.

The policy brief *Using TRIPS Flexibilities to Improve Access to HIV Treatment* (February 15, 2011, http://www .unaids.org/en/media/unaids/contentassets/documents/ policy/2011/JC2049_PolicyBrief_TRIPS_en-1.pdf) by UNAIDS, the WHO, and the United Nations Development Programme (UNDP) details the annual price per person of first-line drug regimens (the first antiretroviral drugs that are given to control HIV infection) and of second-line drug regimens (the second antiretroviral drugs that are given when resistance to first-line drugs occurs) in low, lower-middle, and upper-middle income countries. In low income countries first-line drugs range from $136 to $243; in lower-middle income countries the range is $116 to $667; and in upper-middle income countries the range is from $161 to $1,033. Second-line regimens are costlier. In low-income countries they range from $572 to $803; in lower-middle income countries the range is $818 to $1,545; and in upper-middle income countries the range is from $3,393 to $3,647.

The policy brief explains how countries can interpret the World Trade Organization Agreement on Trade-Related Aspects of Intellectual Property Rights (TRIPS, which was negotiated in 1994 and governs intellectual property considerations of international trade agreement) to expand access to HIV treatment. UNAIDS, the WHO, and the UNDP believe that the TRIPS agreement should be interpreted "in a manner supportive of WTO Members' right to protect public health and, in particular, to promote access to medicines for all."

Increasing Access to HIV/AIDS Drugs in Developing Countries

The Clinton Health Access Initiative (CHAI; http:// www.clintonfoundation.org/what-we-do/clinton-health-access-initiative; until January 1, 2010, this initiative was known as the Clinton Foundation HIV/AIDS Initiative) was founded by President Bill Clinton (1946–) to assist countries to implement large-scale prevention and treatment programs. CHAI works with the governments of countries in Africa, the Caribbean, and Asia and provides technical assistance and human and financial resources to ensure the delivery of quality care and treatment. The initiative also provides access to reduced prices for HIV/AIDS drugs and diagnostics to countries. In total, CHAI represents over 90% of people living with HIV/AIDS in developing countries.

In "What We've Accomplished" (2011, http://www .clintonfoundation.org/what-we-do/clinton-hiv-aids-initiative/ what-we-ve-accomplished), CHAI reports that as of 2011 it had successfully negotiated price reductions for 40 antiretroviral drug formulations and 16 HIV/AIDS diagnostic tests. CHAI's efforts resulted in price reductions of 50% for first-line drug treatment, a 30% reduction for second-line drug treatment, and a 90% reduction for drugs that are used to treat children in low-income countries.

UNITAID is an international drug purchase facility that was established in 2006 by Brazil, Chile, France, Norway, and the United Kingdom. UNITAID is an innovative funding mechanism that focuses on speeding access to quality drugs and diagnostics for HIV/AIDS, malaria, and TB in countries where these diseases pose serious threats to the health of their residents. UNITAID works with CHAI, the WHO, and the United Nations Children's Fund.

UNITAID notes in "HIV/AIDS: Scaling Treatment up, Pushing Prices Down" (2010, http://www.unitaid.eu/en/ projects-mainmenu-3/hivaids-mainmenu-28.html) that in 2010 it granted $156.5 million to CHAI to support the provision of second-line medication for 126,000 people and of AIDS treatment for 300,000 children in 40 developing countries. Philippe Douste-Blazy explains in *UNITAID: Innovative Financing for Health and Development* (June 2011, http://www.unitaid.eu/images/NewWeb/documents/

UNITAID_in_2011/UNITAID_in_2011_EN_June13.pdf) that besides expanding access to, availability, and affordability of antiretroviral drugs, UNITAID's recent accomplishments include the November 2010 creation of the Medicines Patent Pool (MPP), a strategy that compensates pharmaceutical companies and promotes the production of generic drugs, which are more affordable. The intent of the MPP is to "speed up the availability of lower-priced, newer medicines in developing countries."

President's Emergency Plan for AIDS Relief

The President's Emergency Plan for AIDS Relief (PEPFAR) is a U.S. government initiative to help people suffering from HIV/AIDS worldwide. Launched by President George W. Bush (1946–) in 2003, PEPFAR is responsible for saving millions of lives. In "Bush Signs Bill to Triple AIDS Funding" (Associated Press, July 30, 2008), Katharine Euphrat describes the program as "one of the major achievements of the Bush presidency." In 2008 the program was renewed for five years and the controversial requirement that 33% of prevention funds be used for abstinence-until-marriage programs was eliminated.

Abstaining from sexual intercourse does prevent the sexual transmission of HIV, although most experts, who agree that it is not realistic to expect sexual abstinence from many segments of the population, stress that condom use is essential to stop the spread of the disease. Abstinence education remains a key component of PEPFAR, although in 2007 the program's prevention strategy was broadened to include "ABC—Abstain, Be faithful, and correct and consistent Condom use," the prevention of mother-to-child transmission, activities that focus on blood safety, and interventions aimed at IDUs.

PEPFAR was reauthorized by the Tom Lantos and Henry J. Hyde United States Global Leadership against HIV/AIDS, Tuberculosis, and Malaria Reauthorization Act in July 2008. This act extended the program through 2013 and authorized up to $48 billion to wage war against HIV/AIDS, TB, and malaria between fiscal years (FYs) 2009 and 2013. The reauthorization act also stipulates that "in countries with generalized HIV epidemics, at least half of all money directed towards preventing sexual HIV transmission should be for activities promoting abstinence, delay of sexual debut, monogamy, fidelity, and partner reduction," but it does not mandate abstinence-only education and prevention programs as a requirement for receiving funds.

The number of people served by PEPFAR increased dramatically, from less than 2.5 million in 2004 to more than 3.2 million at the close of September 2010. (See

Table 9.1.) The launch of PEPFAR significantly increased U.S. spending to support the fight against the global HIV/AIDS pandemic—it increased from $2.3 billion in FY 2004 to $6.9 billion in FY 2010 and $7 billion in FY 2011. (See Table 9.2.) For FY 2012 President Barack Obama (1961–) requested almost $7.2 billion.

The Kaiser Family Foundation indicates in "Additional Funding Announced for PEPFAR Programs in Africa" (June 17, 2011, http://globalhealth.kff.org/Daily-Reports/2011/June/17/GH-061711-RR-Goosby-Africa-Trip.aspx) that in June 2011 the U.S. secretary of state Hillary Rodham Clinton (1947–) and the U.S. Global AIDS coordinator ambassador Eric Goosby (1953–) traveled to Africa. During the trip Clinton pledged an additional $15 million to support Zambia to achieve its objective of eliminating mother-to-child HIV transmission by 2014. Clinton also introduced a PEPFAR initiative to address gender-based violence, which will be supported with $24 million over three years.

TABLE 9.1

Number of people receiving antiretroviral treatment supported by U.S. government as of September 30, 2010

Country	Number of individuals on antiretroviral treatment
Botswana	12,200
Cambodia	7,300
China	5,500
Côte d'Ivoire	61,200
Democratic Republic of the Congo	1,300
Dominican Republic	5,500
Ethiopia	207,900
Guyana	3,000
Haiti	27,900
India	2,900
Kenya	410,300
Lesotho	45,700
Mozambique	138,800
Namibia	80,300
Nigeria	334,700
Russia	14,700
Rwanda	53,800
South Africa	917,700
Swaziland	38,700
Tanzania	255,500
Uganda	207,900
Vietnam	31,000
Zambia	286,000
Zimbabwe	59,900
Total	**3,209,700**

Numbers may be adjusted as attribution criteria and reporting systems are refined. All numbers greater than 100 have been rounded off to the nearest 100.

SOURCE: "Number of Individuals Directly Supported on Antiretroviral Treatment as of September 30, 2010," in *Saving Lives through Smart Investments: Latest PEPFAR Results*, The United States President's Emergency Plan for AIDS Relief, 2011, http://www.pepfar.gov/documents/organization/153723.pdf (accessed June 27, 2011)

TABLE 9.2

PEPFAR (President's Emergency Plan for AIDS Relief) funding, fiscal years 2004–12

[In millions]

Programs	Fiscal year 2004 enacted	Fiscal year 2005 enacted	Fiscal year 2006 enacted	Fiscal year 2007 enacted	Fiscal year 2008 enacted	Fiscal year 2009 enacted	Fiscal year 2010 enacted	Total enacted[b]	Fiscal year 2011 requested	Fiscal year 2012 requested
Bilateral HIV/AIDS programs[a]	1,643	2,263	2,654	3,699	5,028	5,503	5,574	26,364	5,739	5,599
Global funds	547	347	545	724	840	1,000	1,050	5,053	1,000	1,300
Bilateral TB programs	87	94	91	95	163	177	243	950	251	254
Total Pepfar	**2,277**	**2,705**	**3,290**	**4,518**	**6,031**	**6,680**	**6,867**	**32,367**	**6,989**	**7,154**

TB = Tuberculosis.

[a]Bilateral HIV/AIDS programs includes funding for bilateral country/regional programs, United Nations program on AIDS (UNAIDS), International Vaccine Initiative (IAVI), Microbicides and National Institures of Health HIV/AIDS research.

[b]Includes enacted funding for fiscal years 2004–fiscal year 2011.

Note: All funding amounts have been rounded to the nearest million, so the numbers shown in the table may not sum to the totals.

SOURCE: "FY 2004–FY 2012 PEPFAR Funding ($ in Millions)," in *PEPFAR Funding: Investments That Save Lives and Promote Security (Updated February 2011)*, The United States President's Emergency Plan for AIDS Relief, February 2011, http://www.pepfar.gov/press/80064.htm (accessed June 27, 2011)

CHAPTER 10
KNOWLEDGE, AWARENESS, BEHAVIOR, AND OPINION

CONCERN ABOUT HIV/AIDS

During the first decade of the 21st century the U.S. public appeared less concerned about HIV/AIDS and its impact on health care than ever before. According to the Gallup Organization, the number of Americans who named AIDS as the most urgent health problem facing the country has declined steadily since 1988, when 68% of Americans listed it as number one. It declined to 41% in 1992 and 29% in 1997. (See Figure 10.1.) By 2004 just 5% of Americans considered AIDS the most urgent health problem, and by late 2009 a scant 1% named AIDS as the most urgent health problem. (See Figure 10.1.)

Access to health care and health care costs overshadowed diseases as the most pressing health problems facing the country. (See Table 10.1.) Interestingly, influenza was the most frequently named health problem, outpacing cancer, obesity, heart disease, AIDS, and diabetes.

HIV/AIDS Is No Longer Seen as an Urgent Threat

The publications *Kaiser Family Foundation 2011 Survey of Americans on HIV/AIDS* (June 2011, http://www.kff.org/kaiserpolls/upload/8186-T.pdf) and *HIV/AIDS at 30: A Public Opinion Perspective* (June 2011, http://www.kff.org/kaiserpolls/upload/8186.pdf) describe trends in public opinions, attitudes, knowledge, and awareness of HIV/AIDS and related issues. The 2011 survey was the eighth one conducted by the Kaiser Family Foundation since 1995, so it reveals how Americans' attitudes toward HIV/AIDS have changed over time.

Consistent with the findings of the Gallup Organization, the Kaiser survey finds that the percentage of Americans identifying HIV/AIDS as the "most urgent health problem facing [the] nation" plummeted from 44% in 1995 to 17% in 2006 to 7% in 2011. A slightly higher percentage consider HIV/AIDS as the world's most pressing health problem, but this percentage decreased over time as well, from 34% in 2006 to 21% in 2009 to 13% in 2011. The vast majority (87%) of Americans believed it is possible for people with HIV to lead healthy productive lives, but they were evenly divided about whether to characterize HIV as a manageable chronic disease comparable to diabetes or high blood pressure.

Perhaps concern has diminished because media attention has waned or because other health messages predominate. The Kaiser survey participants reported seeing and hearing less about HIV/AIDS in the United States than they did just five years ago. The proportion claiming to have seen or heard "a lot" or "some" about the problem fell from 70% in 2004 to 40% in 2011. Even the global HIV/AIDS pandemic appears to have receded from Americans' awareness. Seventy-one percent recalled hearing about the magnitude of the problem in Africa in 2004, the first year that the President's Emergency Plan for AIDS Relief (PEPFAR) was funded, but by 2009, 49% said they had heard or read about the global pandemic in the year preceding the survey.

Despite the fact that they have seen or heard less about HIV/AIDS in recent years, between 40% and 50% of Americans felt that the United States is making progress in managing the domestic epidemic. About half (51%) of those surveyed in 2011 said they feel the world is making progress in combating the disease.

Concern about Becoming Infected with HIV

Between 1997 and 2009 the percentage of Americans that described themselves as "very concerned" about becoming infected with HIV has steadily declined. For example, among young adults aged 18 to 29 years, the percentage decreased from 30% in 2000 to 17% in 2009. In 2011, for the first time in more than a decade, the percentage of people personally concerned about becoming infected rose. Among adults aged 18 to 29 years, 24% expressed concern. Likewise, among all adults the percentage expressing concern about becoming infected rose from 13% in 2009 to 18% in 2011.

FIGURE 10.1

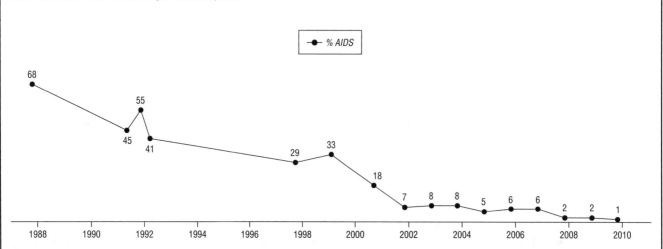

Percent of people naming AIDS as the most urgent health problem, 1988–2010

AIDS—Full trend in mentions as most urgent U.S. health problem

SOURCE: Lydia Saad, "AIDS—Full Trend in Mentions As Most Urgent U.S. Health Problem," in *"Most Urgent U.S. Health Problem" Still Access to Healthcare*, The Gallup Organization, November 23, 2009, http://www.gallup.com/poll/124460/Urgent-Health-Problem-Access-Healthcare.aspx#1 (accessed June 28, 2011). Copyright © 2011 by The Gallup Organization. Reproduced by permission of the Gallup Organization.

TABLE 10.1

Public opinion on the most urgent health problem facing the country, November 2005–November 2009

WHAT WOULD YOU SAY IS THE MOST URGENT HEALTH PROBLEM FACING THIS COUNTRY AT THE PRESENT TIME?

[Open-ended]

	2009 Nov 5–8	2008 Nov 13–16	2007 Nov 11–14	2006 Nov 9–12	2005 Nov 7–10
	%	%	%	%	%
Access	32	30	30	22	17
Costs	18	25	26	29	25
Flu	16	—	1	1	10
Cancer	9	11	14	14	15
Obesity	8	12	10	8	9
Heart disease	2	2	1	3	4
AIDS	1	2	2	6	6
Diabetes	1	2	2	1	1
Finding cures for diseases	*	1	1	1	1
Smoking	*	1	*	*	1
Drug/Alcohol abuse	—	*	1	1	1
Bioterrorism	—	—	—	*	*
Other	3	4	4	6	3
No opinion	10	10	9	8	7

*Less than 0.5%

SOURCE: Lydia Saad, "What Would You Say Is the Most Urgent Health Problem Facing This Country at the Present Time?" in *"Most Urgent U.S. Health Problem" Still Access to Healthcare*, The Gallup Organization, November 23, 2009, http://www.gallup.com/poll/124460/Urgent-Health-Problem-Access-Healthcare.aspx#2 (accessed June 28, 2011). Copyright © 2011 by The Gallup Organization. Reproduced by permission of the Gallup Organization.

Because African-Americans have been disproportionately affected by HIV/AIDS, it is not surprising that in 2011 they were three times as likely to perceive HIV/AIDs as an urgent problem in their community and twice as likely to be concerned about becoming infected. Furthermore, they were nearly four times as likely as whites to be "very concerned" about becoming infected—40% of African-Americans compared to 11% of whites. Concern was highest among African-Americans under the age of 30 years— more than half (51%) said they are "very concerned" about becoming infected.

Hispanics, who are also disproportionately affected by the epidemic, perceive HIV/AIDS as a serious threat to their community and as a personal threat to their health. Nearly two-thirds (61%) viewed it as a serious problem in 2011 and 27% were "very concerned" about becoming infected.

Nevertheless, knowledge and awareness about HIV transmission have not improved since the late 1990s and misperceptions persist. In 2011, 25% of Americans mistakenly believed that HIV can be transmitted by sharing a drinking glass or were unsure whether HIV is transmitted this way. Another 16% believed that HIV can be transmitted via shared toilet seats and 12% thought swimming in a pool with a person who is infected may transmit HIV. The Kaiser Family Foundation finds that one out of three survey respondents gave an incorrect answer when queried about these three ways that HIV cannot be transmitted.

In contrast, some knowledge about HIV treatment had increased by 2011. For example, 53% of all respondents knew that medication can effectively prevent mother-to-child transmission. More than three-quarters (76%) of African-American women under the age of 30 years were aware that drug treatment can prevent mother-to-child transmission of the virus.

HIV Testing

The revised Centers for Disease Control and Prevention guidelines in Bernard M. Branson et al.'s "Revised Recommendations for HIV Testing of Adults, Adolescents, and Pregnant Women in Health-Care Settings" (*Morbidity and Mortality Weekly Report*, vol. 55, RR-14, September 22, 2006) essentially changed HIV testing from an opt-in diagnostic test to an opt-out test that is a routine part of medical practice. Based on the findings of the 2011 Kaiser Family Foundation survey, this change has not, as might have been anticipated, translated into more people being tested for HIV.

The rates of testing have remained relatively unchanged since 2000. In 2011 almost half (48%) of adults said they have been tested for HIV, including 18% who reported testing within the 12 months before the survey. The majority (77%) of those tested said they chose to be tested because "it just seemed like a good idea." People aged 18 to 29 years (26%) were the most likely to have been tested in the past 12 months.

In 2011, 64% of survey respondents who had never been tested for HIV said they had not obtained testing because they did not believe they were at risk of contracting the virus. Twenty-nine percent said their physician had never recommended testing, 12% claimed they did not know where to obtain testing, 7% said their worries about confidentiality prevented them from getting tested, and 3% said they were afraid they would test positive for the virus.

KNOWLEDGE AND TOLERANCE GROW, BUT MISCONCEPTIONS PERSIST

In the three decades since HIV/AIDS was first identified, aggressive community health education and awareness programs have sought to increase the public's knowledge about the prevention, transmission, and treatment of HIV/AIDS. Based on the findings of the 2011 Kaiser Family Foundation survey, even though public understanding and awareness have improved in many areas, misconceptions and stigmatizing attitudes about HIV/AIDS persist.

There is, however, an understanding that the U.S. HIV epidemic has had a profound effect on U.S. culture and society as well as on personal behaviors. Historically, the Kaiser Family Foundation surveys and other polling organizations have found that about half of Americans feel there has been considerable discrimination against people with AIDS. However, the results of the 2011 survey indicate that some, but not all, of the stigmas and discrimination that are associated with HIV/AIDS may be diminishing. About half (49%) of Americans said they would feel comfortable working with someone with HIV/AIDS, up from 32% in 1997. Regardless, 45% said they would be uncomfortable having their food prepared by someone who is HIV positive and 36% would be uncomfortable having an HIV-positive roommate. In general, older adults aged 65 years and older reported more discomfort with the idea of having food prepared by (62%), rooming with (56%), or working with (33%) a person who is HIV positive.

Some of these changing attitudes and declining stigmas may be attributable to how widespread HIV/AIDS has become. More than four out of 10 (42%) Americans, and nearly six out of 10 (57%) African-Americans, said they had personal contact with HIV/AIDS—either they knew someone who is infected with HIV, someone who has AIDS, or someone who has died from the disease.

Still, significant stigmas and negative attitudes persist. Twenty-nine percent, down from 40% in 2002, of survey respondents agreed with the statement, "In general, it's people's own fault if they get AIDS," and 16%, down from 26% in 2002, concurred with the statement, "I sometimes think that AIDS is punishment for the decline in moral standards." Men are more likely than women to assign blame—34% of men said they agree with the notion that "it's people's own fault if they get AIDS," compared to 24% of women.

THE PRIMARY SOURCE OF INFORMATION ABOUT HIV/AIDS IS THE MEDIA

In 2011 the media continued to be the primary source of information about HIV/AIDS. However, just a little over half (54%) of Americans reported having heard about HIV in the year preceding the survey, down from 83% in 2004 and 65% in 2009. Two-thirds (66%) of whites named the media as their principal source of information, compared to 53% of African-Americans. Among whites, doctors or nurses were the primary source of information (15%), followed by friends and family (12%).

Interestingly, even though 55% of African-Americans reported hearing about HIV/AIDS in church, just 4% identified the church as their principal source of information. African-Americans and Hispanics expressed more interest in learning more about HIV/AIDS than did whites—73% of African-Americans and 66% of Hispanics wanted to know more about how to prevent the spread of HIV, 71% each of African-Americans and Hispanics wanted to know how to talk with children about the virus, and 63% of African-Americans and 62% of Hispanics wanted to know who should get tested for HIV. In contrast, 37% of whites reported any interest in learning more about prevention, 39% in talking with children, and 34% in knowing who should get tested.

Among young adults aged 18 to 29 years, about one-third (35%) said school is their primary source of information about HIV/AIDS. More specifically, just 20% of young African-Americans and 33% of young Hispanics named school as a primary source of information, compared to 39% of whites. Almost two-thirds (62%) of young African-Americans felt that schools should be doing more "to help solve the problem of HIV/AIDS in this country" than did Latinos (48%) or whites (46%).

Spending for HIV/AIDS in the United States

Since 1997, when the Kaiser Family Foundation began surveying Americans about HIV/AIDS, the majority of survey respondents have felt that too little money is being devoted to combating HIV/AIDS domestically. In 2011, despite continuing economic uncertainty and instability that remained following the recession (which lasted from late 2007 to mid-2009), support for spending on HIV/AIDS was strong, with more than half (53%) of survey respondents saying that the federal government is spending too little to combat the domestic epidemic. When asked to compare HIV/AIDS funding and spending to expenditures for other diseases such as cancer and heart disease, more than a third (39%) felt that spending is too low and a similar proportion (38%) felt that the current level of spending is about right.

Even though the 2011 survey finds continued support for spending on HIV/AIDS prevention and treatment, Americans were divided about the outcomes of such spending. About half felt spending will produce significant progress and slow the epidemic, but a full 40% felt HIV/AIDS prevention programs will make no difference and 44% felt the same way about HIV/AIDS treatment.

Identifying a Champion for the Cause

The survey finds that Americans are unable to identify a leader in the battle against HIV/AIDS. Three-quarters of respondents were unable to name a national leader. Magic Johnson (1959–) was the most frequently named leader, at 8%, followed by Elizabeth Taylor (1932–2011), at 5%, and President Barack Obama (1961–), at 2%. One percent of respondents named the former presidents Bill Clinton (1946–) and George W. Bush (1946–) and the rock star/activist Bono (1960–).

The majority of Americans wanted to see greater involvement in HIV/AIDS initiatives and efforts from Congress (63%), state governments (61%), congressional representatives (60%), state representatives (57%), corporate and business leaders (56%), local government (54%), and the media (53%). About half felt religious leaders, community leaders, President Obama and his administration, pharmaceutical companies, and public schools should do more to help solve the HIV/AIDS problem in the United States. Even though 42% of Americans thought nonprofit organizations are doing enough to combat HIV/AIDS, 35% felt these organizations could be doing more.

HIV/AIDS AWARENESS EFFORTS

Many national and global initiatives and observances are conducted in an effort to inform the public, heighten awareness, and improve understanding of the HIV/AIDS pandemic. This section describes some of the activities, individuals, and groups that are involved in the ongoing effort to educate, motivate, and mobilize people to prevent the spread of HIV and to assist those who are living with HIV/AIDS.

The U.S. Department of Health and Human Services (2011, http://www.hhs.gov/aidsawarenessdays/) designates the annual observation of HIV/AIDS Awareness Days. These include:

- February 7, National Black HIV/AIDS Awareness Day—this annual awareness day was created by a community-based coalition to raise awareness among African-Americans about HIV/AIDS and its disproportionate and devastating impact on African-American communities.

- March 10, National Women and Girls HIV/AIDS Awareness Day—this day aims to raise awareness of the increasing impact of HIV/AIDS on the lives of women and girls.

- March 20, National Native HIV/AIDS Awareness Day—this day was created to increase awareness of the impact of HIV/AIDS on Native Americans, Alaskan natives, and native Hawaiians.

- May 18, HIV Vaccine Awareness Day—this day recognizes and acknowledges the people who are working to help find an HIV preventive vaccine, such as the clinical trial volunteers, the nurses, the community educators/recruiters, and the researchers.

- May 19, National Asian and Pacific Islander HIV/AIDS Awareness Day—this awareness day intends to increase awareness among Asians and Pacific Islanders in the United States about the ruinous impact of HIV/AIDS.

- June 8, Caribbean American HIV/AIDS Awareness Day—this day is a national mobilization effort that is designed to encourage Caribbean-American and Caribbean-born individuals across the United States and its territories to become better informed and educated and to obtain testing and seek treatment.

- June 27, National HIV Testing Day—this day aims to provide opportunities for testing, especially for those who have never been tested or who have engaged in high-risk behavior since their last test, and to help dispel the myths and stigmas that are associated with HIV.

- September 18, National HIV/AIDS and Aging Awareness Day—this day aims to heighten awareness of the impact of HIV/AIDS on older adults. It intends to focus on HIV prevention, care, and treatment of people aged 50 years and older.

- September 27, National Gay Men's HIV/AIDS Awareness Day—this day aims to regain and refocus the attention of a community that has been disproportionately affected by the HIV/AIDS epidemic at a time when the United States confronts the simultaneous challenges of a resurgence of new HIV infections among gay men and growing complacency about HIV/AIDS among gay men.

- October 15, National Latino AIDS Awareness Day—this awareness day marks an opportunity to communicate the devastating and disproportionate effects AIDS is having on the Hispanic community.

- December 1, World AIDS Day—started by the World Health Organization in 1988, this day serves to focus global attention on the HIV/AIDS pandemic. Observance of this day provides an opportunity for governments, national AIDS programs, churches, community organizations, and individuals to demonstrate the importance of the fight against HIV/AIDS.

The AIDS Memorial Quilt

The AIDS Memorial Quilt is not only an ongoing community art project that pays tribute to and commemorates the lives claimed by AIDS but also serves as a powerful visual way to inform, educate, and heighten awareness of the lives lost in this pandemic. The AIDS Memorial Quilt notes in "History of the Quilt" (2011, http://www .aidsquilt.org/history.htm) that the quilt consists of cloth panels that have been designed and made by friends and families of people who died from AIDS. Cleve Jones, a San Francisco, California, gay rights activist, had the idea for the quilt in November 1985 and the quilt was "born" in June 1987, when Jones and a group of his friends in San Francisco decided to memorialize people who had died from AIDS-related illnesses.

The first public display of the quilt was at the National Mall in Washington, D.C., in October 1987. It contained 1,920 panels and was larger than a football field. The quilt, and enthusiasm for it, grew quickly. One year later the quilt had grown to 8,288 panels. Each time the quilt was displayed the names of those honored by it were read aloud by celebrities, politicians, family members, and friends.

In "Quilt Facts" (2011, http://www.aidsquilt.org/quilt facts.htm), the AIDS Memorial Quilt states that over 18 million people have seen the nearly 1.3-million-square-foot (120,000-square-m) quilt, which weighs more than 54 tons (49 t) and contains over 91,000 names. The names on the quilt represent about 17.5% of all AIDS deaths in the United States. The quilt has traveled around the world, raising awareness and money (more than $4 million) for AIDS-related research and programs. It has been the subject of stories, papers, articles, and books and was nominated for a Nobel Peace Prize in 1989. That same year a feature-length documentary about it, *Common Threads: Stories from the Quilt*, won an Academy Award.

AIDS Activists

AIDS activists have been credited with raising awareness and attracting money and media attention to the pandemic. Many groups, individuals, and celebrities have taken on the cause and become champions of HIV/AIDS research, prevention, and treatment. Others have agitated to change the course of national and government policy and to improve access to and availability of quality care, especially affordable drug treatment. Still others have defended the rights of people living with HIV and AIDS in an effort to counter stigmatization and discrimination. Using a variety of approaches—from fund-raising campaigns and political lobbying to protests and guerilla theater (dramatization of a social issue, often performed outdoors in a park or on the street)—AIDS activists have raised their voices and the consciousness of people around the world.

Even though there are many groups and organizations engaged in AIDS activism, the most effective and vibrant organization is probably the AIDS Coalition to Unleash Power (ACT UP). ACT UP (2011, http://www.actupny .org/) describes itself as "a diverse, non-partisan group of individuals united in anger and committed to direct action to end the AIDS crisis." It states, "We advise and inform. We demonstrate. We are not silent. Silence = Death." ACT UP has thousands of members in more than 70 chapters in the United States and worldwide. The organization advocates nonviolent direct action through vocal demonstrations and acts of civil disobedience that are intended to make the public aware of the crucial issues of the AIDS crisis. During a span of more than 20 years, ACT UP members have staged scores of protests and demonstrations and have often been arrested, usually for civil disobedience.

AIDS United (2011, http://www.aidsaction.org/about-aids-action-mainmenu-187), another national organization, has as its slogan "Every Person, Every Community," which conveys the group's commitment to end the HIV epidemic "through national, regional and local policy/advocacy, strategic grantmaking, and organizational capacity building. With partners throughout the country, we will work to ensure that people living with and affected by HIV/AIDS have access to the prevention and care services they need and deserve." AIDS United has played a key role in the development and implementation of public health policies to improve the quality of life for Americans who are HIV positive. It also works with the public health community to enhance HIV prevention programs and care and treatment services.

The AIDS Treatment Activists Coalition is also a national coalition of AIDS activists who work together to end the AIDS epidemic by advancing research on HIV/AIDS. The coalition's mission statement (2011, http://atac-usa.org/about/mission-goals.htm) describes its goals as:

- To encourage greater and more effective involvement of people with HIV/AIDS in the decisions that affect their lives by identifying, mentoring and empowering treatment activists in all communities affected by the epidemic

- To develop within all communities affected by HIV/AIDS and related coinfections the leadership to provide the knowledge and skills needed to advocate for improved research, treatment and access to care

- To enable treatment activists to speak with a united, powerful voice to provide meaningful input into issues concerning HIV disease and related complications and coinfections

- To facilitate communications and set agenda items…between HIV/AIDS treatment activists and government, industry and academia in matters affecting research, treatment and access [and] among HIV/AIDS treatment activists and the larger HIV community in keeping up to date with the latest developments in research, treatment and access

CELEBRITIES SHINE A SPOTLIGHT ON HIV/AIDS. When celebrities endorse or lend their name to charitable causes, the causes often benefit from increased media attention and visibility. When celebrities actively work to promote their chosen causes, the results can be even more dramatic. For example, the United Nations Children's Fund notes in "Business People, Celebrities, and Officials Join Forces to Raise Awareness about AIDS in China" (May 18, 2006, http://www.unicef.org/people/people_10165.html) that many celebrities—from the late Diana, Princess of Wales (1961–1997), President Clinton, the business executive Ted Turner (1938–), and the Microsoft chairman Bill Gates (1955–), to the actors Richard Gere (1949–), Sharon Stone (1958–), Catherine Deneuve (1943–), and Ashley Judd (1968–), and to the musician Elton John (1947–)—have made outstanding contributions of time, energy, and money to combat the HIV/AIDS pandemic.

Many young celebrities have also taken up the cause. The article "Celebs Promote AIDS Awareness" (CNN.com, November 29, 2010) indicates that to celebrate World AIDS Day on December 1, 2010, the singers Usher (1978–), Jennifer Hudson (1981–), and Alicia Keys (1981–), the actors Kim Kardashian (1980–), Elijah Wood (1981–), Willow Smith (2000–), and Jaden Smith (1998–), and the television show host Ryan Seacrest (1974–) participated in fund-raising efforts to support orphans and others who have been affected by HIV/AIDS in Africa and India. In "Lady Gaga Dresses Like a Condom to Promote AIDS Awareness" (MTV.com, February 17, 2011), Gil Kaufman reports that in February 2011 Lady Gaga (1986–) appeared on a broadcast of the ABC show *Good Morning America* dressed in a "latex-condom-inspired outfit" to promote safe sex and raise HIV/AIDS awareness.

Bono uses his celebrity to champion the fight against HIV/AIDS. In 2002 he formed the organization Debt AIDS Trade Africa (DATA), an advocacy organization that was dedicated to eradicating extreme poverty and AIDS in Africa. In 2005 Bono was named *Time*'s Person of the Year along with Bill Gates and Melinda Gates (1964–). The following year he was nominated for a Nobel Peace Prize.

In January 2008 DATA merged with ONE (http://www.one.org/us/), a global antipoverty organization that pursues high-level global advocacy in concert with grassroots mobilization efforts. Like DATA, ONE's (2011, http://www.one.org/c/us/faq/) mission is to "fight extreme poverty and preventable disease in the poorest places on the planet, particularly in Africa." ONE (2011, http://www.one.org/us/partners/) partners with other global relief and HIV/AIDS initiatives, including CARE, Save the Children, Oxfam America, the Bill and Melinda Gates Foundation, Islamic Relief, Malaria No More, Bread for Life, Physicians for Peace, The White Ribbon Alliance for Safe Motherhood, and (RED).

(RED) (2011, http://www.joinred.com/red/) involves the private and public sectors in a joint fund-raising initiative. Companies whose products carry the (RED) insignia pledge to contribute a significant percentage of their sales or a portion of their profits from those products to the Global Fund to finance AIDS programs in Africa, with an emphasis on the health of women and children. The Global Fund (2011, http://www.joinred.com/aboutred), which is supported by the funds that (RED) generates, is the world's leading financer of programs to fight AIDS, tuberculosis, and malaria. Since its launch in 2002, the Global Fund has earmarked $21.7 billion for programs in 150 countries. Since 2003 PEPFAR and the Global Fund have provided funding for free antiretroviral drugs to countries where they are urgently needed.

In 2011 American Express, Apple, Bugaboo, Converse, Dell, Emporio Armani, Gap, Hallmark, Microsoft, Nike, Penfolds, Penguin Classics, and Starbucks were participating in (RED). MySpace.com was the program's first media sponsor in the United Kingdom. In the press release "The Latest Results from (RED) & the Global Fund" (2011, http://www.joinred.com/red/#impact_364), (RED) indicates that more than 7.5 million people have been reached through programs supported by Global Fund–financed grants that (RED) supports. In the five years since its inception in 2006, (RED) has raised over $170 million for the Global Fund. (RED) provides funding for programs in Ghana, Lesotho, Rwanda, South Africa, Swaziland, and Zambia that promote HIV/AIDS prevention, administer antiretroviral therapy for people with HIV infection, educate children who have been orphaned by AIDS, and supply antiretroviral therapy to prevent mother-to-child transmission.

IMPORTANT NAMES AND ADDRESSES

ACT UP/New York
332 Bleecker St., Ste. G5
New York, NY 10014
URL: http://www.actupny.org/

AIDS Treatment Activists Coalition
611 Broadway, Ste. 308
New York, NY 10012
(646) 284-3801
E-mail: etr@atac-usa.org
URL: http://www.atac-usa.org/

AIDS United
1424 K St. NW, Ste. 200
Washington, DC 20005
(202) 408-4848
FAX: (202) 408-1818
URL: http://www.aidsunited.org/

American Foundation for AIDS Research
120 Wall St., 13th Floor
New York, NY 10005-3908
(212) 806-1600
FAX: (212) 806-1601
URL: http://www.amfar.org/

Center for Women Policy Studies
1776 Massachusetts Ave. NW, Ste. 450
Washington, DC 20036
(202) 872-1770
FAX: (202) 296-8962
E-mail: cwps@centerwomenpolicy.org
URL: http://www.centerwomenpolicy.org/

Centers for Disease Control and Prevention
1600 Clifton Rd.
Atlanta, GA 30333
1-800-232-4636
URL: http://www.cdc.gov/

Human Rights Campaign
1640 Rhode Island Ave. NW
Washington, DC 20036-3278
(202) 628-4160
1-800-777-4723
FAX: (202) 347-5323
URL: http://www.hrc.org/

Joint United Nations Program on HIV/AIDS
20 Ave. Appia
CH-1211 Geneva 27 Switzerland
(011-41-22) 791-3666
FAX: (011-41-22) 791-4187
URL: http://www.unaids.org/

Kaiser Family Foundation
2400 Sand Hill Rd.
Menlo Park, CA 94025
(650) 854-9400
FAX: (650) 854-4800
URL: http://www.kff.org/

National Association of People with AIDS
8401 Colesville Rd., Ste. 505
Silver Spring, MD 20910
(240) 247-0880
1-866-846-9366
FAX: (240) 247-0574
URL: http://www.napwa.org/

National Association of Public Hospitals and Health Systems
1301 Pennsylvania Ave. NW, Ste. 950
Washington, DC 20004
(202) 585-0100
FAX: (202) 585-0101
URL: http://www.naph.org/

National Hemophilia Foundation
116 W. 32nd St., 11th Floor
New York, NY 10001
(212) 328-3700
1-800-424-2634
FAX: (212) 328-3777
E-mail: handi@hemophilia.org
URL: http://www.hemophilia.org/

National Institute of Allergy and Infectious Diseases
6610 Rockledge Dr., MSC 6612
Bethesda, MD 20892-6612
(301) 496-5717
1-866-284-4107
FAX: (301) 402-3573
URL: http://www.niaid.nih.gov/

National Minority AIDS Council
1931 13th St. NW
Washington, DC 20009-4432
(202) 483-6622
FAX: (202) 483-1135
E-mail: communications@nmac.org
URL: http://www.nmac.org/

National Prevention Information Network
PO Box 6003
Rockville, MD 20849-6003
(404) 679-3860
1-800-458-5231
FAX: 1-888-282-7681
E-mail: info@cdcnpin.org
URL: http://www.cdcnpin.org/scripts/index.asp

National Women's Health Network
1413 K St. NW, Fourth Floor
Washington, DC 20005
(202) 682-2640
FAX: (202) 682-2648
URL: http://www.nwhn.org/

ONE
1400 Eye St. NW, Ste. 600
Washington, DC 20005
(202) 495-2700
URL: http://www.one.org/us/

U.S. Department of Health and Human Services AIDSinfo
PO Box 6303
Rockville, MD 20849-6303
1-800-448-0440
FAX: (301) 315-2818
E-mail: contactus@aidsinfo.nih.gov
URL: http://aidsinfo.nih.gov/

U.S. Food and Drug Administration
10903 New Hampshire Ave.
Silver Spring, MD 20993-0002
1-888-463-6332
URL: http://www.fda.gov/cder

RESOURCES

The Centers for Disease Control and Prevention (CDC) provides the most current accounting of the HIV/AIDS epidemic in the United States. Publications cited in this text include "HIV Testing among Men Who Have Sex with Men—21 Cities, United States, 2008" (Alexandra M. Oster et al., June 2011), "CDC Responds to HIV/AIDS" (April 2011), "Are Health Care Workers at Risk of Getting HIV on the Job?" (March 2011), "Disparities in Diagnoses of HIV Infection between Blacks/African Americans and Other Racial/Ethnic Populations—37 States, 2005–2008" (February 2011), *Changing Patterns of HIV Epidemiology United States—2011* (John T. Brooks, 2011), *Trends in Sexually Transmitted Diseases in the United States: 2009 National Data for Gonorrhea, Chlamydia, and Syphilis* (November 2010), "The Role of STD Detection and Treatment in HIV Prevention—CDC Fact Sheet" (September 2010), *HIV Testing Implementation Guidance for Correctional Settings* (January 2009), "HIV/AIDS among Persons Aged 50 and Older" (February 2008), "Revised Recommendations for HIV Testing of Adults, Adolescents, and Pregnant Women in Health-Care Settings" (Bernard M. Branson et al., September 2006), "Point-of-Care Rapid Tests for HIV Antibody" (Bernard M. Branson et al., September 2006), "Updated U.S. Public Health Service Guidelines for the Management of Occupational Exposures to HIV and Recommendations for Postexposure Prophylaxis" (Adelisa L. Panlilio et al., September 2005), and "Recommendations for Preventing Transmission of Human Immunodeficiency Virus and Hepatitis B Virus to Patients during Exposure-Prone Invasive Procedures" (July 1991).

HIV/AIDS Surveillance Reports are prepared by the CDC and describe and quantify transmission categories, risk factor combinations, demographics, and people living with HIV/AIDS. Other CDC publications that were used to prepare this publication include "Surveillance of Occupationally Acquired HIV/AIDS in Healthcare Personnel, as of December 2010" (May 2011), *HIV Surveillance Report:*

Diagnoses of HIV Infection and AIDS in the United States and Dependent Areas, 2009 (February 2011), "Syringe Exchange Programs—United States, 2008" (November 2010), *HIV Testing Implementation Guidance for Correctional Settings* (January 2009), and "Revised Surveillance Case Definitions for HIV Infection among Adults, Adolescents, and Children Aged <18 Months and for HIV Infection and AIDS among Children Aged 18 Months to <13 Years—United States, 2008" (Eileen Schneider et al., December 2008).

The CDC National Center for Health Statistics publishes findings from the Youth Risk Behavior Surveys, the National HIV Behavioral Surveillance System, the *National Vital Statistics Reports*, and the *Morbidity and Mortality Weekly Report*.

The National Institute of Allergy and Infectious Diseases fact sheet "HIV Infection in Infants and Children" (September 2008) describes immunodeficiency in infected infants during their first year of life and distinguishes three distinct patterns of disease progression among HIV-infected children.

The U.S. Department of Justice's *HIV in Prisons, 2007–08* (Laura M. Maruschak, December 2009) provides information on HIV/AIDS in U.S. prisons and jails, inmate deaths from HIV/AIDS, and testing policies for the virus antibody by states.

Information about the worldwide effects of HIV/AIDS, as well as global projections, were provided by reports including *Guidelines for Intensified Tuberculosis Case-Finding and Isoniazid Preventive Therapy for People Living with HIV in Resource-Constrained Settings* (2011) and *HIV Transmission through Breastfeeding: A Review of Available Evidence, 2007 Update* (2008) by the World Health Organization; *Children and AIDS: Second Stocktaking Report* (April 2008), *Children and AIDS: Fifth Stocktaking Report, 2010* (November 2010), and *Opportunity in*

Crisis: Preventing HIV from Early Adolescence to Early Adulthood (June 2011) by the United Nations Children's Fund; and *Global Report: UNAIDS Report on the Global AIDS Epidemic, 2010* (2010), *Global and Regional Trends* (June 2011), and *HIV and Tuberculosis: Ensuring Universal Access and Protection of Human Rights* (March 2010) by the Joint United Nations Program on HIV/AIDS.

Medical and scientific journals provide a wealth of information about the HIV/AIDS pandemic. Articles cited in this publication were published in *AIDS, AIDS and Behavior, AIDS Research and Therapy, AIDS Research and Treatment, AIDS Reviews, American Journal of Epidemiology, American Journal of Men's Health, American Journal of Public Health, Annals of Internal Medicine, Antiviral Chemistry and Chemotherapy, Archives of Internal Medicine, Brain, Behavior, and Immunity, British Medical Journal, BMC International Health and Human Rights, BMC Public Health, Canadian Journal of Neurological Sciences, Clinical Infectious Diseases, Clinics in Perinatology, Cochrane Database of Systematic Reviews, Current Opinions in Oncology, Drugs, Expert Review of Anti-infective Therapy, Hematology, HIV Clinical Trials, HIV Medicine, Human Vaccines, Indian Journal of Experimental Biology, International Journal of Gynecology and Obstetrics, International Journal of STD and AIDS, Issues in Mental Health Nursing, Journal of Adolescent Health, Journal of Acquired Immune Deficiency Syndrome, Journal of the American Medical Association, Journal of Experimental Medicine, Journal of Managed Care Pharmacy, Journal of the National Cancer Institute, Journal of Telemedicine and Telecare, Journal of Urban Health, Journal of Virology, Lancet, Lancet Infectious Diseases, Maternal and Child Health Journal, Medical Care, Medical Decision Making, Medscape Medical News, Nature, Nature Medicine, New England Journal of Medicine, Obstetrics and Gynecology, Pediatric Research, PLoS Medicine, PLoS ONE, PLoS Pathogens, Postgraduate Medical Journal, Proceedings of the American Thoracic Society, Public Health, Science, Science Translational Research, Scientific American, Sexually Transmitted Infections, Southeast Asian Journal of Tropical Medicine and Public Health,* and *Substance Abuse Treatment, Prevention, and Policy.*

Timely information about many facets of HIV/AIDS may be found at the website TheBody.com. The National Coalition for the Homeless, the National AIDS Housing Coalition, and the U.S. Department of Housing and Urban Development provided information on housing opportunities for people with HIV/AIDS.

The Kaiser Family Foundation publications *Kaiser Family Foundation 2011 Survey of Americans on HIV/AIDS* (June 2011), *HIV/AIDS at 30: A Public Opinion Perspective* (June 2011), and "U.S. Federal Funding for HIV/AIDS: The President's FY 2012 Budget Request" (March 2011) were used to prepare this publication. The Kaiser Family Foundation also provides daily updates about a variety of issues that are related to HIV/AIDS on its website (http://www.kff.org/).

We are grateful to the Gallup Organization for permitting us to present the results of its renowned opinion polls and graphics depicting Americans' feelings and concerns about HIV/AIDS.

INDEX

Armour Pharmaceuticals, 64

Arroyo-Cobo, J. M., 128

Ashe, Arthur, 99

Asia

    Cambodia, 129–130

    Central Asia, 121

    China, 130–131

    HIV transmission in, 124

    HIV/AIDS in, 128–129

    India, 130

    Thailand, 129

Asian-Americans

    AIDS cases by race/ethnicity, 43

    in AIDSvax trial, 97

    National Asian and Pacific Islander HIV/AIDS Awareness Day, 138

Asimov, Isaac, 101

"Assessment of Mother-to-Child HIV-1 and HIV-2 Transmission: An AIDS Reference Laboratory Collaborative Study" (Pádua), 122–123

Atlanta, Georgia, 84–85

Atripla

    cost of, 82

    price increase for, 88

Autoimmune response, 6

AVERT, 92

Azidothymidine (AZT)

    effectiveness of, 20

    HIV testing debate and, 107

    See also Zidovudine

B

B cells, 5

Bacterial infections, 65

Badley, Andrew D., 11

Bahamas, HIV/AIDS in, 131

Bailey, Robert, 116

Baker, David R., 97

Ball, Andrew, 58

Banerjee, Ritu, 11

Bangkok, Thailand, 129

Bangladesh, 121

Barekzai, Sabrina, 59–60

Barré-Sinoussi, Françoise, 1

Barton v. American Red Cross, 64

"Basic Statistics" (Centers for Disease Control and Prevention), 115

Basketball, 99

Bazoes, Alexandra, 12

Bebell, Lisa M., 127

Bedimo, Roger J., 18–19

Behavior, 123

Behavioral interventions, 117

Bell, David M., 87–88

Benjamin, Regina, 120

Berenson, Berry, 100

Bermuda, HIV/AIDS in, 131

Bernard, Antoine, 4

"Best-Evidence Interventions: Findings from a Systematic Review of HIV Behavioral Interventions for US Populations at High Risk, 2000–2004" (Lyles et al.), 117

"Best-Evidence Risk Reduction Interventions" (Centers for Disease Control and Prevention), 117

Beth Israel Medical Center (BIMC), 117–118

Black Death (bubonic plague), 21

Bleach, 58

Blood

    blood/transplant procedures, safety of, 22–23

    CDC guidelines for prevention of HIV transmission, 86–87

    donating, HIV contact and, 22

    gene therapy, HIV-resistant blood cells, 95–96

    hemophiliacs and HIV/AIDS, 60–64

    HIV attack on immune system, 8

    HIV spread through, 1

    HIV testing of health care workers and, 113

    HIV transmission through IDU, 52–53

    for home test, 112

    older people with HIV/AIDS from contaminated, 101

    for rapid test, 112

    testing people for HIV, 23–25

"Blood Safety and Availability" (World Health Organization), 23

Blood supply

    decline in AIDS due to blood transfusions, 33

    hemophiliacs and HIV/AIDS, 60–64

    testing people for HIV and, 24

    U.S., safety of, 22–23

Blood transfusions

    decline in AIDS due to, 33

    HIV transmission via, 21, 49

Blood-screening tests, 22

Bloodstream, HIV in, 9

Bodily fluids, 21

Body fluid tests, 24–25

Bone marrow, 9

Bongaarts, John, 122

Bono, 138, 140

Botswana, 72

Bower, Mark, 12

Bowers, Rebecca, 116

Bozzette, Samuel A., 81

Brain

    HIV in, 9

    HIV-associated dementia and, 18

    primary brain lymphoma, 10, 12

    toxoplasmosis attack on, 21

Branson, Bernard M.

    on HIV testing, 108

    on rapid-response tests, 25

    revised recommendations for HIV testing, 27, 137

Brazil, HIV/AIDS in, 131

Breastfeeding

    HIV transmission via, 21, 54

    prevention of mother-to-child transmission, 69–70

    risks of HIV transmission through, 67, 68

Breitbart, William, 105

"Broad Diversity of Neutralizing Antibodies Isolated from Memory B Cells in HIV-Infected Individuals" (Scheid et al.), 97

Brooks, John T., 3

Brown, Timothy Rae, 95

Bubonic plague, 94

Burki, Talha Khan, 131

Burkitt's lymphoma, 10

Burris, Scott, 118

Bush, George H. W., 99

Bush, George W.

    as leader for HIV/AIDS cause, 138

    Medicaid coverage of HIV/AIDS care, 82

    PEPFAR and, 133

"Bush Signs Bill to Triple AIDS Funding" (Euphrat), 133

"Business People, Celebrities, and Officials Join Forces to Raise Awareness about AIDS in China" (UNICEF), 140

C

Caldwell, M. Blake, 112

California

    percentage of AIDS cases, 31

    prisoners with HIV/AIDS in, 57

    San Francisco's model of hospital care, 84

"Calypte Appoints Distributor for Its HIV-1 Urine Test in People's Republic of China" (Business Wire), 24

"Calypte Biomedical Announces Successful Conclusion of Internal Trials" (Reuters), 25

Calypte Biomedical Corporation, 24–25

Cambodia, HIV/AIDS in, 129–130

"Cambodia: Country Situation" (UNAIDS), 129

"Cambodia's AIDS Strategy Could Fail without Sustainable Financing" (Moszynski), 130

"Can Community Health Workers Improve Adherence to Highly Active Antiretroviral Therapy in the USA? A Review of the Literature" (Kenya et al.), 14

"Can Routine Neonatal Circumcision Help Prevent Human Immunodeficiency Virus Transmission in the United States?" (Xu et al.), 116

"Can You Afford Your HIV Treatment?" (Vann), 81

Canada

    HIV tainted blood supply in, 23

    rapid-response test kit manufactured in, 25

from HIV/AIDS, 1, 3, 30

HIV/AIDS deaths attributable to IDU, 52

in India from AIDS, 130

inmate deaths in state prisons by age, race/ethnicity, 60(*t*4.11)

mortality from AIDS, 49–50

of people with HIV attributable to TB, 123

prisoner deaths from AIDS, 56, 57

suicide, 105–106

from tuberculosis, 11

worldwide HIV/AIDS deaths, projections about, 122

"Deaths: Preliminary Data for 2009" (Kochanek et al.), 1, 49–50

Debt AIDS Trade Africa (DATA), 140

Delaney, Martin, 92

Delaware, AIDS cases in, 32

Dementia, 17–18

Deneuve, Catherine, 140

Deoxyribonucleic acid (DNA)

HIV and, 4

HIV vaccine and, 96

NRTIs and, 70, 92

recombinant DNA technology/vaccine development, 96*f*

"Department of Defense: Instruction" (U.S. Department of Defense), 112

Depression

of people with HIV/AIDS, 104

suicide and, 105

"Detection of Drug Resistance Mutations at Low Plasma HIV-1 RNA Load in a European Multicentre Cohort Study" (Prosperi et al.), 27

"Determination That a Demonstration Needle Exchange Program Would be Effective in Reducing Drug Abuse and the Risk of Acquired Immune Deficiency Syndrome Infection among Intravenous Drug Users" (Benjamin), 120

Diagnosis

adults/adolescents living with diagnosed AIDS, 32*f*

adults/adolescents living with diagnosed HIV infection, 30*f*

of AIDS, impact of, 102–103

AIDS cases/deaths/persons living with AIDS, 18*f*

AIDS diagnoses among adult/adolescent females, 54*f*

AIDS diagnoses among adult/adolescent females by race/ethnicity, 54*t*

AIDS diagnoses by age, 33*t*

AIDS diagnoses by transmission category, 43*f*

AIDS diagnoses by year of diagnosis, 36*t*–37*t*

AIDS diagnoses/deaths, 49*f*

AIDS-defining conditions, 17(*t*2.2)

cancer and HIV, 18–19

children under 13 years of age living with diagnosed AIDS, 38*f*

children under 13 years of age living with diagnosed HIV infection, 31*f*

dementia as symptom of AIDS, 17–18

diagnosed HIV infection, by age, race/ethnicity, and transmission category, 46*t*–47*t*

diagnosed HIV infection, by race/ethnicity, 48*t*

emotions, dealing with, 104

females living with diagnosed AIDS, rates of, 55*f*

HIV diagnoses among adult/adolescent females by race/ethnicity, 53(*t*4.4)

HIV diagnoses by state/U.S. dependent areas, 108*t*

HIV diagnoses by year of diagnosis, 34*t*–35*t*

of HIV/AIDS, 16–17

HIV/AIDS case definition for children and, 66–67

life expectancy after HIV diagnosis, 20

number of AIDS cases diagnosed each year, 30–31

persons with HIV infection, persons with undiagnosed HIV infection, 19*t*

Diamondstone, Laura S., 61–62

Diana, Princess of Wales, 140

Didanosine, 71, 92

Dideoxycytosine, 92

Diet, 104

Disabled employees, 103

Disclosure, 112

Discrimination

in China, 131

coping with, 103–104

HIV in Thailand and, 129

HIV testing of health care workers and, 113

against people with AIDS, public opinion about, 137

"Discrimination against People with HIV Persists in China" (Burki), 131

Disease progression, 102–103

"Disparities in Diagnoses of HIV Infection between Blacks/African Americans and Other Racial/Ethnic Populations—37 States, 2005–2008" (Centers for Disease Control and Prevention), 43, 49

District of Columbia

AIDS cases in, 32

AIDS cases of children in, 33

HIV/AIDS in women in, 55

DNA. *See* Deoxyribonucleic acid

Doctor-Assisted Suicide Is Moral Issue Dividing Americans Most (Saad), 106

DOD (U.S. Department of Defense), 112

Dominican Republic, HIV/AIDS in, 131

Douglas, John F., 59

Douste-Blazy, Philippe, 132–133

"Dream Team," 99

Droplet nuclei, 11

Drug resistance

among children, 71

highly drug-resistant tuberculosis, 123–124

Drug treatments

access to in developing countries, 132–133

antiretroviral treatment supported by U.S. government, number of people receiving, 133*t*

azidothymidine, 20

for children, 70–71

cost of AIDS treatment research, 90–91

cost of HIV/AIDS drugs, worldwide, 132

cost of, rise in, 88

costs of, 81

decline in AIDS deaths from use of, 3

early medication, benefits of, 104

FDA-approved drugs, 92–93

FDA-approved drugs for HIV/AIDS, 92–93

HAART, effectiveness/adherence, 13–14

HAART and decline in AIDS-related cancers, 12

for infants of HIV-infected mothers, 67

multidrug-resistant tuberculosis, 123–124

PPACA and, 84

protease inhibitors, 9

state programs to provide HIV/AIDS drugs, 82–83

for treatment of PCP, 10

zidovudine for perinatal HIV infection, 68

Drug use

AIDS rates in metropolitan areas and, 33

among prisoners, 58

HIV infection patterns among adolescents/young adults, 76

HIV infections by transmission category, 52(*t*4.1)

HIV testing debate and, 107

HIV transmission via, 21, 49

injection drug users, HIV transmission among, 52–53

percentage of AIDS cases attributable to, 51

syringe exchange programs, 117–120

See also Injection drug use

Dufoix, Georgina, 23

E

"Early HIV Therapy Protects against Virus Spread" (Associated Press), 104

Early Treatment for HIV Act, 82

Eastern Europe

HIV/AIDS in, 128

rise of HIV incidence in, 121

Easy-E (rapper), 100–101

programs, key objectives of, 114

syringe exchange programs, 117–120

of tuberculosis, 123

Uganda's efforts at, 126–127

of worldwide HIV/AIDS, 121, 124

ZDV for reduction of perinatal infection, 68

"Price, Performance, and the FDA Approval Process: The Example of Home HIV Testing" (Paltiel & Pollack), 25

Primary brain lymphoma, 10, 12

"Primary Care Delivery Is Associated with Greater Physician Experience and Improved Survival among Persons with AIDS" (Kitahata et al.), 85

Primary care physicians, 85

Prisoners

AIDS cases in general population and among state/federal prisoners, 57(t4.7)

AIDS-related deaths among all deaths in state prisons/U.S. general population, percentage of, 57(t4.8)

AIDS-related deaths in state prisons/U.S. general population, ratio of, 58t

drug/needle use among, 58

HIV testing, circumstances under which they received, 63t

HIV testing policies in U.S. prisons, 113

with HIV/AIDS, geographic differences, 57

with HIV/AIDS, sex, racial, age differences, 57–58

with HIV/AIDS by jurisdiction, 59t–60t

with HIV/AIDS by sex/jurisdiction, 61t–62t

HIV/AIDS cases among, 56

HIV/AIDS cases among, by gender, 56t

inmate deaths in state prisons by age, race/ethnicity, 60(t4.11)

prevention of HIV infection in U.S. prison systems, 58–60

"Prisons to Offer Inmates HIV Testing" (Barekzai), 59–60

Privacy

HIV testing of pregnant women, newborns and, 112

reporting of HIV-positive patients by name, 107–108

Productivity, 90–91

"Profound Early Control of Highly Pathogenic SIV by an Effector Memory T-cell Vaccine" (Hansen et al.), 13

"Prognostic Factors for All-Cause Mortality among Hemophiliacs Infected with Human Immunodeficiency Virus" (Diamondstone et al.), 61–62

Projections, of global AIDS epidemic, 121–122

"Projections of Global Mortality and Burden of Disease from 2002 to 2030" (Mathers & Loncar), 121–122

Prosperi, Mattia C. F., 27

Protease inhibitors (PIs)

aggressive treatment, 93

for children, 70

development of, 9

drug resistance of children, 71

effectiveness of, 20, 92

FDA-approved drugs for HIV/AIDS, 92

as morning-after treatment, 95

state programs to provide HIV/AIDS drugs, 82

WHO guidelines for use of in children, 73

"Protein in Saliva Found to Block AIDS Virus in Test Tube Study" (Altman), 21

Protein xCT, 10

"Provider Response to a Rare but Highly Publicized Transmission of HIV Through Solid Organ Transplantation" (Kucirka et al.), 88

Prudential, 90

Psycho (film), 100

Psychosocial stress, 102–103

Public figures, with HIV/AIDS, 99–101

Public Financing and Delivery of HIV/AIDS Care: Securing the Legacy of Ryan White (Institute of Medicine), 82

"Public Health Gains from Health in Prisons in Spain" (Arroyo-Cobo), 128

Public opinion

AIDS as most urgent health problem, percent of people naming, 136f

concern about HIV/AIDS, 135–137

on HIV testing, 137

knowledge, tolerance, misconceptions about HIV/AIDS, 137

on leader for HIV/AIDS cause, 138

media as primary source of information about HIV/AIDS, 137–138

on most urgent health problem facing the country, 136t

on physician-assisted suicide, 106, 106f

on spending for HIV/AIDS in U.S., 138

Puerto Rico

HIV/AIDS in, 32–33, 131

HIV/AIDS in women in, 55

Pulmonary TB, 11

PWAs (People with AIDS), 84

Q

Qiu, Jane, 131

Queen (British rock band), 101

"Quilt Facts" (AIDS Memorial Quilt), 139

R

Race/ethnicity

AIDS cases by, 31–32, 38, 43, 49

AIDS diagnoses among adult/adolescent females by, 54t

CCR5 gene and, 94

children with HIV infection and, 71

concern about getting HIV infection by, 136

diagnosed HIV infection by, 46t–47t, 48t

heterosexual contact, risks of, 51–52

high school students taught in school about HIV/AIDS by, 78(f5.4)

high school students tested for HIV by, 78(f5.5)

HIV diagnoses among adult/adolescent females by race/ethnicity, 53(t4.4)

inmate deaths in state prisons by age, race/ethnicity, 60(t4.11)

knowledge about HIV/AIDS and, 137–138

women with HIV/AIDS, 54

Raltegravir, 71, 93

Rapid progressors, 74

Rapid testing

FDA-approved tests, 26t

for HIV prevention, 114

overview of, 111

Rapid-response tests

by Calypte Biomedical Corporation, 24–25

description of, 25, 27

Reality (female condom), 116

Reasonable accommodation, 103

Recombinant DNA technology, 96, 96f

"Recommendations for Preventing Transmission of Human Immunodeficiency Virus and Hepatitis B Virus to Patients during Exposure-Prone Invasive Procedures" (Centers for Disease Control and Prevention), 86–87

(RED), 140

"Reducing the Price of HIV/AIDS Treatment" (AVERT), 92

"Reduction of Maternal-Infant Transmission of Human Immunodeficiency Virus Type 1 with Zidovudine Treatment" (Connor et al.), 68

Reed, Kasim, 59

Region

adults/adolescents living with diagnosed AIDS, 32f

AIDS cases, regional differences, 32–33

Replication cycle, HIV, 7f

Reporting

of AIDS cases, surveillance case definition and, 16

HIV/AIDS prevalence rates and, 51

of HIV-positive patients by name, 107–108

Reproduction

cell-to-cell spread of HIV through CD4-mediated fusion of infected cell with uninfected cell, 8f

HIV, how it attaches to immune cell and reproduces, 6f

HIV replication cycle, 7f

Research

AIDS Treatment Activists Coalition for, 139–140

Weinberg, Peter D., 63–64

Western blot test
  description of, 24
  rapid-response tests and, 25, 111

Western Europe, HIV/AIDS in, 127–128

"What We've Accomplished" (CHAI), 132

When Someone Close Has AIDS: Acquired Immunodeficiency Syndrome (Judd), 102

Whitaker, Barbee I., 22–23

White, Ryan
  legacy of, 78
  life, work of, 88

White blood cells
  healthy, work of, 5
  HIV attacks/destroys, 1

Whites
  AIDS cases by race/ethnicity, 43
  CCR5 gene among, 94
  concern about getting HIV infection, 136
  knowledge about HIV/AIDS, 137
  women with HIV/AIDS, 54

Whitmore, Suzanne K., 71

Whitney, Craig R., 23

WHO. *See* World Health Organization

"WHO and UNAIDS Announce Recommendations from Expert Consultation on Male Circumcision for HIV Prevention" (WHO & UNAIDS), 116

Widows, 126

Wiener, Lori, 75

"Wife inheritance," 126

"Will I? Won't I? Why Do Men Who Have Sex with Men Present for Post-exposure Prophylaxis for Sexual Exposures?" (Sayer et al.), 95

Window period
  antibody-based tests and, 24
  NAT screening of plasma donors and, 22

Wiysonge, Charles Shey, 116–117

Women. *See* Females; Mothers

Wood, Elijah, 140

World AIDS Day, 139, 140

"A World First: Vaccine Helps Prevent HIV Infection" (Associated Press), 98

World Health Organization (WHO)
  on breastfeeding by HIV-positive mothers, 69, 70
  on circumcision, 116
  on cost of HIV/AIDS drugs, 132
  on dementia and AIDS, 17–18
  global outlook for children and HIV/AIDS, 72–73
  HIV data from, 124
  on HIV testing in China, 24
  on HIV transmission through breastfeeding, 21
  nevirapine recommendation of, 71
  on prevention of HIV infection in prisons, 58
  on reduction of mother-to-child transmission, 68
  on safety of blood supply, 23
  stages of HIV infection, 17(*t*2.3)
  surveillance case definition for HIV/AIDS, 16
  on tuberculosis, 123–124
  vaccine report, 98
  on worldwide HIV/AIDS, number of people with, 121

World Trade Organization, 132

Worldwide HIV/AIDS
  Africa, 124–127
  antiretroviral treatment supported by U.S. government, number of people receiving, 133*t*
  Asia, 128–131
  Caribbean, 131
  Central and South America, 131
  controversies, 131–133
  Europe, 127–128
  global HIV infection in young people, 75
  global outlook for children with HIV/AIDS, 72–73
  highly drug-resistant tuberculosis, 123–124
  HIV transmission, geographic differences, 124
  HIV-1 and HIV-2, 122–123
  interactions and HIV transmission, 123
  number of people living with HIV/AIDS, 3
  patterns of infection, 122

PEPFAR funding, 134*t*
  scope of problem, 121–122

Wren, Leia, 13

X

XDR-TB (extensively drug-resistant TB), 11–12, 123–124

Xu, Xiao, 116

Y

Yemen, HIV/AIDS in, 124

Young, Taryn, 95

Young adults
  as AIDS activists, 78
  HIV infection patterns among, 76
  sexual health education, 115–116
  sexually transmitted diseases and, 76, 78

The Youth Risk Behavior Surveillance System (YRBSS): 2009 (Centers for Disease Control and Prevention), 76

Youth Risk Behavior Surveys, 116

Z

Zambia
  funding for HIV prevention in, 133
  HIV prevalence rate in, 125
  HIV testing of expectant mothers, 72

ZDV. *See* Zidovudine

Zhang, Xinjian, 71

Zidovudine (ZDV)
  didanosine and, 71
  effectiveness of, 20, 92
  as FDA-approved drug for HIV/AIDS, 92
  HIV testing debate and, 107
  for infants of HIV-infected mothers, 67
  overview of, 68–70
  for PEP for health care workers, 87
  for prevention of perinatal HIV infection, 54, 68
  state programs to provide HIV/AIDS drugs, 82

Zimbabwe, HIV prevalence rate in, 125

Zolfo, Maria, 85–86

Zur Hausen, Harald, 1